Digestive Endoscopy: Inside the Evidence and Outside

Digestive Endoscopy: Inside the Evidence and Outside

Editors

Andrea Anderloni
Cecilia Binda

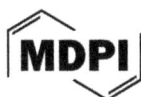

Basel • Beijing • Wuhan • Barcelona • Belgrade • Novi Sad • Cluj • Manchester

Editors

Andrea Anderloni
Gastroenterology and
Endoscopy Unit
Fondazione IRCCS Policlinico
San Matteo
Pavia, Italy

Cecilia Binda
Gastroenterology and
Digestive Endoscopy Unit,
Forlì-Cesena Hospitals
AUSL ROMAGNA
Forlì-Cesena, Italy

Editorial Office
MDPI
St. Alban-Anlage 66
4052 Basel, Switzerland

This is a reprint of articles from the Special Issue published online in the open access journal *Medicina* (ISSN 1648-9144) (available at: https://www.mdpi.com/journal/medicina/special_issues/Digestive_Endoscopy_2022).

For citation purposes, cite each article independently as indicated on the article page online and as indicated below:

Lastname, A.A.; Lastname, B.B. Article Title. *Journal Name* **Year**, *Volume Number*, Page Range.

ISBN 978-3-0365-9684-6 (Hbk)
ISBN 978-3-0365-9685-3 (PDF)
doi.org/10.3390/books978-3-0365-9685-3

© 2023 by the authors. Articles in this book are Open Access and distributed under the Creative Commons Attribution (CC BY) license. The book as a whole is distributed by MDPI under the terms and conditions of the Creative Commons Attribution-NonCommercial-NoDerivs (CC BY-NC-ND) license.

Contents

Irina Florina Cherciu Harbiyeli, Daniela Elena Burtea, Mircea-Sebastian Serbanescu, Carmen Daniela Nicolau and Adrian Saftoiu
Implementation of a Customized Safety Checklist in Gastrointestinal Endoscopy and the Importance of Team Time Out—A Dual-Center Pilot Study
Reprinted from: *Medicina* **2023**, *59*, 1160, doi:10.3390/medicina59061160 1

Landry Hakiza, Adrian Sartoretto, Konstantin Burgmann, Vivek Kumbhari, Christoph Matter, Frank Seibold and Dominic Staudenmann
Transoral Outlet Reduction (TORe) for the Treatment of Weight Regain and Dumping Syndrome after Roux-en-Y Gastric Bypass
Reprinted from: *Medicina* **2023**, *59*, 125, doi:10.3390/medicina59010125 13

Omero Alessandro Paoluzi, Edoardo Troncone, Elena De Cristofaro, Mezia Sibilia, Giovanni Monteleone and Giovanna Del Vecchio Blanco
Hemostatic Powders in Non-Variceal Upper Gastrointestinal Bleeding: The Open Questions
Reprinted from: *Medicina* **2023**, *59*, 143, doi:10.3390/medicina59010143 21

Aurelio Mauro, Francesca Lusetti, Davide Scalvini, Marco Bardone, Federico De Grazia, Stefano Mazza, et al.
A Comprehensive Review on Bariatric Endoscopy: Where We Are Now and Where We Are Going
Reprinted from: *Medicina* **2023**, *59*, 636, doi:10.3390/medicina59030636 35

Stefan Stojkovic, Milica Bjelakovic, Milica Stojkovic Lalosevic, Milos Stulic, Nina Pejic, Nemanja Radivojevic, et al.
Accidental Sewing Pin Ingestion by a Tailor: A Case Report and Literature Review
Reprinted from: *Medicina* **2023**, *59*, 1566, doi:10.3390/medicina59091566 53

Cecilia Binda, Carlo Felix Maria Jung, Stefano Fabbri, Paolo Giuffrida, Monica Sbrancia, Chiara Coluccio, et al.
Endoscopic Management of Postoperative Esophageal and Upper GI Defects—A Narrative Review
Reprinted from: *Medicina* **2023**, *59*, 136, doi:10.3390/medicina59010136 61

Adriana Ortega Larrode, Sergio Farrais Villalba, Claudia Guerrero Muñoz, Leonardo Blas Jhon, Maria Jesus Martin Relloso, Paloma Sanchez-Fayos Calabuig, et al.
Detection of Neuroendocrine Tumours by Enteroscopy: A Case Report
Reprinted from: *Medicina* **2023**, *59*, 1469, doi:10.3390/medicina59081469 79

Elia Armellini, Antonio Facciorusso and Stefano Francesco Crinò
Efficacy and Safety of Endoscopic Ultrasound-Guided Radiofrequency Ablation for Pancreatic Neuroendocrine Tumors: A Systematic Review and Metanalysis
Reprinted from: *Medicina* **2023**, *59*, 359, doi:10.3390/medicina59020359 87

Koji Takahashi, Hiroshi Ohyama, Yuichi Takiguchi, Yu Sekine, Shodai Toyama, Nana Yamada, et al.
Efficacy and Safety of Electrohydraulic Lithotripsy Using Peroral Cholangioscopy under Endoscopic Retrograde Cholangiopancreatography Guidance in Older Adults: A Single-Center Retrospective Study
Reprinted from: *Medicina* **2023**, *59*, 795, doi:10.3390/medicina59040795 99

Hayato Kurihara, Francesca M. Bunino, Alessandro Fugazza, Enrico Marrano, Giulia Mauri, Martina Ceolin, et al.
Endosonography-Guided Versus Percutaneous Gallbladder Drainage Versus Cholecystectomy in Fragile Patients with Acute Cholecystitis—A High-Volume Center Study
Reprinted from: *Medicina* **2022**, *58*, 1647, doi:10.3390/medicina58111647 . . . . **109**

Cecilia Binda, Alessandro Fugazza, Stefano Fabbri, Chiara Coluccio, Alessandro Repici, Ilaria Tarantino, et al.
The Use of PuraStat® in the Management of Walled-Off Pancreatic Necrosis Drained Using Lumen-Apposing Metal Stents: A Case Series
Reprinted from: *Medicina* **2023**, *59*, 750, doi:10.3390/medicina59040750 . . . . **121**

Olga Mandic, Igor Jovanovic, Mirjana Cvetkovic, Jasmina Maksimovic, Tijana Radonjic, Maja Popovic, et al.
Factors Predicting Malignant Occurrence and Polyp Recurrence after the Endoscopic Resection of Large Colorectal Polyps: A Single Center Experience
Reprinted from: *Medicina* **2022**, *58*, 1440, doi:10.3390/medicina58101440 . . . . **133**

Yi Liu, Zhihao Chen, Lizhou Dou, Zhaoyang Yang and Guiqi Wang
Solitary Rectal Ulcer Syndrome Is Not Always Ulcerated: A Case Report
Reprinted from: *Medicina* **2022**, *58*, 1136, doi:10.3390/medicina58081136 . . . . **145**

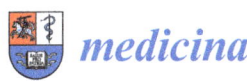

Article

Implementation of a Customized Safety Checklist in Gastrointestinal Endoscopy and the Importance of Team Time Out—A Dual-Center Pilot Study

Irina Florina Cherciu Harbiyeli [1], Daniela Elena Burtea [1,*], Mircea-Sebastian Serbanescu [2], Carmen Daniela Nicolau [3] and Adrian Saftoiu [1]

[1] Research Centre of Gastroenterology and Hepatology, University of Medicine and Pharmacy of Craiova, 200638 Craiova, Romania; cherciuirina@gmail.com (I.F.C.H.); adriansaftoiu@gmail.com (A.S.)
[2] Department of Medical Informatics and Biostatistics, University of Medicine and Pharmacy of Craiova, 200638 Craiova, Romania; mircea_serbanescu@yahoo.com
[3] Lotus Image Medical Center, Actamedica SRL, 540084 Targu Mures, Romania; carmen.nicolau@gmail.com
* Correspondence: dana.burtea26@gmail.com

Abstract: *Background and Objectives:* Checking and correctly preparing the patient for endoscopic procedures is a mandatory step for the safety and quality of the interventions. The aim of this paper is to emphasize the importance and necessity of a "team time out" as well as the implementation of a customized "checklist" before the actual procedure. *Material and Methods:* We developed and implemented a checklist for the safe conduct of endoscopies and for the entire team to thoroughly know about the patient's medical history. The subjects of this study were 15 physicians and 8 endoscopy nurses who performed overall 572 consecutive GI endoscopic procedures during the study period. *Results:* This is a prospective pilot study performed in the endoscopy unit of two tertiary referral medical centers. We customized a safety checklist that includes the steps to be followed before, during and after the examination. It brings together the whole team participating in the procedure in order to check the key points during the following three vital phases: before the patient falls asleep, before the endoscope is inserted and before the team leaves the examination room. The perception of team communication and teamwork was improved after the introduction of the checklist. The checklist completion rates, identity verification rates of patients by the endoscopist, adequate histological labeling management and explicit recording of follow-up recommendations are some of the parameters that improved post-intervention. *Conclusions:* Using a checklist and adapting it to local conditions is a high-level recommendation of the Romanian Ministry of Health. In a medical world where safety and quality are essential, a checklist could prevent medical errors, and team time out can ensure high-quality endoscopy, enhance teamwork and offer patients confidence in the medical team.

Keywords: GI endoscopy; safety checklist; team time out; patient safety

1. Introduction

Endoscopic procedures represent an important part of daily practice for both gastroenterologists and nurses, enabling the timely diagnosis and precise treatment of digestive diseases. In the past 20 years, the possibilities of diagnosing and treating digestive diseases have increased considerably; GI (gastro-intestinal) endoscopy procedures have become more complicated and varied, hence, the concerns about the quality of medical care and patient safety have increased [1]. In recent years, there has been a growing interest in the possibilities of preventing errors in diagnostic and interventional endoscopy suites. The knowledge about and awareness of patient safety risk factors are essential in order to improve and enhance the GI endoscopy team, the working environment and, finally, the endoscopic performance.

The diversity of digestive pathology as well as the fast growth of the therapeutic endoscopic opportunities led to more evolved and complex procedures. The practical challenges of advanced endoscopy are approaching the complexity of a surgery. An advanced endoscopy is similar to surgery in terms of the technical complexity and invasiveness. This contains a higher risk of adverse events associated with the therapeutic interventions [2]. The patients count on the endoscopy team to execute the GI endoscopy procedures in a secure, rigorous and standardized manner. Given the growing number of GI endoscopic procedures, many of which are technically complex, as well as the aging patient population and its increased prevalence of comorbidities, the GI endoscopy safety checklists have become more popular in recent years. Regardless of the wide acknowledgement of the significance of GI endoscopy safety checklists, there is little information regarding the actual implementation among the GI endoscopy units [3–5].

A modern endoscopy unit needs extremely competent leaders, supported by excellent teams who can handle a high volume of procedures safely, efficiently and for the benefit of the patient. In gastroenterology, quality and safety are crucial issues that are motivated by a shared desire to advance best practices and make it easier for patients to receive evidence-based care. Patient safety should not be compromised in light of the development of endoscopic practice, and efforts to uphold and enhance GI endoscopy safety should always be made [6,7]. Additionally, it is very important that the team understand and accept that some of the endoscopic procedures, especially advanced GI endoscopic procedures, have a higher risk of adverse events compared to regular endoscopies [1,8].

The advanced endoscopy team is part of a bigger service that provides access to therapeutic intervention, and the staff should already have experience, planned strategies and skills to deal with potential adverse events or failed procedures. If the adverse events result from inadequate planning of the intervention rather than a lack of technical skills, quality improvement initiatives may help to reduce such complications [9,10].

The results are determined not only by the skills of the endoscopist, but by the effectiveness of the team.

An effective endoscopy service depends on the following [7]:

- The endoscopy team;
- Team leaders;
- The institution where the service operates;
- The political context.

The team itself consists of nurses, technical staff, administrative staff, anesthesiologists and endoscopic physicians. Some of the endoscopists may spend half a day or one day per week in the endoscopy department. The temporary nature of some team members can affect the team dynamics, leading to an increased disruption in the workplace. As a result, the team may not function efficiently. Providing a modern endoscopy service requires effective leadership and teamwork [11,12].

Each endoscopy unit has the possibility to draw up its own checklist, either in a printed or electronic version. Most checklists in digestive endoscopy do not specifically address advanced procedures; therefore, they need to be nuanced/individualized [13,14]. According to the World Health Organization, the implementation of customized safety checklists can improve procedural outcomes and reduce human errors [15]. Several studies state that the implementation of a GI endoscopy safety checklist significantly improved endoscopy team communication and teamwork. It is possible to extrapolate that with improved team communication, medical errors may be reduced, thereby preventing adverse events [2,14]. However, there is no guidance on how best to implement GI endoscopy checklists or solid high-level data regarding any measure of their usefulness including mortality rates, adverse event rates or endoscopy completion rates. Hence, there is a real need for more studies centered on assessing not only the usefulness of an endoscopy safety checklist, but also for identifying the best implementation strategies.

In this paper, we aim to formally evaluate the feasibility of successfully implementing a customized safety checklist in our dual center GI endoscopy units, to identify strategies and address barriers for facilitating checklist compliance and to summarize the impact on team communication and commitment to patients' safety culture.

2. Material and Methods

This is a prospective pilot study performed in the endoscopy unit of two tertiary referral medical centers (Research Center of Gastroenterology and Hepatology, Craiova, Romania and Lotus Image Medical Center, Targu Mures, Romania).

This initiative was designed and approved as a quality improvement study, with the study subjects set to be the endoscopy staff comprising gastroenterology and anesthesia physicians and endoscopy nurses. The subjects from both endoscopy teams were enrolled at the same time in October 2021. The endoscopy staff members were included in the present study if they performed at least one endoscopy procedure and took part in each phase of the study. No patient information was collected during this study, hence, the exempt of approval from the Local Institutional Ethical Committee. The authors did not have access to information that could identify individual participants during or after data collection.

The case diversity included elective inpatients and outpatients who underwent diagnostic and therapeutic endoscopies. All procedures were performed with the patients under propofol sedation, administered by an anesthesiologist.

Real-time observation of each endoscopic procedure was performed by one designated staff member, and data were collected from October 2021 to the end of September 2022, as described in Figure 1. The observations were performed on random consecutive days, with the aim of observing the widest range of physician–nurse combinations. There was no established scale to rate the difficulty of the endoscopy procedures. Rather, it was a personal evaluation made by each physician. The person responsible for completing the checklist asked the physicians "Do you consider the procedure difficult?" and they had the option to provide a Yes or No answer. The difficulty of the endoscopic procedure was assessed by each physician according to their knowledge and experience. It took into consideration factors such as poor bowel preparation; anatomical gastrointestinal alterations; the existence of tumors challenging to be traversed with the endoscope; polyps, which are hard to resect due to the size, number and location (characterized by using the SMSA classification); chronic alcoholic patients requiring higher sedation doses and breaks during the procedure due to the agitated status; etc.

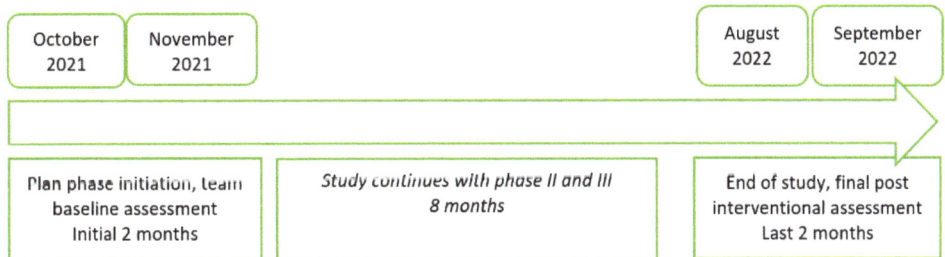

Figure 1. Study timeline.

The observational studies were prospectively conducted and reported following the STROBE statement. Initially, the baseline compliance rates were inspected during the first 2 months of the study. The final data were cross-checked by the multidisciplinary team established in both institutions, and the final assessment was performed during the last 2 months. Pre- and post-intervention staff compliance rates were compared. Team satisfaction and perception of the checklist was assessed by conducting a 5-question survey, after the quality improvement interventions were applied. The staff was asked if the checklist either caused time delay, improved patients' safety, proved to be useful if they were to have an endoscopy or if, overall, they were satisfied with the checklist implementation process.

The framework for the implementation of the safety checklist is described in Figure 2. Firstly, the scarce existing literature regarding the topic of this paper was consulted, and a personalized checklist was developed in order to be used in our two centers. After reaching an agreement regarding the final form of the checklist, we proceeded to the implementation stage, all with the goals to safely conduct endoscopies and for the entire team to thoroughly know the patient's medical history.

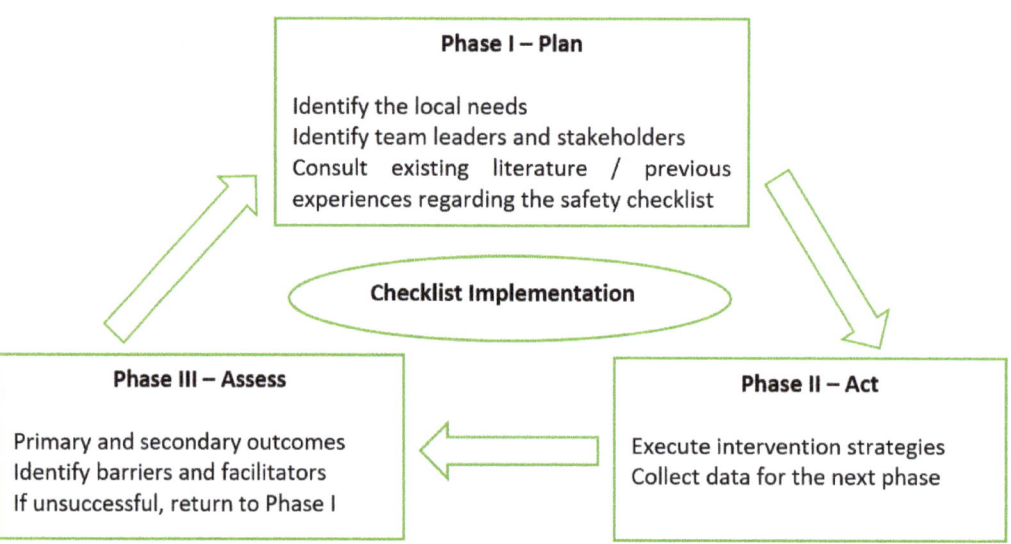

Figure 2. Study design.

Intervention strategies for the implementation of our prospectively developed checklist are as follows:

a. Development and adjustment of the endoscopy checklist;
b. Checklist introduction seminars;
c. Team training sessions mandatory for all endoscopy staff;
d. Physical reminders spread around the endoscopy department;
e. Printed paper-based checklists available in a clear designated area;
f. Advocating the use of a safety checklist as part of the endoscopy department policy;
g. Mandating a single individual (physician or nurse) to lead the checklist process;
h. Actively engaging the entire endoscopy team to contribute to all phases of the checklist.

Primary and secondary outcomes expected to be analyzed during the study included the following: (a) checklist completion rate, (b) identity verifications of patients, (c) validity of the endoscopy procedure appropriateness, (d) colonic preparation (Boston Bowel Preparation Scale—BBPS was used for the assessment of the colonic preparation), (e) colonoscopy completion rate and adenoma detection rate, (f) staff satisfaction and perception about the checklist, (g) peri-procedural complications (bleeding, perforation, cardiovascular events, death), (h) adequate histological labeling management, (i) explicit recording of follow-up recommendations (post-polypectomy surveillance, follow-up interval after colonoscopy with inadequate preparation, colorectal cancer screening, follow-up endoscopy for varices for patients with cirrhosis, follow-up after EUS for pancreatic lesions, etc.).

Statistical Analysis

As all collected data were categorical, comparisons between groups (nurses versus physicians) were performed using chi-square test and, alternatively, Fisher's exact test, when not all the parameters of the chi-square test were fulfilled. A *p*-value of <0.05 was considered to be significant.

For the staff questionnaires, the frequencies and proportions of responses were computed including only the response alternatives "Yes" and "No", and ignoring the "Hesitant" responses.

Data collection was performed using Microsoft Office Excel 2019, (Microsoft Corp.; Redmond, WA, USA), while the statistical assessment was carried out using MATLAB 2021a (MathWorks Inc.; Natick, MA, USA).

3. Results

Based on the existing checklists published in the literature and the constant feedback received during the study, we developed a personalized checklist that includes the steps to be followed before, during and after the endoscopic examination (Figure 3). Although only one designated person was responsible to physically tick the required information and lead the process (either a physician or a nurse), the checklist drew together the whole team participating in the procedure in order to check the key points during the following three vital and equally important phases: before the patient falls asleep ("Sign in"), before the endoscope is inserted ("Team out") and before the team leaves the examination room ("Sign out").

Team Time Out for Endoscopy
Criteria to be checked

Patient							
Sign in - upon arrival in endoscopy	✓	Team Time out -before the procedure	✓	Sign out -after the procedure	✓		
Patient identification data Name, date of birth	☐	Confirmation that the patient is aware of the procedure	☐	Completion of documents, including instructions for recovery	☐		
Informed consent	☐	Patient and procedure confirmation	☐	Samples	☐		
Relevant documents available	☐	Indications, planning procedure/steps	☐	Documented patient condition	☐		
Risk assessment							
Morbidity classification	☐	Is the necessary equipment ready?	☐				
Cardiological conditions?	yes no	Airway monitoring, medication and equipment	☐	Were there any problems during the procedure?	yes no		
Allergies?	yes no						
Infections?	yes no	Is endoscopy difficult? Additional preparations	yes no	Any special patient information to pass on?	yes no		
Anticoagulants?	yes no						
Glaucoma?	yes no	Special aspects for sedation and patient position?	yes no	Any special patient information to release?	yes no		
Proper preparation?	yes no						
Signature		Signature		Signature			

Figure 3. Our customized endoscopy checklist.

The "Sign in" phase starts once the patient enters the endoscopy room and comprises the following: (a) verification of patient's identity, (b) completion of the informed consent forms, (c) verification of patient's relevant medical documents, (d) morbidity classification according to the American Society of Anesthesiologists score, (e) assessment of relevant co-morbidities (cardiopulmonary risks, presence of implantable medical devices, etc.), (f) any known allergies (including medication or previous difficulties with sedation/anesthesia), (g) usage of anticoagulant/antiplatelet medications, (h) a review of known infections (hepatitis, HIV, tuberculosis, COVID-19, etc.) and (i) confirmation of proper bowel preparation.

The "Time out" phase occurs before the endoscope is inserted and/or before the induction of sedation/general anesthesia. It includes the following: (a) confirmation that the patient is aware of the planned endoscopic procedure, (b) patient and procedure validation, (c) confirmation of indications, aims, potential limitations and summary of each step of the procedure, (d) confirmation that all required endoscopy equipment, endoscope(s) and accessories are available and properly functioning, (e) confirmation that the patient monitoring equipment is prepared and operational (functioning intravenous access, pulse oximetry, blood pressure, cardiac monitor), (f) inspection of any special aspects regarding sedation or patient position and (g) assessment of whether the endoscopic procedure is difficult and whether additional preparations are required.

The "Sign out" phase takes place in between the end of the endoscopic procedure and prior to the team exiting the endoscopy lab. This phase includes the following: (a) confirmation that the endoscopy report is accurate, including post-procedure instructions for patient's recovery and eventual follow-up procedures that could be indicated, (b) confirmation that all histological samples collected during the endoscopy procedure are correctly labelled and documented, (c) documentation of patient's post-procedure status and if any problems occurred during the procedure and (d) confirmation that all the necessary documents and information were passed on to the patient.

A mixed team dedicated to quality improvement reviewed both the local and already published data in order to identify the barriers and facilitators which might influence the checklist compliance (Table 1). In consequence, an implementation strategy was developed for overcoming the potential barriers. Within the strategy, we established a target for the checklist adherence rate (>75%). Supporting the team members who consistently used the checklist and debriefing the non-cooperative staff were important parts of achieving our target.

Table 1. Facilitators and barriers to the implementation of endoscopy safety checklist.

Facilitators	Barriers
✔ Concise and specific safety checklist ✔ Rising awareness among the entire team regarding quality control and safety in endoscopy ✔ Senior physician/professor leadership ✔ Endoscopic procedures performed during the first part of the working day ✔ Daily nomination of a team member responsible for checklist ✔ The young age of the person nominated to be responsible for the checklist ✔ Minimize distractions in the endoscopy room ✔ Immediate targeted feedback ✔ Constant checklist reassessment and fast adjustments in the daily practice	✔ Irrelevant safety checklist items ✔ The additional time required to complete the checklist ✔ Fear that additional time spent per procedure will lead to less funding ✔ Deficient patient safety culture ✔ Team resistance to change ✔ Loss of physician autonomy ✔ Lack of leadership ✔ Lack of a designated member responsible for the checklist ✔ Fear of accentuating patient anxiety

The study's outcome rates were calculated after completing 572 consecutive endoscopic procedures, including 126 procedures during the baseline period and 446 procedures until the end of the study period. The assessment of the checklist implementation is presented in Table 2. There was a significant increase in the checklist completion rate (25% to 89%) after the intervention procedures. The identity verification of patients by the endoscopist also reached a significant increase (15% at baseline up to 90%) and remained high among nurses (98% at baseline to 99% at the end of the study). The baseline adenoma detection rate was 0.36, and the post-intervention rate was 0.39, hence, there was no significant statistical difference. The adequate histological labeling management and explicit recording of the follow-up recommendations are two parameters which had statistically significant improvements post-intervention, similar with the documentation of the colonic preparation and the assessment of the procedure validity.

Table 2. Study outcome rates, n = numeric value; 126 baseline procedures, 446 post-intervention procedures.

Study Outcomes	Baseline Rates (Yes %)	Yes n/126	No n/126	Post-Intervention Rates (Yes%)	Yes n/446	No n/446	p-Value
Checklist completion rate	24.60	31	95	89.01	397	49	The chi-square statistic is 216.37. The p-value is <0.01. The result is significant at $p < 0.05$.
Patient's identity verification (by nurse)	97.62	123	3	98.88	441	5	The chi-square statistic is 1.1308. The p-value is 0.28. The result is not significant at $p < 0.05$.
Patient's identity verification (by endoscopist)	15.87	20	106	90.13	402	44	The chi-square statistic is 280.04. The p-value is <0.01. The result is significant at $p < 0.05$.
Validity of the procedure appropriateness	87.30	110	16	93.95	419	27	The chi-square statistic is 6.23. The p-value is 0.012. The result is significant at $p < 0.05$.
Documented proper colonic preparation	76.98	97	29	90.81	405	41	The chi-square statistic is 17.47. The p-value is <0.01. The result is significant at $p < 0.05$.
Colonoscopy completion rate	97.62	123	3	98.88	441	5	The chi-square statistic is 17.47. The p-value is <0.01. The result is significant at $p < 0.05$.
Peri-procedural complications	0.79	1	125	0.45	2	444	The chi-square statistic is 0.22. The p-value is 0.63. The result is not significant at $p < 0.05$.
Adequate histological labeling management	48.67	110	16	93.72	418	28	The chi-square statistic is 180.79. The p-value is <0.01. The result is significant at $p < 0.05$.
Explicit recording of follow-up recommendations	69.84	88	38	95.07	424	22	The chi-square statistic is 66.58. The p-value is <0.01. The result is significant at $p < 0.05$.

The subjects of this study were 15 physicians (gastroenterologists and anesthesiologists) and 8 endoscopy nurses who worked at the endoscopy units in varying degrees of frequency and performed, overall, 572 consecutive GI endoscopic procedures during the study period. When assessing the compliance rates of the physicians versus the nurses, at baseline and post-intervention, an increase from 20% to 83% ($p < 0.05$) was noted among the physicians, and from 42% to 91% ($p < 0.05$) among nurses (Figure 4).

The survey conducted to assess the team satisfaction and perception of the checklist, after the quality improvement intervention, revealed that the perception of team communication and teamwork was improved after the checklist introduction; it denied the initial fears that the checklist might cause an extensive time delay, all the staff agreed that the checklist improves patient safety and the majority of the team would consider the checklist useful if they were to have an endoscopic procedure (Table 3).

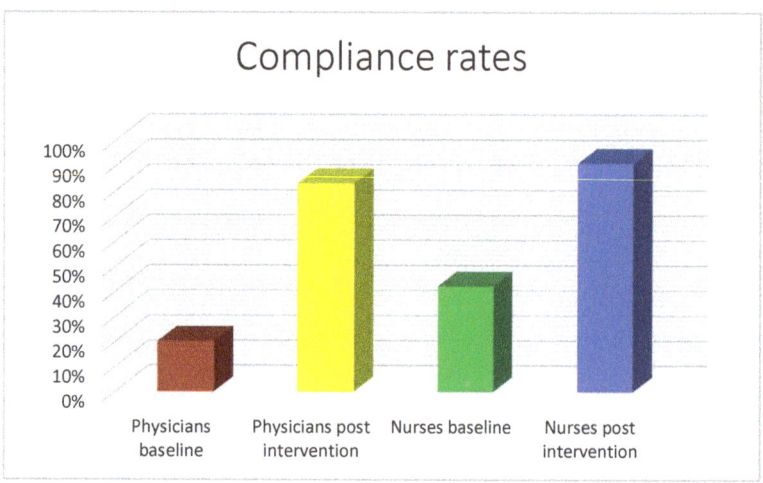

Figure 4. Compliance rates among physicians versus nurses.

Table 3. Staff perception regarding the checklist implementation (physicians n = 15, nurses n = 8).

	Yes n (%)		No n (%)		Hesitant n (%)		p-Value
	Physicians	Nurses	Physicians	Nurses	Physicians	Nurses	
In your opinion, did the checklist cause a time delay?	2 (13.3%)	3 (37.5%)	10 (66.6%)	5 (62.5%)	3 (20%)	0	The chi-square statistic is 1.11. The p-value is 0.29. The result is not significant at $p < 0.05$.
In your opinion, did the checklist improve team communication and teamwork?	11 (73.3%)	7 (87.5%)	1 (6.6%)	0	3 (20%)	1 (12.5%)	The Fisher's exact test statistic value is 1. The result is not significant at $p < 0.05$.
In your opinion, did the checklist improve patient safety?	13 (86.66%)	7 (87.5%)	1 (6.66%)	0	1 (6.66%)	1 (12.5%)	The Fisher's exact test statistic value is 1. The result is not significant at $p < 0.05$.
Would you consider the checklist useful if you were to have an endoscopy?	14 (93.3%)	6 (75%)	0	1 (12.5%)	1 (6.6%)	1 (12.5%)	The Fisher's exact test statistic value is 0.33. The result is not significant at $p < 0.05$.
Would you declare yourself satisfied with the checklist implementation process?	10 (66.6%)	5 (62.5%)	3 (20%)	0	2 (13.3%)	3 (37.5%)	The Fisher's exact test statistic value is 0.52. The result is not significant at $p < 0.05$.

4. Discussions

With increasing indications and more technically advanced gastrointestinal endoscopy techniques, finding strategies to prevent adverse events is an important aspect of the current clinical practice. In many places, the endoscopy has developed in the ad hoc way, following a variety of business models. Although an endoscopy team is a little unusual compared to other diagnostic health services, the team members still need to work in a coordinated and organized way, they must be trained to do their jobs, be motivated to excel, know what is expected from them and know their responsibilities [16].

Communication is important for both the safety and effectiveness of the GI endoscopic procedure. Studies on communication remain limited even in the field of surgery, where there is a much higher flow of complex procedures performed in teams [8,11,17]. An advanced endoscopic intervention would benefit from strong leadership and teamwork skills. One possible way to achieve this is for the endoscopist to adopt conscious verbal competence. An experienced endoscopist could defuse the team by starting a good flow of communication through a full team briefing even before the patient arrives, so that there is no distraction when the procedure begins [18,19].

The concept of verbal conscious competence may be relevant to the expert endoscopist, especially during the team time out process. The complexity of performing a polypectomy, for example, can be classified using the parameters of size, morphology, site and access (SMSA). Furthermore, SMSA classification can be used to estimate the time required to perform an advanced polypectomy along with assessing the difficulty of the procedure as it is mentioned in the Team Time Out phase of the endoscopy checklist. The following would be an illustrative example of performing an endoscopic mucosal resection: Before starting, the endoscopist describes their impression, whether they expect the polypectomy to be simple, moderately challenging or difficult. This first impression may not be definitive and may change during the treatment, at which point the endoscopist should provide an update to the team. The planned technical approach is described, including where the injection needle will be used for mucosal elevation, the intended effect and positioning of the polyp after elevation, the size of the polypectomy loop and the electrical settings for cutting and/or coagulation, etc. The endoscopist continues to discuss the likelihood of adverse events (e.g., bleeding, perforation, or incomplete resection), how these will be solved (e.g., adrenaline, clips, argon plasma, loop tip coagulation, additional cutting, surgical consult, etc.) and once again, asks for team confirmation that all the equipment is available and that the staff is competent and trained [20,21]. It is also recommended that at this point, the endoscopist encourages the team members to state whether they agree with the plan, to express their uncertainties and ask questions or to clearly articulate their opinions. Once a consensus of the whole team is reached and the start is confirmed, the endoscopist gives a verbal signal for the start of the therapy—"let us begin". This is a practical example of how the Team Time Out phase should progress during the process of completing the endoscopy checklist.

Similar to the majority of previous published studies evaluating safety checklists in the GI endoscopy setting [22–24], our study did not find a clear association between the checklist implementation and the clinical outcomes. The staff members were worried that the patients would grow anxious if they were repeatedly asked a lot of questions, but this did not seem to be the case. This was just a secondary observation, considering that the patients were not the subjects of this study, although a questionnaire addressing the patients' perspectives on the safety checklist would bring an added value to the study. As revealed in other published materials, in our study, the compliance rates of the nurses were higher than the physician compliance rates [12,22], but we noticed an increase in the identity checks performed by the physicians, which is an important safety improvement.

Many factors must be taken into account when performing a safe procedure. Although each endoscopy has its own precautions and preparations, many are common and can be divided into the following three major procedural stages: pre-procedure, intra-procedure and post-procedure. While initiating our study, during the baseline phase, it became obvious that adding a checklist to the endoscopy unit's current practices would result in low compliance, hence, intervention methods were required for reaching the goal of a minimum compliance of 75%. As the study continued, we noticed that immediate and targeted feedback seems to be a useful tool for dealing with low compliance. Team feedback in surgery was shown to improve technical performance and reduce adverse events. Post-procedural team feedback is useful, especially in the case of a significant adverse event. In our study, the feedback offered by all team members revealed that the improvement of the checklist implementation is credited to the designated individual assuming ownership for the completion and being accountable for involving the entire multidisciplinary team at each "time out" and "sign in" checklist completion. Even though the results of the staff questionnaire were not statistically significant due to the small number of participants, both physicians and nurses offered consistent and valuable responses, all supporting the usefulness of the endoscopy safety checklist.

The following two main variables of interest were identified in our study: colonic preparation–colonoscopy completion rate and colonic preparation–adenoma detection rate. Both the colonoscopy completion rate and the adenoma detection rate are positively influenced by a proper colonic preparation (Boston Bowel Preparation Scale 2 or 3 for each colonic segment) and, on the other hand, a poor colonic preparation (Boston Bowel Preparation Scale 0 or 1 for each colonic segment) will lead to a poor adenoma detection rate and/or an incomplete colonoscopy evaluation.

Due to a relatively short study period, the compact and constant number of the subjects involved in completing the safety checklist and the staff questionnaire associated with the clear protocol regarding the data collection, we did not register any missing data, which might represent one of the study strengths. A limitation of our study might be the sample size, as the number of GI endoscopy procedures were restricted by the COVID-19 pandemic. An ongoing audit is necessary, ideally with a bigger sample size, to enable subgroup analysis and reveal particular weak points or problematic practices. The baseline measurements included 126 procedures, while post-intervention, 446 procedures were assessed. To strengthen the validity of the findings, it would be advantageous to collect comparable numbers at the study's baseline and post-intervention periods if it were to be conducted again. The "Hawthorne effect," which occurs when team members become aware that they are being watched, is an observation bias and another limitation of the study's scope, as the outcomes might not accurately reflect the everyday surveillance-free practice in the endoscopy lab. The installation of cameras in the endoscopy rooms and using remote video auditing, like in the study of Raphael et al. [22], can help to fight the observation bias. Regarding the survey conducted for assessing the team satisfaction and perception of the checklist, we could think about recall bias, as the questionnaire was handed out to the staff members at the end period of the study. In this case, the memory of the initial experiences with the checklist might be diluted or underestimated versus the more recent and positive experiences after adapting to the checklist requirements. In order to address the potential confirmation bias, the authors of this paper were not included in the observational study as subjects of the GI endoscopy team.

Although the study achieved its objectives, there is still an opportunity for further development. This ought to enable more focused initiatives to lessen the standard-setting variation.

In the end, we acknowledge that a customized approach and patient involvement was necessary for understanding the entire patient experience throughout the GI endoscopy department and how the endoscopy unit performed. Although there were still some items on the checklist that needed to be completed, overall, the compliance rates among the team members increased during the study period, which is very encouraging.

5. Conclusions

Using a checklist and adapting it to local conditions is a high-level recommendation of the Romanian Ministry of Health. In a medical world where safety and quality are essential, a checklist could prevent medical errors, and team time out can ensure high-quality endoscopies, enhance teamwork and offer patients confidence in the medical team. The checklist implementation, in our labs, significantly strengthened the team, flattened hierarchies and improved patient approach and team communication. In a medical world where safety and quality are paramount, a checklist, implemented in all endoscopy services, could prevent procedural errors, streamline teamwork, ensure high-quality work and provide confidence to patients. Hence, standardized methods, such as checklists, promoting patient safety culture and encouraging patient involvement, are strategies for augmented patient safety.

Author Contributions: Conceptualization, A.S. and I.F.C.H.; methodology, I.F.C.H., M.-S.S. and D.E.B.; data curation D.E.B., C.D.N. and M.-S.S.; writing—original draft preparation, I.F.C.H.; writing—review and editing, I.F.C.H.; supervision, A.S. and C.D.N. All authors have read and agreed to the published version of the manuscript.

Funding: This work was supported by a grant of Ministry of Research and Innovation-project number ID P_34_498, within MFE 2014-2020-POC.

Institutional Review Board Statement: This initiative was designed and approved as a quality improvement study with the study subjects set to be the endoscopy staff comprising gastroenterology and anesthesia physicians and endoscopy nurses. No patient information was collected during this study, hence, the exempt of approval from the Local Institutional Ethical Committee.

Informed Consent Statement: Informed consent was obtained from all subjects involved in the study.

Data Availability Statement: All data supporting the study can be located in the archive of the Research Center of Gastroenterology and Hepatology Craiova, Romania and the Lotus Image Medical Center, Actamedica SRL, Targu Mures, Romania.

Conflicts of Interest: The authors declare no conflict of interest.

References

1. Sivak, M.V. Gastrointestinal endoscopy: Past and future. *Gut* **2006**, *55*, 1061–1064. [CrossRef] [PubMed]
2. Borchard, A.; Schwappach, D.; Barbir, A.; Bezzola, P. A systematic review of the effectiveness, compliance, and critical factors for implementation of safety checklists in surgery. *Ann. Surg.* **2012**, *256*, 925–933. [CrossRef] [PubMed]
3. Valori, R.; Cortas, G.; De Lange, T.; Balfaqih, O.S.; De Pater, M.; Eisendrath, P.; Falt, P.; Koruk, I.; Ono, A.; Rustemović, N.; et al. Performance measures for endoscopy services: A European Society of Gastrointestinal Endoscopy (ESGE) quality improvement initiative. *United Eur. Gastroenterol. J.* **2019**, *7*, 21–44. [CrossRef] [PubMed]
4. Haynes, A.B.; Weiser, T.G.; Berry, W.R.; Lipsitz, S.R.; Breizat, A.-H.S.; Dellinger, E.P.; Herbosa, T.; Joseph, S.; Kibatala, P.L.; Lapitan, M.C.M.; et al. A surgical safety checklist to reduce morbidity and mortality in a global population. *N. Engl. J. Med.* **2009**, *360*, 491–499. [CrossRef] [PubMed]
5. Treadwell, J.R.; Lucas, S.; Tsou, A.Y. Surgical checklists: A systematic review of impacts and implementation. *BMJ Qual. Saf.* **2014**, *23*, 299–318. [CrossRef] [PubMed]
6. Gralnek, I.M.; Bisschops, R.; Matharoo, M.; Rutter, M.; Veitch, A.; Meier, P.; Beilenhoff, U.; Hassan, C.; Dinis-Ribeiro, M.; Messmann, H. Guidance for the implementation of a safety checklist for gastrointestinal endoscopic procedures: European Society of Gastrointestinal Endoscopy (ESGE) and European Society of Gastroenterology and Endoscopy Nurses and Associates (ESGENA) Position Statement. *Endoscopy* **2022**, *54*, 206–210. [CrossRef] [PubMed]
7. Valori, R.M.; Johnston, D.J. Leadership and team building in gastrointestinal endoscopy. *Best Pract. Res. Clin. Gastroenterol.* **2016**, *30*, 497–509. [CrossRef]
8. Ching, H.-L.; Lau, M.S.; Azmy, I.A.; Hopper, A.D.; Keuchel, M.; Gyökeres, T.; Kuvaev, R.; Macken, E.J.; Bhandari, P.; Thoufeeq, M.; et al. Performance measures for the SACRED team-centered approach to advanced gastrointestinal endoscopy: European Society of Gastrointestinal Endoscopy (ESGE) Quality Improvement Initiative. *Endoscopy* **2022**, *54*, 712–722. [CrossRef]
9. Bitar, V.; Martel, M.; Restellini, S.; Barkun, A.; Kherad, O. Checklist feasibility and impact in gastrointestinal endoscopy: A systematic review and narrative synthesis. *Endosc. Int. Open* **2021**, *9*, E453–E460. [CrossRef]
10. Gavin, D.R.; Valori, R.M.; Anderson, J.T.; Donnelly, M.T.; Williams, J.G.; Swarbrick, E.T. The national colonoscopy audit: A nationwide assessment of the quality and safety of colonoscopy in the UK. *Gut* **2012**, *62*, 242–249. [CrossRef]
11. Lingard, L.; Espin, S.; Whyte, S.; Regehr, G.; Baker, G.R.; Reznick, R.; Bohnen, J.; Orser, B.; Doran, D.; Grober, E. Communication failures in the operating room: An observational classification of recurrent types and effects. *Hear* **2004**, *13*, 330–334. [CrossRef]
12. Wheelock, A.M.; Suliman, A.M.; Wharton, R.; Babu, E.D.F.; Hull, L.; Vincent, C.; Sevdalis, N.; Arora, S. The Impact of Operating Room Distractions on Stress, Workload, and Teamwork. *Ann. Surg.* **2015**, *261*, 1079–1084. [CrossRef]
13. Kherad, O.; Restellini, S.; Ménard, C.; Martel, M.; Barkun, A. Implementation of a checklist before colonoscopy: A quality improvement initiative. *Endoscopy* **2018**, *50*, 203–210. [CrossRef]
14. Matharoo, M.; Sevdalis, N.; Thillai, M.; Bouri, S.; Marjot, T.; Haycock, A.; Thomas-Gibson, S. The endoscopy safety checklist: A longitudinal study of factors affecting compliance in a tertiary referral centre within the United Kingdom. *BMJ Qual. Improv. Rep.* **2015**, *4*, u206344.w2567. [CrossRef]
15. World Health Organization. WHO Guidelines for Safe Surgery: Safe Surgery Saves Lives. Available online: http://www.who.int/patientsafety/safesurgery/en/ (accessed on 1 January 2020).

16. Mason, M.C.; Griggs, R.K.; Withecombe, R.; Xing, E.Y.; Sandberg, C.; Molyneux, M.K. Improvement in staff compliance with a safety standard checklist in endoscopy in a tertiary centre. *BMJ Open Qual.* **2018**, *7*, e000294. [CrossRef]
17. Calland, J.F.; Turrentine, F.E.; Guerlain, S.; Bovbjerg, V.; Poole, G.R.; Lebeau, K.; Peugh, J.; Adams, R.B. The surgical safety checklist: Lessons learned during implementation. *Am. Surg.* **2011**, *77*, 1131–1137. [CrossRef]
18. Ramanujan, R.; Keyser, D.J.; Sirio, C.A. Making a Case for Organizational Change in Patient Safety Initiatives. In *Advances in Patient Safety: From Research to Implementation*; Defense Technical Information Center: Fort Belvoir, VA, USA, 2005.
19. Kristensen, N.; Nymann, C.; Konradsen, H. Implementing research results in clinical practice—The experiences of healthcare professionals. *BMC Health Serv. Res.* **2016**, *16*, 48. [CrossRef]
20. Kang, H.; Thoufeeq, M.H. Size of colorectal polyps determines time taken to remove them endoscopically. *Endosc. Int. Open* **2018**, *6*, E610–E615. [CrossRef]
21. Sidhu, R.; Turnbull, D.; Newton, M.; Thomas-Gibson, S.; Sanders, D.S.; Hebbar, S.; Haidry, R.J.; Smith, G.; Webster, G. Deep sedation and anaesthesia in complex gastrointestinal endoscopy: A joint position statement endorsed by the British Society of Gastroenterology (BSG), Joint Advisory Group (JAG) and Royal College of Anaesthetists (RCoA). *Front. Gastroenterol.* **2019**, *10*, 141–147. [CrossRef]
22. Raphael, K.; Cerrone, S.; Sceppa, E.; Schneider, P.; Laumenede, T.; Lynch, A.; Sejpal, D.V. Improving patient safety in the endoscopy unit: Utilization of remote video auditing to improve time-out compliance. *Gastrointest. Endosc.* **2019**, *90*, 424–429. [CrossRef]
23. Dubois, H.; Schmidt, P.T.; Creutzfeldt, J.; Bergenmar, M. Person-centered endoscopy safety checklist: Development, implementation, and evaluation. *World J. Gastroenterol.* **2017**, *23*, 8605–8614. [CrossRef] [PubMed]
24. Matharoo, M.; Thomas-Gibson, S.; Haycock, A.; Sevdalis, N. Implementation of an endoscopy safety checklist. *Front. Gastroenterol.* **2013**, *5*, 260–265. [CrossRef] [PubMed]

Disclaimer/Publisher's Note: The statements, opinions and data contained in all publications are solely those of the individual author(s) and contributor(s) and not of MDPI and/or the editor(s). MDPI and/or the editor(s) disclaim responsibility for any injury to people or property resulting from any ideas, methods, instructions or products referred to in the content.

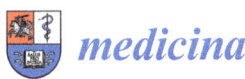

Review

Transoral Outlet Reduction (TORe) for the Treatment of Weight Regain and Dumping Syndrome after Roux-en-Y Gastric Bypass

Landry Hakiza [1,2], Adrian Sartoretto [3], Konstantin Burgmann [1,2], Vivek Kumbhari [4], Christoph Matter [1,2], Frank Seibold [1,2] and Dominic Staudenmann [1,2,*]

1. Gastroenterology Service Intesto, 3012 Bern, Switzerland
2. Gastroenterology Service Intesto, Hôpital Fribourgeois, University of Fribourg, 1700 Fribourg, Switzerland
3. The BMI Clinic, Double Bay, NSW 2028, Australia
4. Division of Gastroenterology and Hepatology, Mayo Clinic, Jacksonville, FL 32224, USA
* Correspondence: staudenmannd@intesto.ch; Tel.: +41-31-302-32-34

Abstract: Obesity is a chronic relapsing disease of global pandemic proportions. In this context, an increasing number of patients are undergoing bariatric surgery, which is considered the most effective weight loss treatment for long-term improvement in obesity-related comorbidities. One of the most popular bariatric surgeries is the Roux-en-Y gastric bypass (RYGB). Despite its proven short- and long-term efficacy, progressive weight regain and dumping symptoms remain a challenge. Revisional bariatric surgery is indicated when dietary and lifestyle modification, pharmaceutical agents and/or psychological therapy fail to arrest weight regain or control dumping. However, these re-interventions present greater technical difficulty and are accompanied by an increased risk of peri- and postoperative complications with substantial morbidity and mortality. The endoscopic approach to gastrojejunal anastomotic revision, transoral outlet reduction (TORe), is used as a minimally invasive treatment that aims to reduce the diameter of the gastrojejunal anastomosis, delaying gastric emptying and increasing satiety. With substantial published data supporting its use, TORe is an effective and safe bariatric endoscopic technique for addressing weight regain and dumping syndrome after RYGB.

Keywords: endoscopic transoral outlet reduction; bariatric endoscopy; obesity; gastric bypass; dumping syndrome; weight regain

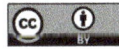

1. Introduction

Obesity is currently one of the greatest public health challenges, with substantial economic implications. According to estimates published by the World Health Organization (WHO) on 4 March 2022, more than one billion people worldwide suffer with obesity— 650 million adults, 340 million adolescents and 39 million children [1]. The WHO estimates that by 2025, approximately 167 million people (adults and children) will become less healthy due to overweight or obesity [1].

The measures implemented against obesity usually include conservative treatment, such as lifestyle modification and drug therapy, as well as bariatric surgery; however, in most patients, sustained weight loss is not achieved [2–4].

Pharmacologic treatments allow an average loss of 10% of body weight (BW), and newer drugs under investigation seem even more promising [5]. However, weight regain is universally observed upon discontinuation of treatment [6].

Contemporary guidelines on the management of morbid obesity recognize bariatric surgery (BS) as the gold standard for weight loss and the improvement of obesity-related comorbidities [7–9]. Patients with obesity are generally considered eligible for BS at a BMI greater than 40 kg/m^2, or greater than 35 kg/m^2 when accompanied by serious weight-related comorbidities, such as type 2 diabetes mellitus, (T2DM) hypertension or obstructive sleep apnea [9].

The two most commonly performed bariatric procedures worldwide are the Roux-en-Y gastric bypass (RYGB) (39.6%) and the sleeve gastrectomy (SG) (45.9%) [9]. Compared to SG, RYGB confers superior clinical efficacy in terms of weight loss and in the remission of comorbidities, particularly T2DM [7,9,10].

2. Methods

A comprehensive search of several English-language databases and conference proceedings from 1990 to 2022 was conducted. The databases included PubMed, MEDLINE, EMBASE, Web of Science databases, Google Scholar and SCOPUS, with PubMed being the main database used. Secondary weight regain after gastric bypass surgery, dumping syndrome after gastric bypass, transoral outlet reduction and endoscopic suturing were used as keywords. Literature screening was independently performed by two authors (L.H. and D.S.), with research focusing on studies with long-term outcomes (from 2 to 5 years post-TORe).

3. TORe for Weight Regain after RYGB

Weight recidivism is a common complication following RYGB surgery. On average, patients regain between 20 and 30 % of lost weight, and moreover, excessive weight gain is experienced by over one third of patients [11,12]. Weight regain after gastric bypass is often multifactorial and can be attributed to eating patterns, and psychological and social factors. However, dilatation or enlargement of the gastrojejunal anastomosis of >30 mm is a significant predictor of weight regain following RYGB [13–15]. Due to the technical complexity of the anatomy, surgical re-intervention is accompanied by a high risk of complications and an increase in postoperative morbidity and mortality [16]. As an alternative, TORe was developed in 2013 as an endoscopic procedure focusing on reducing the size of the gastrojejunal anastomosis (GJA) [17]. The first interventional study included 25 patients with an average weight regain of 24 kg after RYGB [17]. This study described endoscopically reducing the diameter of the anastomosis by an average of 77.3% which was associated with an average weight loss of 11.5 kg, 11.7 kg and 10.8 kg at 3, 6 and 12 months, respectively [17].

Vargas et al. demonstrated in a multicenter study that TORe is a safe, reproducible and effective approach to managing weight recidivism after RYGB [18]. The average weight loss at 6, 12 and 18 months was 9.31 ± 6.7 kg, 7.75 ± 8.4 kg and 8 ± 8.8 kg, respectively, and no serious adverse events were reported [18].

Recently, a five-year outcome study concluded that endoscopic revision of the GJA for weight regain is a durable approach [12]. Total body weight loss (TBWL) of 8.5% at 1 year (n = 276/331 patients), 6.9% at 3 years (n = 211/331), and 8.8% at 5 years after TORe was shown [12]. In addition, the majority of the patients (77%) experienced complete cessation of weight gain and 62% were able to maintain a TBWL of >5% at 5 years [12].

Furthermore, an American group assessed patients' ability to lose weight after TORe and the magnitude of the reduction of the GJA [19]. They demonstrated that patients who had a larger reduction in diameter had a more significant TBWL. After 3 and 5 years following TORe, TBWL was 5.3 ± 9.1 kg and 3.9 ± 13.1 kg, respectively [19].

4. TORe for Dumping Syndrome after RYGB

Dumping syndrome (DS) is a postprandial phenomenon in which patients present with a constellation of gastrointestinal and vasomotor symptoms, including tachycardia, fatigue, syncope, and occasionally, shock and seizures due to profound hypoglycemia [20]. Symptoms may occur early (within 1 h of a meal) or up to 3 h later, the latter being associated with postprandial hypoglycemia. As the name suggests, DS occurs, in part, due to rapid gastric emptying, leading to rapid passage of food into the small intestine [21,22].

The patient's typical history and blood sugar determination inform the diagnosis. The Sigstad score (a score >7 is strongly suggestive of dumping) and questionnaires may also be helpful [21].

A conservative stepwise approach is currently recommended, starting with dietary changes in the form of more frequent meals with increased protein content and lower overall carbohydrate content, favoring complex carbohydrates [23,24]. If dietary measures prove unsuccessful, drug therapy can be initiated with acarbose, calcium antagonists or GLP-1 analogues [25].

However, dietary restrictions and pharmacological treatments are often ineffective or poorly tolerated [21,22]. In these cases, TORe provides a solution by reducing the speed of gastric emptying, however there is no clear consensus in the literature regarding the place of surgical re-intervention in treating dumping syndrome [21,26–28].

A large study involving 115 patients from two large academic centers in the United States and Germany supported TORe as an effective and safe adjuvant therapy to lifestyle and pharmacologic treatment of refractory DS [29]. The Sigstad score reduced significantly after only 3 months post-TORe, with the mean sore changing from 17 ± 6.1 to 2.6 ± 1.9 [29]. Similarly, Brown et al. demonstrated a 90% rate of resolution of DS after only 3 months of revision [30].

A recent retrospective study was published in October 2022, where 83% of the patients had a long-term follow-up at a mean of 3.45 years [31]. This retrospective study also found that the presence of gastro-esophageal reflux disease prior to TORe was a predictor of the resolution of DS following the procedure. While the difference was small, it achieved statistical significance (69% vs. 62%; $p = 0.03$) [31].

In this context, TORe is not only an effective approach to managing weight recidivism after RYGB, but also to treating DS.

5. TORe Technique

TORe is currently the most frequently used technique for the reduction of a dilated GJA (Figure 1A). The intervention is usually performed under general anesthesia. A double-lumen gastroscope is passed through a proprietary overtube of 25 cm in length, and CO_2 is used for insufflation. It can be carried out on an outpatient basis, and it is typically performed with argon plasma coagulation (APC) combined with full-thickness suturing achieved using the OverStitchTM device (Apollo Endosurgery, Austin, TX, USA) [15,32,33]. This combined technique allows for greater durability of anastomotic reduction by inducing fibrosis of the GJA [34,35]. The first step of the procedure is to ablate the gastric rim of the anastomosis via APC (forced APC, 0.8 L/min with 30–70 watts) (Figure 1B), followed by a circumferential, transmural endoscopic suture (Figure 1C). Suturing is mainly performed via the creation of a purse-string, or alternatively, by placing interrupted sutures at the GJA [29]. The purse-string technique is, however, generally favored, as it results in more significant weight loss at one year than interrupted suture patterns [36]. Ideally, a dilation balloon (CRE balloon dilator, Boston Scientific, Marlborough, MA, USA) is introduced through the second channel of the endoscope and inflated to a diameter of 8–10 mm (Figure 1D) to size the GJA before the suture is tightened and cinched over the balloon, allowing the GJA to be precisely sized (Figure 1E and Video S1).

There are several other TORe techniques described in the literature [35,37–40]. Initially, some studies demonstrated efficacy using APC alone in the GJA, which was relatively simple to perform, and even feasible with patients under conscious sedation [41–44]. Jaruvongvanich et al. reported a meta-analysis showing that both full-thickness suturing plus APC (ft-TORe) and argon plasma mucosal coagulation alone (APMC-TORe) offer comparable weight loss outcomes and safety profiles, but the AMPC-TORe technique usually requires multiple endoscopic sessions [35].

Barola et al. performed a two-fold running suture TORe technique with a significant reduction in BMI (5.5 + 5.0%, $p < 0.001$ at mean follow-up of 113.2 ± 75.7 days

(15.4%)); however, 15.4% of the patients developed a gastric stenosis that was treated with balloon dilation [39].

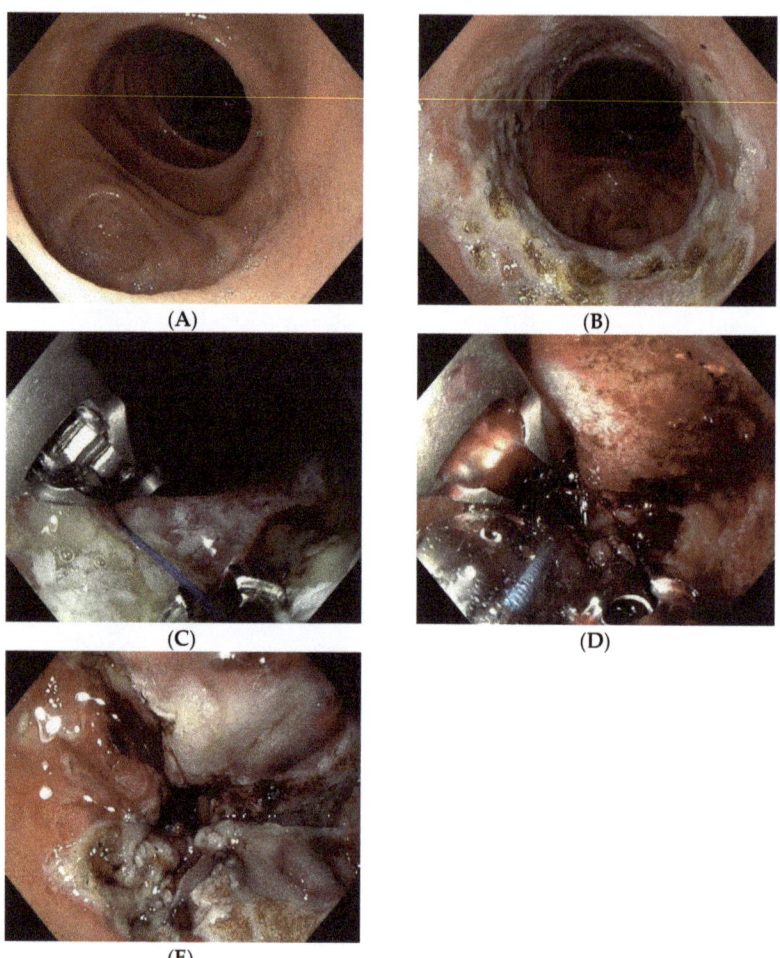

Figure 1. (**A**) Dilated GJA; (**B**) ablation of the gastric rim via APC; (**C**) suturing the anastomosis with the Apollo Overstitch system; (**D**) suture size control using an 8 mm CRE balloon; (**E**) narrowed GJA after TORe.

A new approach combining the restriction component of TORe followed by type 1 surgical distalization of the Roux limb may be another alternative for managing weight regain in high-BMI patients after RYGB; however, this could result in greater malabsorption, leading to greater deficiency syndrome [40].

More recently, we have seen the emergence of a novel, modified technique: first performing an endoscopic submucosal dissection (ESD) before applying endoscopic sutures. This is known as ESD-TORe [37,38]. A retrospective study compared patients who underwent modified ESD-TORe vs. APC -TORe. At 12 months, the ESD-TORe group experienced greater weight loss compared with the traditional TORe group (12.1% ± 9.3% vs. 7.5% ± 3.3% TBWL) [38]. However, this technique resulted in a higher rate of major complications (21.1% for ESD-TORe vs. 8.77% for APC-TORe) which, combined with the technical difficulty of ESD, limits its widespread adoption [34,38].

On the other hand, the TORe procedure has demonstrated a high degree of safety, with only minor intraprocedural adverse effects (AE) such as superficial lacerations of the esophageal mucosa due to the use of the overtube [12,17–19,29–33,45–47]. Additional postprocedural serious AEs include bleeding from marginal ulceration and GJA stenosis [20–22,25,30–34,40–42]. In general, AEs can be successfully managed endoscopically without the need for surgery.

6. Discussion

Despite the efficacy and durability of RYGB, weight regain and the return of comorbid conditions, as well as DS, is of major concern [15,18,29,31,45,46,48]. The underlying causes are multifactorial, and therefore, its management requires a multidisciplinary approach, in collaboration with general practitioners, surgeons, dietitians, endocrinologists, psychiatrists or psychologists and gastroenterologists [49,50]. One of the most common factors contributing to weight regain and DS after RYGB is a dilated GJA [15,18,19,32,33,46]. Initially, this was treated with revisional bariatric surgery such as pyloric reconstruction, the conversion of Billroth II to Billroth I anastomoses, jejunal interposition and Roux-en-Y conversion [51]. However, the surgical approach is associated with increased risk and limited effectiveness [21,26–28].

The TORe technique has now repeatedly demonstrated its efficacy, safety and favorable long term results for up to 5 years in the management of weight regain after RYGB [12,13,15,19,32,38]. Patients are able to maintain a TBWL of 12.5% at 5 years [19,38,45]. Recent studies have also shown that it can be used as a minimally invasive treatment for refractory DS, demonstrating an 80% and 84% resolution of DS at 2- and 3.5-year follow-ups, respectively [30,31]. Moreover, it has been illustrated that TORe is accompanied by a very low risk of serious adverse events, and no deaths have been causally associated with the procedure [12,19,31,52]. Given the very low risk of severe complications, TORe is easily repeatable if necessary [29,45]. This growing body of evidence supports the role of TORe as an emerging standard of care in the treatment of weight regain and DS in patients with prior RYGB, now superseding surgical intervention.

7. Conclusions

TORe represents an endoscopic bariatric technique that has been proven to be safe and durably efficacious in managing weight regain, as well as DS, post-RYGB. While first-line treatment for these conditions remains lifestyle and pharmacologic therapies delivered in a multidisciplinary setting, TORe has effectively replaced revisional surgery as a first-line interventional therapy owing to its superior safety profile, lower resource requirement and demonstrated clinically meaningful efficacy.

Supplementary Materials: The following supporting information can be downloaded at: https://www.mdpi.com/article/10.3390/medicina59010125/s1, Video S1: The transoral outlet reduction (TORe) endoscopy procedure.

Author Contributions: Conceptualization, all authors; methodology, L.H. and D.S.; writing—original draft preparation, L.H. and D.S.; writing—review and editing, A.S., V.K., D.S., L.H., K.B., F.S. and C.M.; supervision, D.S. and A.S. All authors have read and agreed to the published version of the manuscript.

Funding: This research received no external funding.

Institutional Review Board Statement: Not applicable.

Informed Consent Statement: Not applicable.

Data Availability Statement: Not applicable.

Conflicts of Interest: The authors declare no conflict of interest.

References

1. World Health Organisation. Acceleration Action to Stop Obesity. Available online: https://www.who.int/news/item/04-03-2022-world-obesity-day-2022-accelerating-action-to-stop-obesity (accessed on 26 October 2022).
2. Knowler, W.C.; Fowler, S.E.; Hamman, R.F.; Christophi, C.A.; Hoffman, H.J.; Brenneman, A.T.; Brown-Friday, J.O.; Goldberg, R.; Venditti, E.; Nathan, D.M. 10-year follow-up of diabetes incidence and weight loss in the Diabetes Prevention Program Outcomes Study. *Lancet* **2009**, *374*, 1677–1686. [PubMed]
3. Christou, N.v.; Look, D.; MacLean, L.D. Weight Gain After Short- and Long-Limb Gastric Bypass in Patients Followed for Longer than 10 Years. *Ann Surg.* **2006**, *244*, 734–740. [CrossRef] [PubMed]
4. Magro, D.O.; Geloneze, B.; Delfini, R.; Pareja, B.C.; Callejas, F.; Pareja, J.C. Long-term Weight Regain after Gastric Bypass: A 5-year Prospective Study. *Obes. Surg.* **2008**, *18*, 648–651. [CrossRef] [PubMed]
5. Knerr, P.J.; Mowery, S.A.; Douros, J.D.; Premdjee, B.; Hjøllund, K.R.; He, Y.; Hansen, A.M.K.; Olsen, A.K.; Perez-Tilve, D.; DiMarchi, R.D.; et al. Next generation GLP-1/GIP/glucagon triple agonists normalize body weight in obese mice. *Mol. Metab.* **2022**, *63*, 101533. [CrossRef]
6. Vosoughi, K.; Atieh, J.; Khanna, L.; Khoshbin, K.; Prokop, L.J.; Davitkov, P.; Murad, M.H.; Camilleri, M. Association of glucagon-like peptide 1 analogs and agonists administered for obesity with weight loss and adverse events: A systematic review and network meta-analysis. *Eclinicalmedicine* **2021**, *42*, 101213. [CrossRef]
7. Wharton, S.; Lau, D.C.; Vallis, M.; Sharma, A.M.; Biertho, L.; Campbell-Scherer, D.; Adamo, K.; Alberga, A.; Bell, R.; Boulé, N.; et al. Obesity in adults: A clinical practice guideline. *Can. Med. Assoc. J.* **2020**, *192*, E875–E891. [CrossRef]
8. Powell-Wiley, T.M.; Poirier, P.; Burke, L.E.; Després, J.-P.; Gordon-Larsen, P.; Lavie, C.J.; Lear, S.A.; Ndumele, C.E.; Neeland, I.J.; Sanders, P.; et al. Obesity and Cardiovascular Disease: A Scientific Statement from the American Heart Association. *Circulation* **2021**, *143*, e984–e1010. [CrossRef]
9. Welbourn, R.; Hollyman, M.; Kinsman, R.; Dixon, J.; Liem, R.; Ottosson, J.; Ramos, A.; Våge, V.; Al-Sabah, S.; Brown, W.; et al. Bariatric Surgery Worldwide: Baseline Demographic Description and One-Year Outcomes from the Fourth IFSO Global Registry Report 2018. *Obes. Surg.* **2019**, *29*, 782–795. [CrossRef]
10. McTigue, K.M.; Wellman, R.; Nauman, E.; Anau, J.; Coley, R.Y.; Odor, A.; Tice, J.; Coleman, K.J.; Courcoulas, A.; Pardee, R.E.; et al. Comparing the 5-Year Diabetes Outcomes of Sleeve Gastrectomy and Gastric Bypass. *JAMA Surg.* **2020**, *155*, e200087. [CrossRef]
11. Cooper, T.C.; Simmons, E.B.; Webb, K.; Burns, J.L.; Kushner, R.F. Trends in Weight Regain Following Roux-en-Y Gastric Bypass (RYGB) Bariatric Surgery. *Obes. Surg.* **2015**, *25*, 1474–1481. [CrossRef]
12. Jirapinyo, P.; Kumar, N.; AlSamman, M.A.; Thompson, C.C. Five-year outcomes of transoral outlet reduction for the treatment of weight regain after Roux-en-Y gastric bypass. *Gastrointest. Endosc.* **2020**, *91*, 1067–1073. [CrossRef] [PubMed]
13. Ramadan, M.; Loureiro, M.; Laughlan, K.; Caiazzo, R.; Iannelli, A.; Brunaud, L.; Czernichow, S.; Nedelcu, M.; Nocca, D. Risk of Dumping Syndrome after Sleeve Gastrectomy and Roux-en-Y Gastric Bypass: Early Results of a Multicentre Prospective Study. *Gastroenterol. Res. Pract.* **2016**, *2016*, 2570237. [CrossRef] [PubMed]
14. Abu Dayyeh, B.K.; Lautz, D.B.; Thompson, C.C. Gastrojejunal Stoma Diameter Predicts Weight Regain after Roux-en-Y Gastric Bypass. *Clin. Gastroenterol. Hepatol.* **2011**, *9*, 228–233. [CrossRef] [PubMed]
15. Kumar, N.; Thompson, C.C. Transoral outlet reduction for weight regain after gastric bypass: Long-term follow-up. *Gastrointest. Endosc.* **2016**, *83*, 776–779. [CrossRef] [PubMed]
16. Mann, J.P.; Jakes, A.D.; Hayden, J.D.; Barth, J.H. Systematic Review of Definitions of Failure in Revisional Bariatric Surgery. *Obes. Surg.* **2015**, *25*, 571–574. [CrossRef]
17. Jirapinyo, P.; Slattery, J.; Ryan, M.B.; Abu Dayyeh, B.K.; Lautz, D.B.; Thompson, C.C. Evaluation of an endoscopic suturing device for transoral outlet reduction in patients with weight regain following Roux-en-Y gastric bypass. *Endoscopy* **2013**, *45*, 532–536. [CrossRef]
18. Vargas, E.J.; Bazerbachi, F.; Rizk, M.; Rustagi, T.; Acosta, A.; Wilson, E.B.; Wilson, T.; Neto, M.G.; Zundel, N.; Mundi, M.S.; et al. Transoral outlet reduction with full thickness endoscopic suturing for weight regain after gastric bypass: A large multicenter international experience and meta-analysis. *Surg. Endosc.* **2018**, *32*, 252–259. [CrossRef] [PubMed]
19. Callahan, Z.M.; Su, B.; Kuchta, K.; Linn, J.; Carbray, J.; Ujiki, M. Five-year results of endoscopic gastrojejunostomy revision (transoral outlet reduction) for weight gain after gastric bypass. *Surg. Endosc.* **2020**, *34*, 2164–2171. [CrossRef]
20. Van Beek, A.P.; Emous, M.; Laville, M.; Tack, J. Dumping syndrome after esophageal, gastric or bariatric surgery: Pathophysiology, diagnosis, and management. *Obes. Rev.* **2017**, *18*, 68–85. [CrossRef]
21. Scarpellini, E.; Arts, J.; Karamanolis, G.; Laurenius, A.; Siquini, W.; Suzuki, H.; Ukleja, A.; Van Beek, A.; Vanuytsel, T.; Bor, S.; et al. International consensus on the diagnosis and management of dumping syndrome. *Nat. Rev. Endocrinol.* **2020**, *16*, 448–466. [CrossRef]
22. Tack, J.; Arts, J.; Caenepeel, P.; De Wulf, D.; Bisschops, R. Pathophysiology, diagnosis and management of postoperative dumping syndrome. *Nat. Rev. Gastroenterol. Hepatol.* **2009**, *6*, 583–590. [CrossRef] [PubMed]
23. Ukleja, A. Dumping Syndrome: Pathophysiology and Treatment. *Nutr. Clin. Pract.* **2005**, *20*, 517–525. [CrossRef]
24. Banerjee, A.; Ding, Y.; Mikami, D.J.; Needleman, B.J. The role of dumping syndrome in weight loss after gastric bypass surgery. *Surg. Endosc.* **2013**, *27*, 1573–1578. [CrossRef] [PubMed]
25. Moreira, R.O.; Moreira, R.B.M.; Machado, N.A.M.; Gonçalves, T.B.; Coutinho, W.F. Post-prandial Hypoglycemia after Bariatric Surgery: Pharmacological Treatment with Verapamil and Acarbose. *Obes. Surg.* **2008**, *18*, 1618–1621. [CrossRef] [PubMed]

26. Lakdawala, M.; Limas, P.; Dhar, S.; Remedios, C.; Dhulla, N.; Sood, A.; Bhasker, A.G. Laparoscopic revision of Roux-en-Y gastric bypass to sleeve gastrectomy: A ray of hope for failed Roux-en-Y gastric bypass. *Asian J. Endosc. Surg.* 2016, 9, 122–127. [CrossRef] [PubMed]
27. Campos, G.M.; Ziemelis, M.; Paparodis, R.; Ahmed, M.; Davis, D.B. Laparoscopic reversal of Roux-en-Y gastric bypass: Technique and utility for treatment of endocrine complications. *Surg. Obes. Relat. Dis.* 2014, 10, 36–43. [CrossRef]
28. Tran, D.D.; Nwokeabia, I.D.; Purnell, S.; Zafar, S.N.; Ortega, G.; Hughes, K.; Fullum, T.M. Revision of Roux-En-Y Gastric Bypass for Weight Regain: A Systematic Review of Techniques and Outcomes. *Obes. Surg.* 2016, 26, 1627–1634. [CrossRef]
29. Vargas, E.J.; Dayyeh, B.K.; Storm, A.C.; Bazerbachi, F.; Matar, R.; Vella, A.; Kellogg, T.; Stier, C. Endoscopic management of dumping syndrome after Roux-en-Y gastric bypass: A large international series and proposed management strategy. *Gastrointest. Endosc.* 2020, 92, 91–96. [CrossRef]
30. Brown, M.; Zaman, J.; Arellano, J.; Binetti, B.; Singh, T.P. Sa2011 Endoscopic Gastrojejunostomy Revision Following Roux-En-Y Gastric Bypass: Outcomes at 2-Year Follow-Up. *Gastrointest. Endosc.* 2017, 85, AB275. [CrossRef]
31. Petchers, A.; Walker, A.; Bertram, C.; Feustel, P.; Singh, T.P.; Zaman, J. Evaluation of endoscopic gastrojejunostomy revision after Roux-en-Y gastric bypass for treatment of dumping syndrome. *Gastrointest. Endosc.* 2022, 96, 639–644. [CrossRef]
32. Dhindsa, B.S.; Saghir, S.M.; Naga, Y.; Dhaliwal, A.; Ramai, D.; Cross, C.; Singh, S.; Bhat, I.; Adler, D.G. Efficacy of transoral outlet reduction in Roux-en-Y gastric bypass patients to promote weight loss: A systematic review and meta-analysis. *Endosc. Int. Open* 2020, 8, E1332–E1340. [CrossRef]
33. Brunaldi, V.O.; Jirapinyo, P.; de Moura, D.T.H.; Okazaki, O.; Bernardo, W.M.; Neto, M.G.; Campos, J.M.; Santo, M.A.; de Moura, E.G.H. Endoscopic Treatment of Weight Regain Following Roux-en-Y Gastric Bypass: A Systematic Review and Meta-analysis. *Obes. Surg.* 2018, 28, 266–276. [CrossRef] [PubMed]
34. Wong, S.K.H. Endoscopic full-thickness transoral outlet reduction with endoscopic submucosal dissection or argon plasma coagulation: Does it make a difference? *Endoscopy* 2019, 51, 617–618. [CrossRef]
35. Jaruvongvanich, V.; Vantanasiri, K.; Laoveeravat, P.; Matar, R.H.; Vargas, E.J.; Maselli, D.B.; Alkhatry, M.; Fayad, L.; Kumbhari, V.; Fittipaldi-Fernandez, R.J.; et al. Endoscopic full-thickness suturing plus argon plasma mucosal coagulation versus argon plasma mucosal coagulation alone for weight regain after gastric bypass: A systematic review and meta-analysis. *Gastrointest. Endosc.* 2020, 92, 1164–1175.e6. [CrossRef] [PubMed]
36. Schulman, A.R.; Kumar, N.; Thompson, C.C. Transoral outlet reduction: A comparison of purse-string with interrupted stitch technique. *Gastrointest. Endosc.* 2018, 87, 1222–1228. [CrossRef] [PubMed]
37. Hollenbach, M.; Selig, L.; Lellwitz, S.; Beer, S.; Feisthammel, J.; Rosendahl, J.; Schaumburg, T.; Mössner, J.; Hoffmeister, A. Endoscopic full-thickness transoral outlet reduction with semicircumferential endoscopic submucosal dissection. *Endoscopy* 2019, 51, 684–688. [CrossRef] [PubMed]
38. Jirapinyo, P.; de Moura, D.T.; Thompson, C.C. Endoscopic submucosal dissection with suturing for the treatment of weight regain after gastric bypass: Outcomes and comparison with traditional transoral outlet reduction (with video). *Gastrointest. Endosc.* 2020, 91, 1282–1288. [CrossRef]
39. Barola, S.; Agnihotri, A.; Hill, C.; Dunlap, M.K.; Ngamruengphong, S.; Chen, Y.-I.; Singh, V.; Khashab, M.A.; Kumbhari, V. Sa2017 Transoral Outlet Reduction Post Roux-En-Y Gastric Bypass: Evaluation of a Treatment Algorithm Using Two-Fold Running Sutures. *Gastrointest. Endosc.* 2017, 85, AB278–AB279. [CrossRef]
40. Abu Dayyeh, B.; Portela, R.; Mahmoud, T.; Ghazi, R.; Ghanem, O.M. A novel approach for weight regain after Roux-en-Y gastric bypass: Staged transoral outlet reduction (TORe) followed by surgical type 1 distalization. *VideoGIE* 2022, 7, 135–137. [CrossRef]
41. Jirapinyo, P.; Moura, D.; Dong, W.Y.; Farias, G.; Thompson, C.C. Dose response for argon plasma coagulation in the treatment of weight regain after Roux-en-Y gastric bypass. *Gastrointest. Endosc.* 2020, 91, 1078–1084. [CrossRef]
42. Jirapinyo, P.; Kroner, P.T.; Thompson, C.C. Argon Plasma Coagulation is Effective in Roux-En-Y Gastric Bypass Patients that do not Achieve Weight Loss Goals after Sutured Transoral Outlet Reduction (TORe). *Gastroenterology* 2017, 152, S635. [CrossRef]
43. Baretta, G.A.P.; Alhinho, H.C.A.W.; Matias, J.E.F.; Marchesini, J.B.; de Lima, J.H.F.; Empinotti, C.; Campos, J.M. Argon Plasma Coagulation of Gastrojejunal Anastomosis for Weight Regain After Gastric Bypass. *Obes. Surg.* 2015, 25, 72–79. [CrossRef] [PubMed]
44. Moon, R.C.; Teixeira, A.F.; Neto, M.G.; Zundel, N.; Sander, B.Q.; Ramos, F.M.; Matz, F.; Baretta, G.A.; de Quadros, L.G.; Grecco, E.; et al. Efficacy of Utilizing Argon Plasma Coagulation for Weight Regain in Roux-en-Y Gastric Bypass Patients: A Multi-center Study. *Obes. Surg.* 2018, 28, 2737–2744. [CrossRef]
45. Relly, R.; Mati, S.; Aviv, C.N.; Fishman, S. Endoscopic trans-oral outlet reduction after bariatric surgery is safe and effective for dumping syndrome. *Surg. Endosc.* 2021, 35, 6846–6852. [CrossRef] [PubMed]
46. Tsai, C.; Steffen, R.; Kessler, U.; Merki, H.; Zehetner, J. Endoscopic Gastrojejunal Revisions Following Gastric Bypass: Lessons Learned in More Than 100 Consecutive Patients. *J. Gastrointest. Surg.* 2019, 23, 58–66. [CrossRef]
47. Stier, C.; Chiappetta, S. Endoluminal Revision (OverStitch TM, Apollo Endosurgery) of the Dilated Gastroenterostomy in Patients with Late Dumping Syndrome after Proximal Roux-en-Y Gastric Bypass. *Obes. Surg.* 2016, 26, 1978–1984. [CrossRef]
48. Wing, R.R.; Lang, W.; Wadden, T.A.; Safford, M.; Knowler, W.C.; Bertoni, A.G.; Hill, J.O.; Brancati, F.L.; Peters, A.; Wagenknecht, L.; et al. Benefits of Modest Weight Loss in Improving Cardiovascular Risk Factors in Overweight and Obese Individuals With Type 2 Diabetes. *Diabetes Care* 2011, 34, 1481–1486. [CrossRef] [PubMed]

49. Cambi, M.P.C.; Baretta, G.A.P.; Magro, D.D.O.; Boguszewski, C.L.; Ribeiro, I.B.; Jirapinyo, P.; de Moura, D.T.H. Multidisciplinary Approach for Weight Regain—How to Manage this Challenging Condition: An Expert Review. *Obes. Surg.* **2021**, *31*, 1290–1303. [CrossRef] [PubMed]
50. Ryou, M.; McQuaid, K.R.; Thompson, C.C.; Edmundowicz, S.; Mergener, K. ASGE EndoVators Summit: Defining the role and value of endoscopic therapies in obesity management. *Surg. Endosc.* **2018**, *32*, 1–13. [CrossRef] [PubMed]
51. Hui, C.; Dhakal, A.; Bauza, G.J. Dumping Syndrome. In *StatPearls*; StatPearls Publishing: Treasure Island, FL, USA, 2022.
52. Jirapinyo, P.; Kröner, P.T.; Thompson, C.C. Purse-string transoral outlet reduction (TORe) is effective at inducing weight loss and improvement in metabolic comorbidities after Roux-en-Y gastric bypass. *Endoscopy* **2018**, *50*, 371–377. [CrossRef] [PubMed]

Disclaimer/Publisher's Note: The statements, opinions and data contained in all publications are solely those of the individual author(s) and contributor(s) and not of MDPI and/or the editor(s). MDPI and/or the editor(s) disclaim responsibility for any injury to people or property resulting from any ideas, methods, instructions or products referred to in the content.

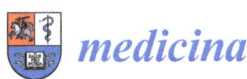

Review

Hemostatic Powders in Non-Variceal Upper Gastrointestinal Bleeding: The Open Questions

Omero Alessandro Paoluzi [1,*], Edoardo Troncone [1], Elena De Cristofaro [1], Mezia Sibilia [2], Giovanni Monteleone [1] and Giovanna Del Vecchio Blanco [1]

[1] Gastroenterology Unit, Department of Systems Medicine, University Tor Vergata, 00133 Rome, Italy
[2] Gastroenterology Unit, Department of Medical Sciences, University Tor Vergata Hospital, 00133 Rome, Italy
* Correspondence: omeroalessandro.paoluzi@ptvonline.it

Abstract: Hemostatic powder (HP) is a relatively recent addition to the arsenal of hemostatic endoscopic procedures (HEPs) for gastrointestinal bleeding (GIB) due to benign and malignant lesions. Five types of HP are currently available: TC-325 (Hemospray™), EndoClot™, Ankaferd Blood Stopper®, and, more recently, UI-EWD (Nexpowder™) and CEGP-003 (CGBio™). HP acts as a mechanical barrier and/or promotes platelet activation and coagulation cascade. HP may be used in combination with or as rescue therapy in case of failure of conventional HEPs (CHEPs) and also as monotherapy in large, poorly accessible lesions with multiple bleeding sources. Although the literature on HP is abundant, randomized controlled trials are scant, and some questions remain open. While HP is highly effective in inducing immediate hemostasis in GIB, the rates of rebleeding reported in different studies are very variable, and conditions affecting the stability of hemostasis have not yet been fully elucidated. It is not established whether HP as monotherapy is appropriate in severe GIB, such as spurting peptic ulcers, or should be used only as rescue or adjunctive therapy. Finally, as it can be sprayed on large areas, HP could become the gold standard in malignancy-related GIB, which is often nonresponsive or not amenable to treatment with CHEPs as a result of multiple bleeding points and friable surfaces. This is a narrative review that provides an overview of currently available data and the open questions regarding the use of HP in the management of non-variceal upper GIB due to benign and malignant diseases.

Keywords: ankaferd blood stopper; CEGP-003; endoclot; gastrointestinal bleeding; hemospray; hemostatic powders; hemostatic procedures; TC-325; UI-EWD; upper gastrointestinal bleeding

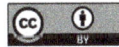

1. Introduction

Upper gastrointestinal bleeding (UGIB) is mostly of non-variceal origin and has an annual incidence rate from 50 to 150 per 100,000 adults [1–3]. Peptic ulcer disease (PUD) is the most common cause of non-variceal UGIB (NVUGIB) and accounts for at least 50% of UGIB. Other frequent benign conditions underlying NVUGIB include gastroduodenal erosions (8–15%), Mallory–Weiss tears (8–15%), and erosive esophagitis (5–15%) [1]. Malignancy causes comprise 1–5% of all NVUGIB [4–6]. GIB is the initial presenting symptom of malignancy in up to 70% of patients [4,5], and the disease is already metastatic in about one-third of them [5]. Gastric cancer is the most common cause of malignancy-related NVUGIB (MR-NVUGIB) [4–7], and about one-third is metastatic [4]; the duodenum is the most frequent site of malignancy involving the small bowel [4,5], usually primary or metastatic from a pancreatic or biliary malignancy. In all NVUGIB related to benign and malignant lesions, upper digestive endoscopy (EGDS) with hemostatic endoscopic procedure (HEP) is the first-choice approach. Conventional HEPs (CHEPs) include injection agents (epinephrine, ethanol, and cyanoacrylate), contact thermal devices (heater probes and multipolar electrocautery probes), noncontact thermal devices (argon plasma coagulation), and mechanical devices (hemostatic graspers, band ligators, clips, and loops) [3]. The use of one or more CHEP, often in combination, induces endoscopic hemostasis in 67–100% of cases, although rebleeding occurs in up to about 25–30% of treated patients [2,3]. In recent years, hemostatic powder (HP) has been proposed and tested for the treatment of acute GIB, arousing growing interest among clinicians. The present narrative review provides an overview of currently available data and the open questions regarding the use of HP in the management of NVUGIB due to benign and malignant diseases.

2. Type, Modality of Action, and Application of Hemostatic Powder

To date, five HPs have been developed for the management of GIB (Table 1). The most diffused agents are TC-325 (Hemospray™; Cook Medical, Winston-Salem, NC, USA), EndoClot™ (EndoClot Plus, Santa Clara, CA, USA), and Ankaferd Blood Stopper® (ABS; Ankaferd Health Products, Istanbul, Turkey); two more recent HPs are UI-EWD (NexPowder™; Nextbiomedical, Incheon, Republic of Korea) and CEGP-003 (CGBio, Seong-Nam, Republic of Korea). All these products are applied using a delivery catheter passed through the working channel of the endoscope to reach the bleeding site (Figures 1–3).

Table 1. Hemostatic powders available on the market.

Trade Name	Market Area	Composition	Action
Hemospray	Canada, Europe, USA	inert mineral	absorption of water, promotion of clotting, coagulation cascade activation, mechanical tamponade
Endoclot	Turkey, Europe, Malaysia Australia	starch-derived polysaccharides	absorption of water promotion of clotting, coagulation cascade activation
Ankaferd Blood Stopper	Turkey	herbal ingredients	protein network promoting erythrocyte aggregation interaction with blood protein
Nexpowder	South Korea, Europe, USA	aldehyde dextran and succinic acid modified ε-poly (l-lysine)	adhesive hydrogel with multiple crosslinks within the hydrogel and between the hydrogel and tissue
CGBio	South Korea	hydroxyethylcellulose, EGF	adhesive seal in which the EGF promotes wound healing

EGF: epidermal growth factor; TGF: transforming growth factor.

Figures 1–3: different lesions with active oozing bleeding and after hemostasis achieved by application of hemostatic powder.

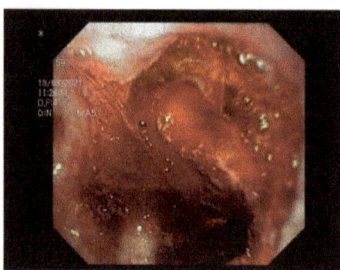 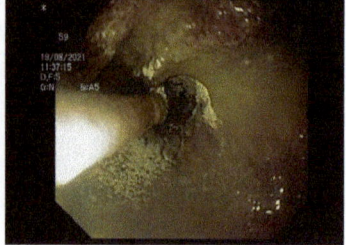

Figure 1. Duodenal cancer.

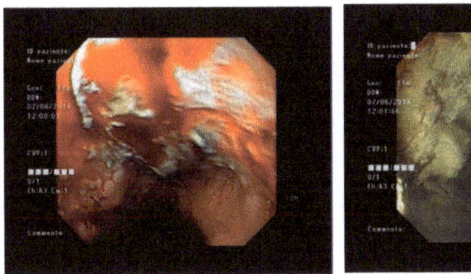
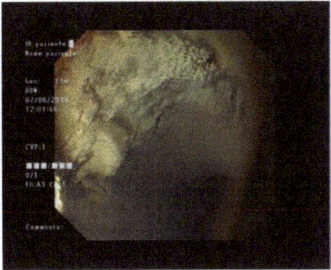

Figure 2. Esophageal cancer.

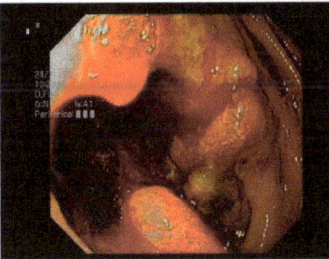
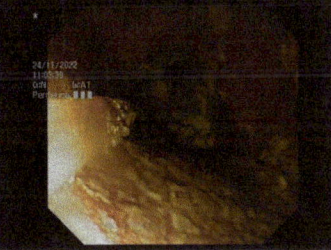

Figure 3. Pancreatic cancer invading duodenum.

TC-325 is compounded by bentonite, a naturally sourced aluminum phyllosilicate clay. This inert powder is propelled through a carbon dioxide pressurized catheter and sprayed at a distance of 1–2 cm from the bleeding site, forming a coat covering the lesion. This coat acts as a mechanical barrier and absorbs water, leading to a concentration of platelets and clotting factors with the activation of platelets and the coagulation cascade [8]. Due to its modality of action, TC-325 should be used in cases of active bleeding, as it is likely poorly or not effective in nonbleeding lesions [9]. Once sprayed over the area of bleeding, TC-325 adheres over the lesion for a limited time: the HP sloughs off the mucosa and is eliminated from the gastrointestinal tract within 24–72 h after application [8].

Endoclot is a starch-derived compound of hemostatic polysaccharides which, in contact with blood, absorbs water, causes a high concentration of platelets, red blood cells, and coagulation proteins at the bleeding site, and accelerates the physiological clotting cascade [8]. An air compressor provides consistent air pressure to propel the HP to the bleeding site. Endoclot also remains over the lesion for a limited time ranging from hours to days [10].

ABS is a plant-based agent that rapidly forms an encapsulated protein network providing focal points for erythrocytes and activated leukocyte aggregation. This network stems from interactions between ABS and blood proteins, such as fibrinogen, inducing protein agglutination. ABS also inhibits fibrinolysis and anticoagulant pathways, promoting wound healing [8].

UI-EWD is a biocompatible natural polymer produced using aldehyde dextran and succinic acid modified ε poly (l-lysine). In the presence of water, the two compounds of the polymer react together, forming a hydrogel with multiple crosslinks resulting in high adhesiveness to the tissue. The hydrogel acts as a mechanical barrier and promotes hemostasis. UI-EWD is delivered via a system based on a liquid coating technology using a fluidized bed granulator. Since UI-EWD does not require clot formation to induce hemostasis, active bleeding is not necessary for this HP to be effective [11].

CEGP-003 powder is a mix of hydroxyethylcellulose and epidermal growth factor (EGF). Due to its adhesive and hygroscopic properties, hydroxyethylcellulose, in contact with water, forms an adhesive gel that acts as a barrier, while the EGF, by binding to EGF receptors, activates the syntheses of hyaluronan and aquaporin-3, both promoting wound healing [12,13].

2.1. Pros

HP is an attractive agent for endoscopic hemostasis in patients with GIB as it is straightforward to use, does not require prolonged training, can be applied to sites poorly accessible by endoscopy and hemostatic devices, can treat extensive areas with multiple bleeding points, and does not need to be in direct contact with the bleeding lesion.

HP is generally safe and well tolerated. Some cases of embolization, bowel obstruction, and perforation have been reported in patients treated with Hemospray®, but, based on an analysis of the literature, the Food and Drug Administration (FDA) declared that Hemospray® is an endoscopic hemostat with a very low-risk profile, with no contraindication except for gastrointestinal endoscopy (active or risk of gastrointestinal perforation) and gastrointestinal fistulas [14]. Endoclot also received a very low-risk profile statement from the FDA [15].

2.2. Cons

- Clogging of the delivery catheter has been reported [16] during the release of TC-325, as it coagulates when in contact with fresh blood. During an emergency endoscopy with active GIB, it is necessary to aspirate blood from the lumen of the digestive tract, and the presence of blood in the working channel may determine the coagulation of HP, causing occlusion of the catheter. This issue may be overcome by a prolonged insufflation following blood aspiration to dry the working channel immediately before the spraying of HP [17]. Clogging seems to be infrequent (3.6%) with UI-EWD due to the system of delivery adopted [18]. Following the application of HP, the visibility of the target lesion is no longer guaranteed as the HP may obscure the endoscopic view.
- TC-325 has a high cost (US list price of USD 2500 in November 2020); this is the reason guidelines suggest that, in countries such as the United States, TC-325 should not be the initial modality used if other therapies can be readily applied [19].

3. Fields of Application of Hemostatic Powder in Nvugib and Evidence on Short- and Long-Term Efficacy

HP is used to induce hemostasis following failure of rescue therapy or together with CHEP (combination therapy) and also alone as a first-choice treatment (monotherapy) in upper and lower GIB related to malignant and benign conditions, including postendoscopic therapeutic procedures such as endoscopic submucosal dissection, sphincterotomy, and polypectomy, as well as to less frequent conditions such as Dieulafoy lesions and lesions due to graft-versus-host disease [17]. Although it has been used also in upper variceal bleeding and lower gastrointestinal bleeding, this article will only address the use of HP in NVUGIB.

Table 2 lists studies on HP published to date, most of which investigate TC-325, likely because this agent is marketed more widely than the others; larger series have been published in recent years. For example, in the French "GRAPHE" registry including 202 patients with UGIB—most commonly related to PUD (37.1%), malignancy (30.2%), and postendoscopic therapy (17.3%)—TC-325 was used as rescue (53.5%) or first-line therapy (46.5%) and achieved an immediate hemostasis rate of 96.5%, with rebleeding in 26.7% and 33.5% of cases at day 8 and day 30, respectively, and the definitive hemostasis rate being 63% [20]. A retrospective nationwide study conducted in Spain involving 219 patients with UGIB—most frequently due to peptic ulcer (28%), malignancy (18.4%), and postendoscopic therapeutic procedures (17.6%)—showed that TC-325 was effective in inducing an immediate hemostasis rate of 93%, with rebleeding rates of 16.1%, 19.9%, and 22.9% at 3, 7, and 30 days, respectively, and a definitive hemostasis rate of 77% [21]. A multicenter European registry of 314 patients with UGIB—mainly due to PUD (53%), malignancy (16%), and postendoscopic procedures (16%)—treated with TC-325 reported immediate hemostasis in 89.5% of cases, with a rebleeding rate of 10.3% and a definitive hemostasis rate of 79.2% [22]. A retrospective study including 86 patients treated with HP as rescue therapy and monotherapy reported a high rate (88.4%) of immediate hemostasis but a cumulative rebleeding rate of 33.7% [23]. Overall, current evidence shows that TC-325 and other HPs can achieve immediate hemostasis in about 80–100% of UGIB regardless of etiology. In contrast, the rates of definitive hemostasis are more widely variable in the different studies, ranging from 40% to 100%. There may be several reasons for this discrepancy. Many published studies are retrospective analyses or case series, a small number are prospective investigations often lacking controls, and there is a paucity of randomized controlled trials (RCTs). Outcomes are variable: immediate hemostasis is almost uniformly defined as the stop of bleeding immediately after application of HP, whilst hemostasis is considered definitive (no relapse following application of HP) at different follow-up times (from 1 to 180 days); some studies evaluated the impact of HP on mortality rather than hemostasis. Lastly, the conditions underlying GIB in the study populations are highly heterogeneous and include GIB related to different malignancies, PUD with active bleeding (Forrest Ia and Ib) and with stigmata of recent but no-longer-active bleeding (Forrest IIa and IIb), postendoscopic therapy (e.g., endoscopic submucosal dissection and sphincterotomy), postsurgery bleeding, or other rarer lesions.

Table 2. Studies on hemostatic powders and outcomes in patients with upper gastrointestinal bleeding.

Author, Year (Reference)	Country	Design	Hemostatic Powder	Indication	Forrest Ia/Ib (%)	Application	Hemostasis
Sung, 2011 [24]	Hong Kong	PC, N = 20	TC-325	PUD	5/95	Mono	I: 95% D: 95% (30 days)
Holster, 2013 [25]	The Netherlands	PC, N = 16	TC-325	MR-GIB, PUD, Other	31/25	Mono, Rescue	I: 81% D: 49.7% (7 days)
Leblanc, 2013 [26]	France	CS, N = 17	TC-325	MR-GIB, Other	NA	Mono, Rescue	I: 100% D: 88% (7 days)
Smith, 2014 [27]	France, Denmark, Germany Italy, Spain, Sweden, UK, The Netherlands	RC, N = 63	TC-325	MR-GIB, PUD, Other	17/25	Mono, Combo	I: 85% D: 70% (7 days)
Sulz, 2014 [28]	Switzerland	CS, N = 16	TC-325	PUD, Other	0/25	Mono, Rescue	I: 94% D: 81% (7 days)
Yau, 2014 [29]	Canada	RC, N = 19	TC-325	UGIB	21/57	Mono, Rescue	I: 93% D: 61% (7 days)
Chen, 2015 [30]	Canada	RC, N = 66	TC-325	UGIB, LGIB	7/23	Mono, Rescue	I: 99% D: 84% (30 days)
Giles, 2016 [31]	New Zealand	CS, N = 36	TC-325	PUD, Other	20/60	Mono, Rescue	I: 100% D: 89% (7 days)
Haddara, 2016 [20]	France	PC, N = 202	TC-325	MR-GIB, PUD, Other	7/21	Mono, Rescue	I: 96.5% D: 63.2% (30 days)
Sinha, 2016 [32]	UK	RC, N = 20	TC-325	PUD	60/40	Rescue, Combo	I: 92–100% D: 75–83% (7 days)
Arena, 2017 [33]	Italy	RC, N = 15	TC-325	MR-UGIB	NA	Mono	I: 93% D: 72% (6 days)
Cahyadi, 2017 [34]	Germany	RC, N = 52	TC-325	MR-GIB, PUD, Other	0/39	Mono, Rescue	I: 98% D: 51% (7 days)
Hagel, 2017 [35]	Germany	RC, N = 25	TC-325	MR-GIB, PUD, Other	ND	Mono, Rescue	I: 96% D: 60% (30 days)
Pittayanon, 2018 [36]	Canada	RC, N = 86	TC-325	MR-GIB	1/94	Mono, Rescue	I: 98% D: 72% (30 days)
Ramírez-Polo, 2019 [37]	Mexico	RC, N = 81	TC-325	MR-GIB, PUD, Other	ND	Mono, Combo	I: 99% D: 79% (5 days)
Rodriguez De Santiago, 2019 [21]	Spain	RC, N = 261	TC-325	MR-GIB, PUD, Other	25/64	Mono, Rescue	I: 93% D: 73% (30 days)
Meng, 2019 [38]	Canada	RC, N = 25	TC-325	MR-GIB	8/76	Mono, Rescue	I: 88%, D: 50% (14 days)
Alzoubaidi, 2020 [22]	France, Germany UK	PC, N = 314	TC-325	MR-GIB, PUD, Other	17/60	Mono, Combo, Rescue	I: 89% D:79% (3 days)
Baracat, 2020 [39]	Brazil	RCT, N = 19 N = 20	TC-325 CHEP	MR-GIB, PUD, Other	16/84 5/95	Mono, Combo	I: 100% D: 74% (7 days) I: 90% D: 75% (7 days)
Chahal, 2020 [23]	Canada	RC, N = 86	TC-325	MR-GIB, PUD, Other	14/53	Mono, Combo	I: 88% D: 55% (30 days)
Chen, 2020 [40]	Canada	RCT, N = 10 N = 10	TC-325 CHEP	UGIB, LGIB	NA	Mono, Rescue	I: 90% D: 70% (180 days) I: 40% D: NA
Hussein, 2021 [41]	France, Germany UK, USA	PC, N = 202	TC-325	PUD	19/58	Mono, Combo, Rescue	I: 88% D: 71% (30 days)

Table 2. Cont.

Author, Year (Reference)	Country	Design	Hemostatic Powder	Indication	Forrest Ia/Ib (%)	Application	Hemostasis
Becq, 2021 [42]	France	RC, N = 152	TC-325	UGIB, LGIB	ND	Mono, Rescue	I: 79% D: 39% (30 days)
Hussein, 2021 [43]	France, Germany Spain, UK, USA	PC, N = 105	TC-325	MR-GIB	NA	Mono, Combo, Rescue	I: 97% D: 82% (30 days)
Kwek, 2017 [44]	Singapore	RCT, N = 20	TC-325 CHEP	PUD	10/40 0/33	Mono	I: 90% D: 67% (4 weeks) I: 100% D: 90% (4 weeks)
Vitali, 2019 [45]	Germany	PC, N = 154	TC-325 EndoClot	MR-GIB, PUD, Other	11/66	Mono, Rescue	I: 81% D: 67% (30 days) I: 81% D: 56% (30 days)
Paoluzi, 2021 [17]	Italy	PC, N = 43	TC-325, Endoclot CHEP	MR-GIB, PUD	16/84 22/78	Mono, Rescue	I: 86–100% D: 45–86% (30 days) I: 42–78%; D: 33–69% (30 days)
Lau, 2022 [46]	Hong Kong, Thailand, Singapore	RCT, N = 224	TC-325 CHEP	MR-GIB, PUD, Other	8/92 11/89	Mono	I: 93%, D: 90% (30 days) I: 91% D: 81% (30 days)
Sung, 2022 [47]	Canada, Hong Kong, The Netherlands, UK	PC, N = 67	TC-325	PUD	16/84	Mono	I: 91% D: 78% (30 days)
Martins, 2022 [48]	Brazil	RCT, N = 59	TC-325 CHEP	MR-UGIB	NA	Mono	I: 100% D: 68% (30 days) I: 100% D: 80% (30 days)
Beg, 2015 [49]	UK	RC, N = 21	EndoClot	PUD, Other	24/76	Rescue	I: 100% D: 95% (30 days)
Prei, 2016 [50]	Germany	PC, N = 70	EndoClot	UGIB, LGIB	1/66	Mono, Rescue	I: 83% D: 72% (3 days)
Kim, 2018 [51]	South Korea	RC, N = 12	EndoClot	MR-GIB	NA	Mono, Rescue	I: 100% D: 84% (3–5 days)
Park, 2018 [52]	South Korea	CC, N = 30	EndoClot	UGIB	17/70	Mono, Combo	I: 97% D: 94% (30 days)
Hagel, 2020 [53]	Germany	RC, N = 43	EndoClot	UGIB	ND	Mono, Rescue	I: 100% D: 76% (1 day)
Kurt, 2010 [54]	Turkey	CS, N = 10	ABS	MR-GIB	NA	Mono	I: 100% D: 100% (7–48 days)
Karaman, 2012 [55]	Turkey	PC, N = 30	ABS	UGIB	ND	Mono, Combo	I: 87% D: 100% (7 days)
Gungor, 2012 [56]	Turkey	PC, N = 26	ABS	UGIB	15/85	Mono, Combo	I: 73% D: 53% (2 days)
Bang, 2018 [13]	South Korea	RCT, N = 35	CEGP-003 CHEP	UGIB	0/86 0/81	Mono	I: 89% D: 86% (3 days)
Park, 2019 [18]	South Korea	PC, N = 17	UI-EWD	UGIB	12/88	Rescue	I: 94% D: 75% (30 days)
Park, 2019 [11]	South Korea	RC, N = 56	UI-EWD	UGIB	0/64	Mono	I: 96% D: 92% (7 days)
Shin, 2021 [57]	South Korea	RC, N = 41	UI-EWD	MR-GIB	71–93	Mono, Rescue	I: 97% D: 67% (28 days)

CS: case series; D: definitive; I: immediate; LGIB: lower gastrointestinal bleeding; MR-GIB: malignancy-related gastrointestinal bleeding; PC: prospective cohort; PUD: peptic ulcer disease; RC: retrospective cohort; RCT: randomized controlled trial; UGIB: upper gastrointestinal bleeding; NA: not applicable; ND: not defined.

To better determine the efficacy of HP in GIB, two systematic reviews with meta-analysis were recently published. Facciorusso et al. [58] reviewed and included in a meta-analysis 24 studies, 3 of which were RCTs and 21 of which were retrospective investigations; 19 studies used TC-325, 4 used Endoclot, and 1 used CGEP-003, with a total of 1063 patients. Immediate hemostasis was achieved in 95.3% of patients, with a success rate of 91.9% in spurting bleeding; the rebleeding rate was 17.9% and 16.9% at 7 and 30 days, respectively, and, according to treatment strategy, the overall rebleeding rate was 13.5% and 24.8% in monotherapy and combined/rescue therapy, respectively. Although useful, this first meta-analysis has several limitations, such as the high heterogeneity of populations in the different studies (sample size and geographic areas), source of bleeding (PUD, other benign conditions, malignancies, and, in three studies, liver cirrhosis), study protocol (retrospective/prospective and time of rebleeding), and type of HP applied. A subsequent meta-analysis by Mutneja et al. [59] of 11 prospective studies (3 of which were RCTs) investigating different etiologies of GIB (2 on PUD only, 3 on variceal bleeding only, 2 on malignancies only, 3 on mixed benign and malignant tumors without variceal bleeding, and 1 on mixed conditions including variceal bleeding) in a total of 609 patients treated with TC-325 reported a pooled immediate hemostasis rate of 93.0% regardless of etiology and 95.3% in malignancy-related GIB (MR-GIB); the overall 12 h–30 days rebleeding rate was 14.4%, and the MR rebleeding rate was 21.9%. A separate analysis of the three RCTs on NVUGIB revealed that the probability of achieving immediate hemostasis was more than three times higher with TC-325 than with CHEP. However, statistical significance was not reached, likely due to the limited number of RCTs. Although the strength of this meta-analysis lies in the selection of only prospective studies using the same type of HP, the findings are to some extent underpowered by statistical and clinical heterogeneity due to the different sources of GIB, different rebleeding times, selection biases, and lack of controls.

A very recent noninferiority RCT compared the efficacy of TC-325 monotherapy versus CHEP (thermocoagulation or clipping with/without epinephrine injection) in 224 adult patients with NVUGIB due to malignancy and nonmalignant lesions [46]. The primary endpoint was control of bleeding within 30 days, defined as endoscopic hemostasis by the assigned treatment modality during the first endoscopy and no recurrent bleeding after endoscopic hemostasis. Secondary endpoints included failure to control bleeding during the first endoscopy and recurrent bleeding after hemostasis, combined with a lack of recurrent bleeding, with secondary outcomes including further interventions, transfusion, and death. Bleeding was controlled within 30 days in 90.1% of cases in the TC-325 group and in 81.4% in the CHEP group. Recurrent bleeding within 30 days did not differ between groups (8.1% versus 8.8%, respectively). Additional interventions, length of stay, and death were similar between groups. The limitations of this study were the heterogeneity of lesions, an unbalanced allocation of patients with malignancy, attending endoscopists not blinded to study treatments, and a low rate of Forrest Ia lesions.

Despite the limitations described above, data currently available indicate that HP can induce immediate hemostasis in the majority of treated patients, but rebleeding in the following days should be kept in mind. It has not yet been fully established whether the limited time of persistence of HP over the lesion may reduce long-term hemostasis and contribute to the occurrence of a late (7–30 days) rebleeding. Taking into account the time of elimination from the gastrointestinal tract, recent guidelines suggest the use of TC-325 as a temporizing intervention that should be followed by a second definitive HEP [60] in patients with persistent bleeding refractory to CHEPs [61] or conditionally in peptic ulcer bleeding [19].

4. Open Questions

4.1. Peptic-Ulcer-Related NVUGIB: HP Only as Rescue Therapy and Combination Therapy or Also as Monotherapy?

The efficacy of HP in combination or rescue therapy is well demonstrated, and this noncontact hemostatic technique should now be considered an indispensable part of the standard therapeutic armamentarium in emergency endoscopy. However, the use of HP as monotherapy means excluding CHEPs, which are routinely used in the endoscopy room and well known to be effective in stopping NVUGIB in 85–95% of cases, reducing the need for surgery and lowering mortality rates [47]. Therefore, before using HP as monotherapy instead of CHEPs, it should be certain that HP is highly effective in bleeding PUD. An early prospective single-arm pilot study by Sung et al. investigating the use of HP in NVUGIB-related PUD in 20 patients with Forrest Ia (1 patient) or Forrest Ib (19 patients) PUD revealed that TC-325 as monotherapy achieved immediate and definitive hemostasis rates of 95% and 89.5%, respectively [24]. In another prospective study of 20 patients with PUD, randomized to receive either TC-325 (10 patients) or CHEP (10 patients), Kwek et al. reported immediate hemostasis rates of 90% and 100% and definitive hemostasis rates of 67% and 90%, respectively [44]. However, only 8 (3 in the TC-325 arm and 5 in the CHEP arm) out of 20 patients (40%) had Forrest Ia or Ib PUD, while the remaining 12 had nonbleeding Forrest IIa or IIb PUD. As TC-325 may be active only in cases of active bleeding, these findings are difficult to assess. Holster et al. prospectively treated eight patients with PUD (four with Forrest Ia and four with Forrest Ib) with TC-325 as monotherapy (six patients), achieving immediate and definitive hemostasis rates of 83% and 67%, respectively [25]. The largest case series published to date is a prospective single-arm multicenter study of 202 patients with PUD-related NVUGIB, 156 patients with active bleeding (39 patients (19%) with Forrest Ia and 117 patients (58%) with Forrest Ib), and 46 patients with nonactive bleeding (25 patients (12%) with Forrest IIa and 21 patients (10%) with Forrest IIb) treated with TC-325 as combination therapy (101 patients), rescue therapy (51 patients), and monotherapy (50 patients), showing an overall immediate hemostasis rate of 88% and a definitive hemostasis rate of 71% [41]. According to its application, TC-325 achieved immediate and definitive hemostasis rates of 89% and 74% as combination therapy, 86% and 64% as rescue therapy, and 88% and 72% as monotherapy. Taking into account only patients with active bleeding, the immediate hemostasis rate was 85% in the Forrest group (87% Forrest Ia and 85% Forrest Ib); however, only a small proportion of these patients ($\leq$25%) received TC-325 as monotherapy, and the outcome was not specified.

Two prospective studies on TC-325 administered as monotherapy in PUD-related NVUGIB were very recently published. In a prospective, single-arm, multicenter study, Sung et al. evaluated the efficacy of TC-325 as monotherapy in 67 patients with actively bleeding PUD (11 patients (16%) with Forrest Ia and 55 patients (84%) with Forrest Ib) who had not already undergone another HEP [47]. Patients received up to three canisters of TC-325 (20 g per canister) and, if unresponsive, were treated with a CHEP according to the physician's preference. Persistent or recurrent bleeding within the first 72 h (early rebleeding) was the primary endpoint; recurrent bleeding between 72 h and 30 days (late rebleeding), adverse events, and mortality within 30 days were additional outcome measures. In one patient, TC-325 was not administered due to the occlusion of two consecutive catheters, and CHEP was performed. TC-325 achieved initial hemostasis in 60/66 (91%) treated patients, and early and late rebleeding were endoscopically confirmed in 5 and 3 patients (7.6% and 4.5%), respectively, with an overall recurrent bleeding rate of 12.1% and a definitive hemostasis rate of 79%. Two patients with Forrest Ia in whom TC-325 achieved initial hemostasis died (mortality rate: 3%). Multiple logistic regression revealed that Forrest classification was the only variable associated with recurrent bleeding, where the highest risk was associated with Forrest Ia. In a noninferiority RCT by Lau et al. including 224 patients with NVUGIB due to malignant and nonmalignant conditions, 68 patients with PUD (all Forrest Ia or Ib) were randomized to TC-325 versus a combination of CHEPs (contact thermocoagulation or hemoclipping with or without prior injection of diluted epinephrine), with immediate hemostasis rates of 95.6% and 83.8% and definitive (30 days) hemostasis rates of 83.8% and 73.5%, respectively [46].

The latter two studies provide robust data in support of the efficacy of TC-325 when used as monotherapy. HP may be considered as one of the first-choice techniques, in addition to being used in combination with CHEPs or as rescue therapy, in the management of NVUGIB due to PUD-related oozing bleeding. In contrast, the efficacy of HP as monotherapy in inducing definitive hemostasis in NVUGIB due to Forrest Ia PUD still seems to need definitive validation by further research, as already suggested [19], ideally in RCTs including large populations. Spurting active bleeding due to Forrest Ia PUD is much less common than oozing [21,47,62]. However, it may be massive and life-threatening, especially in patients with clinical conditions compromised by other comorbidities and hemodynamic instability, and is likely the main reason for the recurrence of NVUGIB [21,47]. In this context, in our opinion, CHEPs remain the gold standard approach to Forrest Ia PUD except when the lesion is not easy to reach, the operator is not familiar with CHEPs, or there is a risk of perforation in the case of contact-based thermal procedures. This risk seems to be increased in patients with recurrent bleeding when treated with a second consecutive thermal contact therapy, such as heater probe [19,63]. As alternative forms of hemostatic therapy are suggested in the event of rebleeding if thermal contact was used at the initial endoscopy [19], HP may be a possible choice. In the absence of conditions in which HP seems a suitable approach, it is reasonable to question why HP should be used to treat a bleeding lesion that can be controlled by a CHEP. Another reason to use HP only when necessary is the high cost.

4.2. Is HP a Possible Gold Standard in Malignancy-Related NVUGIB?

There is currently no gold-standard treatment for MR-NVUGIB, and the choice of CHEP depends on the characteristics of the tumor, such as location, size, consistency of surface, and pathological angiogenesis. Malignant lesions often have a friable surface with multiple bleeding points, negatively affecting the effectiveness of CHEPs, and mechanical contact-based HEP carries the risk of worsening the bleed or perforation. Nonlesion-related conditions influencing hemostasis include underlying coagulopathy, disease burden, and severity of hemorrhage [6,61]. In these cases, the success of CHEPs in MR-NVUGIB is variable, with immediate hemostasis achieved in about 30–40% of patients but with a short-term rebleeding rate of about 40–80% and 90-day mortality of about 95%, mainly due to the preterminal stage [36,64]. Based on the possibility of its application on large surfaces, argon plasma coagulation is frequently used in clinical practice but with temporary efficacy and high recurrent bleeding rates in MR-NVUGIB [65,66]. HP could be the ideal procedure of choice in the management of MR-NVUGIB, as it acts in the absence of mechanical contact and can also be sprayed over a large surface, allowing the simultaneous treatment of multiple bleeding points. To date, data regarding the use of HP in patients with MR-UGIB derive mainly from retrospective studies analyzing heterogeneous series (mixed lesions) and prospective studies lacking controls (Table 2). Hussein et al. [43] evaluated the efficacy of TC-325 in a prospective study including 105 patients who received HP either as monotherapy (67%) or in combination with or as rescue therapy after failure of CHEPs (25%). The decision to use TC-325 was at the discretion of the endoscopist. Overall, TC-325 achieved immediate hemostasis in 97% of patients, with a 30-day rebleeding rate of 15% and a definitive hemostasis rate of 82%. Immediate and definitive hemostasis rates were 100% and 85%, respectively, when TC-325 was used as monotherapy and 88% and 70% when used as combination therapy. Regarding possible factors influencing rebleeding due to malignancy, a univariable analysis conducted by Pittayanon et al. found that poor performance status, an Eastern Cooperative Oncology Group (ECOG) score ≥ 3, and INR > 1.3 were significantly associated with increased early recurrent bleeding, while definitive hemostatic treatment subsequent to TC-325 use was predictive of less delayed recurrent bleeding [36]. However, in a multivariable analysis, no significant prognostic factor for delayed recurrent bleeding was identified [36]. In contrast, good performance status (ECOG score 0–2), cancer stage 1–3, and achievement of definitive hemostatic treatment (surgery, chemotherapy, radiotherapy, and embolization) were significantly associated with greater survival. In a retrospective cohort of 41 patients with MR-UGIB, classified as Forrest Ib in 93% of cases, Shin et al. evaluated the efficacy of UI-EWD (Nexpowder) as monotherapy (23 patients, 56%) or rescue therapy (18 patients, 44%) [57]. In this study, UI-EWD achieved overall immediate and definitive hemostasis rates of 97.5% and 67.5%, respectively; as monotherapy only, the immediate and definitive success rates were 100% and 73.9%, respectively. Our study of HP in MR-GIB involved 23 patients, 14 with primary and 9 with metastatic cancer, in a series including other conditions, all treated with HP or CHEPs [17]. The source of bleeding was the stomach in 15 patients, the duodenum in 6 patients, and the colon/rectum in 2 patients; in all cases, the bleeding was oozing from multiple sites. Considering only patients with UGIB, HP was used as monotherapy in 9 patients and as rescue therapy in 7 patients (TC-325 in 14 patients and Endoclot in 2 patients), with immediate hemostasis rates of 100% and 85.7% and definitive hemostasis rates of 50% and 100%, respectively, significantly higher than those in patients treated with CHEPs (immediate hemostasis: 41.7%; definitive hemostasis: 33.3%). Of the 21 patients with MR-UGIB, 16 had an advanced unresectable tumor, 11 were discharged for palliative treatment, and 5 died from MR complications other than GIB, while the 5 remaining patients underwent elective (4 patients) or emergency surgery (1 patient) due to failure of hemostatic procedures.

To date, only two RCTs have been published on the use of TC-325 in MR-NVUGIB. In a pilot RCT, Chen et al. compared the efficacy of TC-325 versus CHEPs in upper (17 patients) and lower (3 patients) GIB, with 10 patients allocated to each group; crossover to the other treatment was permitted in patients not responding to the assigned therapy [40]. TC-325 achieved immediate hemostasis in 9/10 patients (90%) when used as monotherapy and in 4/5 patients (80%) unresponsive to CHEPs (rescue therapy); the definitive hemostasis rate at 180 days was 70% and 40% in the TC-325 and CHEP group, respectively. In a very recent RCT, Martins et al. compared the efficacy of TC-325 in monotherapy versus CHEPs in 68 patients with NVUGIB due to primary or metastatic malignancy who had not already undergone any HEPs [48]. In the control arm, a CHEP was not mandatory but could be applied if the attending endoscopist judged that hemostatic treatment might benefit the patient. TC-325 was always used in the presence of active bleeding; if bleeding was nonactive but stigmata were present, endoscopic washing of the tumor surface with a water jet was performed to remove the clot and reactivate bleeding or to induce brisk bleeding so that TC-325 could adhere to the tumor surface and promote coagulation. Immediate hemostasis was achieved in 100% of patients treated in both groups, with not-statistically-different 30-day rebleeding rates (32.1% in the TC-325 group and 19.4% in the control group) and 30-day mortality rates (28.6% in the TC-325 group and 19.4% in the control group). The difference between long-term outcomes, specifically late rebleeding rates, in the two groups was not statistically significant, likely because this study was underpowered due to incomplete (62%) enrollment of the planned population. Nevertheless, this is the first RCT with a very large series of patients evaluating the efficacy of HP in MR-NVUGIB, and the findings support the hypothesis that HP is more effective than CHEPs.

Karna et al. very recently conducted a systematic review and meta-analysis of the literature aimed at assessing the efficacy of topical hemostatic agents (TC-325, Endoclot, ABS, and UI-EWD) in the management of MR-NVUGIB [67]. The authors excluded studies reporting variceal bleeding or other nontumoral bleeding, studies performed in pediatric populations, those reporting data in <10 patients, case reports, case series, letters to the editor, review articles, and editorials. In the case of overlapping cohorts, the study providing the most recent results and/or the study with the largest sample size was included. Due to these strict selection criteria, from an initial pool of 355 investigations, the final analysis included 16 studies, 2 RCTs [40,68], and 14 observational studies [20,21,30,33,36–38,42,43, 51,54,57,69,70]. In this meta-analysis, immediate hemostasis was achieved in 94.1% of patients, early rebleeding was observed in 13.9%, and delayed rebleeding in 11.4%, with an aggregate rebleeding of 24.2%. A subgroup analysis revealed similar immediate hemostasis rates in the TC-325 and non-TC-325 cohorts (93.9% versus 96.7%, respectively). All-cause mortality was 33.1%, while GIB-related mortality was 5.9%. Despite the large number of patients included in the investigation, this meta-analysis has the limitation of including both retrospective and prospective studies, some of which combine bleeding and nonbleeding (adherent clot and visible vessel) lesions, and only two RCTs.

The paucity of studies comparing HP with CHEPs does not provide sufficient data to draw a definitive conclusion as to whether HP may be considered a gold-standard procedure in MR-NVUGIB. Multicenter comparative studies on larger populations are necessary to confirm this potential role and to determine in which kind of malignant lesions HP can be most effective. However, before further controlled findings are available, current data allow us to make some observations regarding the use of HP as monotherapy in MR-NVUGIB. First, as previously mentioned, HP can be used to simultaneously treat multiple bleeding sites in large lesions often difficult to reach or to treat with no risk of perforation as with the traumatic action of contact-based CHEPs. HP was highly effective in inducing immediate hemostasis in the majority of cases of NVUGIB in which it was used as monotherapy or rescue therapy. Second, it is possible that different types of HP, namely TC-325 and non-TC-325, may have similar efficacy in the treatment of MR-NVUGIB [45,67].

This hypothesis needs confirmation in comparative studies, particularly with newer types of HP that do not require active bleeding to perform their action. Third, HP is a temporary and palliative intervention in GIB related to advanced diseases, the so-called preterminal stage, and cannot affect the outcome. In malignancies, progressive tissue destruction and necrosis contribute to rebleeding GIB even following treatment with TC-325 [35]. However, HP may play a bridging role toward a more definitive management of diseases still amenable to treatment. Albeit for a short period, the achievement of hemostasis by HP, when used as monotherapy and to a much greater extent as rescue therapy, provides valuable time to stabilize the patient's cardiovascular functions and/or recover coagulation parameters when impaired, make blood transfusions, and carry out elective surgery, radiological procedures, or other definitive interventions [35]. HP should therefore be considered a first-choice hemostatic technique, as it is highly effective in MR-NVUGIB.

5. Conclusions

HP is highly effective in patients with NVUGIB when used either in combination with or as rescue therapy in the event of failure of CHEPs. Recent robust evidence supports the efficacy of TC-325 as monotherapy in NVUGIB due to spurting or oozing (Forrest Ia and Ib) PUD, but it cannot be regarded as an alternative to CHEPs as first-line treatment. Additional randomized comparative studies are necessary to define the role of HP as monotherapy and to establish whether it may be considered a gold standard in MR-NVUGIB. The potential role of new formulations, such as UI-EWD, in preventing bleeding during postendoscopic procedures and rebleeding following an early HEP needs to be confirmed by further investigations.

Author Contributions: Conceptualization, writing-original draft, review and editing, O.A.P. and G.D.V.B.; literature analysis and original draft preparation, E.T. and E.D.C.; literature search and iconographic resources, M.S.; supervision and review, G.M. All authors have read and agreed to the published version of the manuscript.

Funding: This research received no external funding.

Institutional Review Board Statement: Not applicable.

Informed Consent Statement: Not applicable.

Data Availability Statement: Not applicable.

Conflicts of Interest: The authors declare no conflict of interest.

References

1. Szura, M.; Pasternak, A. Upper non-variceal gastrointestinal bleeding—Review the effectiveness of endoscopic hemostasis methods. *World J. Gastrointest. Endosc.* **2015**, *7*, 1088–1095. [CrossRef]
2. Hearnshaw, S.A.; Logan, R.F.A.; Lowe, D.; Travis, S.P.L.; Murphy, M.F.; Palmer, K.R. Acute upper gastrointestinal bleeding in the UK. Patient characteristics, diagnoses and outcomes in the 2007 UK audit. *Gut* **2011**, *60*, 1327–1335. [CrossRef]
3. Fukuda, S.; Shimodaira, Y.; Watanabe, K.; Takahashi, Y.; Sugawara, K.; Suzuki, Y.; Watanabe, N.; Koizumi, S.; Matsuhashi, T.; Iijima, K. Risks for rebleeding and in-hospital mortality after gastrointestinal bleeding in a tertiary referral center in Japan. *Digestion* **2020**, *101*, 31–37. [CrossRef]
4. Schatz, R.A.; Rockey, D.C. Gastrointestinal bleeding due to gastrointestinal tract malignancy: Natural history, management, and outcomes. *Dig. Dis. Sci.* **2017**, *62*, 491–501. [CrossRef]
5. Sheibani, S.; Kim, J.J.; Chen, B.; Park, S.; Saberi, B.; Keyashian, K.; Buxbaum, J.; Laine, L. Natural history of acute upper GI bleeding due to tumours: Short-term success and long-term recurrence with or without endoscopic therapy. *Aliment. Pharmacol. Ther.* **2013**, *38*, 144–150. [CrossRef]
6. Kim, Y.I.; Choi, I.J. Endoscopic Management of Tumor Bleeding from Inoperable Gastric Cancer. *Clin. Endosc.* **2015**, *48*, 121–127. [CrossRef]
7. Savides, T.J.; Jensen, D.M.; Cohen, J.; Randall, G.M.; Kovacs, T.O.; Pelayo, E.; Cheng, S.; Jensen, M.E.; Hsieh, H.Y. Severe upper gastrointestinal tumor bleeding: Endoscopic findings, treatment, and outcome. *Endoscopy* **1996**, *28*, 244–248. [CrossRef]
8. Bustamante-Balén, M.; Plumé, G. Role of hemostatic powders in the endoscopic management of gastrointestinal bleeding. *World J. Gastrointest. Pathophysiol.* **2014**, *5*, 284–292. [CrossRef]

9. Chen, Y.I.; Barkun, A.N. Hemostatic powders in gastrointestinal bleeding: A systematic review. *Gastrointest. Endosc. Clin. N Am.* **2015**, *25*, 535–552. [CrossRef]
10. Polymer Technology. Available online: https://endoclot.com/technology.html (accessed on 4 January 2023).
11. Park, J.S.; Kim, H.K.; Shin, Y.W.; Kwon, K.S.; Lee, D.H. Novel hemostatic adhesive powder for nonvariceal upper gastrointestinal bleeding. *Endosc. Int. Open* **2019**, *7*, e1763–e1767. [CrossRef]
12. Jiang, S.X.; Chahal, D.; Ali-Mohamad, N.; Kastrup, C.; Donnellan, F. Hemostatic powders for gastrointestinal bleeding: A review of old, new, and emerging agents in a rapidly advancing field. *Endosc. Int. Open* **2022**, *10*, E1136–E1146. [CrossRef]
13. Bang, B.W.; Lee, D.H.; Kim, H.K.; Kwon, K.S.; Shin, Y.W.; Hong, S.J.; Moon, J.H. CEGP-003 Spray has a similar hemostatic effect to epinephrine injection in cases of acute upper gastrointestinal bleeding. *Dig. Dis. Sci.* **2018**, *63*, 3026–3032. [CrossRef]
14. Available online: https://www.accessdata.fda.gov/cdrh_docs/reviews/DEN170015.pdf (accessed on 4 January 2023).
15. Available online: https://www.accessdata.fda.gov/cdrh_docs/pdf19/K190677.pdf (accessed on 4 January 2023).
16. Barkun, A. New topical hemostatic powders in endoscopy. *Gastroenterol. Hepatol.* **2013**, *9*, 744–746.
17. Paoluzi, O.A.; Cardamone, C.; Aucello, A.; Neri, B.; Grasso, E.; Giannelli, M.; Di Iorio, L.; Monteleone, G.; Del Vecchio Blanco, G. Efficacy of hemostatic powders as monotherapy or rescue therapy in gastrointestinal bleeding related to neoplastic or non-neoplastic lesions. *Scand. J. Gastroenterol.* **2021**, *56*, 1506–1513. [CrossRef]
18. Park, J.S.; Bang, B.W.; Hong, S.J.; Lee, E.; Kwon, K.S.; Kim, H.K.; Shin, Y.W.; Lee, D.H. Efficacy of a novel hemostatic adhesive powder in patients with refractory upper gastrointestinal bleeding: A pilot study. *Endoscopy* **2019**, *51*, 458–462. [CrossRef]
19. Laine, L.; Barkun, A.N.; Saltzman, J.R.; Martel, M.; Leontiadis, G.I. ACG clinical guideline: Upper gastrointestinal and ulcer bleeding. *Am. J. Gastroenterol.* **2021**, *116*, 899–917. [CrossRef]
20. Haddara, S.; Jacques, J.; Lecleire, S.; Branche, J.; Leblanc, S.; Le Baleur, Y.; Privat, J.; Heyries, L.; Bichard, P.; Granval, P.; et al. A novel hemostatic powder for upper gastrointestinal bleeding: A multicenter study (the "GRAPHE" registry). *Endoscopy* **2016**, *48*, 1084–1095. [CrossRef]
21. Rodriguez de Santiago, E.; Burgos-Santamaria, D.; Perez-Carazo, L.; Brullet, E.; Ciriano, L.; Riu Pons, F.; de Jorge Turrión, M.A.; Prados, S.; Pérez-Corte, D.; Becerro-Gonzalez, I.; et al. Hemostatic spray powder TC-325 for GI bleeding in a nationwide study: Survival and predictors of failure via competing risks analysis. *Gastrointest. Endosc.* **2019**, *90*, 581–590.e6. [CrossRef]
22. Alzoubaidi, D.; Hussein, M.; Rusu, R.; Napier, D.; Dixon, S.; Rey, J.W.; Steinheber, C.; Jameie-Oskooei, S.; Dahan, M.; Hayee, B.; et al. Outcomes from an international multicenter registry of patients with acute gastrointestinal bleeding undergoing endoscopic treatment with Hemospray. *Dig. Endosc.* **2020**, *32*, 96–105. [CrossRef]
23. Chahal, D.; Lee, J.G.; Ali-Mohamad, N.; Donnellan, F. High rate of re-bleeding after application of Hemospray for upper and lower gastrointestinal bleeds. *Dig. Liver Dis.* **2020**, *52*, 768–772. [CrossRef]
24. Sung, J.J.Y.; Luo, D.; Wu, J.C.Y.; Ching, J.Y.L.; Chan, F.K.L.; Lau, J.Y.W.; Mack, S.; Ducharme, R.; Okolo, P.; Canto, M.; et al. Early clinical experience of the safety and effectiveness of Hemospray in achieving hemostasis in patients with acute peptic ulcer bleeding. *Endoscopy* **2011**, *43*, 291–295. [CrossRef]
25. Holster, I.L.; Kuipers, E.J.; Tjwa, E.T.T.L. Hemospray in the treatment of upper gastrointestinal hemorrhage in patients on antithrombotic therapy. *Endoscopy* **2013**, *45*, 63–66. [CrossRef]
26. Leblanc, S.; Vienne, A.; Dhooge, M.; Coriat, R.; Chaussade, S.; Prat, F. Early experience with a novel hemostatic powder used to treat upper GI bleeding related to malignancies or after therapeutic interventions (with videos). *Gastrointest. Endosc.* **2013**, *78*, 169–175. [CrossRef]
27. Smith, L.A.; Stanley, A.J.; Bergman, J.J.; Kiesslich, R.; Hoffman, A.; Tjwa, E.T.; Kuipers, E.J.; von Holstein, C.S.; Oberg, S.; Brullet, E.; et al. Hemospray application in nonvariceal upper gastrointestinal bleeding: Results of the Survey to Evaluate the Application of Hemospray in the Luminal Tract. *J. Clin. Gastroenterol.* **2014**, *48*, e89–e92. [CrossRef]
28. Sulz, M.C.; Frei, R.; Meyenberger, C.; Bauerfeind, P.; Semadeni, G.M.; Gubler, C. Routine use of Hemospray for gastrointestinal bleeding: Prospective two-center experience in Switzerland. *Endoscopy* **2014**, *46*, 619–624. [CrossRef]
29. Yau, A.H.L.; Ou, G.; Galorport, C.; Amar, J.; Bressler, B.; Donnellan, F.; Ko, H.H.; Lam, E.; Enns, R.A. Safety and Efficacy of Hemospray® in Upper Gastrointestinal Bleeding. *Can. J. Gastroenterol. Hepatol.* **2014**, *28*, 72–76. [CrossRef]
30. Chen, Y.-I.; Barkun, A.; Nolan, S. Hemostatic powder TC-325 in the management of upper and lower gastrointestinal bleeding: A two-year experience at a single institution. *Endoscopy* **2015**, *47*, 167–171. [CrossRef]
31. Giles, H.; Lal, D.; Gerred, S.; Casey, P.; Patrick, A.; Luo, D.; Ogra, R. Affiliations expand. Efficacy and safety of TC-325 (Hemospray™) for non-variceal upper gastrointestinal bleeding at Middle-more Hospital: The early New Zealand experience. *N. Z. Med. J.* **2016**, *129*, 38–43.
32. Sinha, R.; Lockman, K.A.; Church, N.I.; Plevris, J.N.; Hayes, P.C. The use of hemostatic spray as an adjunct to conventional hemostatic measures in high-risk nonvariceal upper GI bleeding (with video). *Gastrointest. Endosc.* **2016**, *84*, 900–906.e3. [CrossRef]
33. Arena, M.; Masci, E.; Eusebi, L.H.; Iabichino, G.; Mangiavillano, B.; Viaggi, P.; Morandi, E.; Fanti, L.; Granata, A.; Traina, M.; et al. Hemospray for treatment of acute bleeding due to upper gastrointestinal tumours. *Dig. Liver Dis.* **2017**, *49*, 514–517. [CrossRef]
34. Cahyadi, O.; Bauder, M.; Meier, B.; Caca, K.; Schmidt, A. Effectiveness of TC-325 (Hemospray) for treatment of diffuse or refractory upper gastrointestinal bleeding—A single center experience. *Endosc. Int. Open* **2017**, *05*, E1159–E1164. [CrossRef] [PubMed]
35. Hagel, A.F.; Albrecht, H.; Nägel, A.; Vitali, F.; Vetter, M.; Dauth, C.; Neurath, M.F.; Raithel, M. The Application of Hemospray in gastrointestinal bleeding during emergency endoscopy. *Gastroenterol. Res. Pract.* **2017**, *2017*, e3083481. [CrossRef]

36. Pittayanon, R.; Rerknimitr, R.; Barkun, A. Prognostic factors affecting outcomes in patients with malignant GI bleeding treated with a novel endoscopically delivered hemostatic powder. *Gastrointest. Endosc.* **2018**, *87*, 994–1002. [CrossRef] [PubMed]
37. Ramírez-Polo, A.I.; Casal-Sánchez, J.; Hernández-Guerrero, A.; Castro-Reyes, L.M.; Yáñez-Cruz, M.; De Giau-Triulzi, L.F.; Vinageras-Barroso, J.; Téllez-Ávila, F.I. Treatment of gastrointestinal bleeding with hemostatic powder (TC-325): A multicenter study. *Surg. Endosc.* **2019**, *33*, 2349–2356. [CrossRef]
38. Meng, Z.W.; Marr, K.J.; Mohamed, R.; James, P.D. Long-term effectiveness, safety and mortality associated with the use of TC-325 for malignancy-related upper gastrointestinal bleeds: A multicentre retrospective study. *J. Can. Assoc. Gastroenterol.* **2019**, *2*, 91–97. [CrossRef] [PubMed]
39. Baracat, F.I.; de Moura, D.T.H.; Brunaldi, V.O.; Tranquillini, C.V.; Baracat, R.; Sakai, P.; Guimarães Hourneaux de Moura, E. Randomized controlled trial of hemostatic powder versus endoscopic clipping for non-variceal upper gastrointestinal bleeding. *Surg. Endosc.* **2020**, *34*, 317–324. [CrossRef]
40. Chen, Y.; Wyse, J.; Lu, Y.; Martel, M.; Barkun, A.N. TC-325 hemostatic powder versus current standard of care in managing malignant GI bleeding: A pilot randomized clinical trial. *Gastrointest. Endosc.* **2020**, *91*, 321–328.e1. [CrossRef]
41. Hussein, M.; Alzoubaidi, D.; Lopez, M.-F.; Weaver, M.; Ortiz-Fernandez-Sordo, J.; Bassett, P.; Rey, J.W.; Hayee, B.H.; Despott, E.; Murino, A.; et al. Hemostatic spray powder TC-325 in the primary endoscopic treatment of peptic ulcer-related bleeding: Multicenter international registry. *Endoscopy* **2021**, *53*, 36–43. [CrossRef]
42. Becq, A.; Houdeville, C.; Tran Minh, M.-L.; Steuer, N.; Danan, D.; Guillaumot, M.A.; Ali, E.A.; Barret, M.; Amiot, A.; Carbonell, N.; et al. Experience with the use of a hemostatic powder in 152 patients undergoing urgent endoscopy for gastrointestinal bleeding. *Clin. Res. Hepatol. Gastroenterol.* **2021**, *45*, 101558. [CrossRef]
43. Hussein, M.; Alzoubaidi, D.; O'Donnell, M.; de la Serna, A.; Bassett, P.; Varbobitis, I.; Hengehold, T.; Ortiz Fernandez-Sordo, J.; Rey, J.W.; Hayee, B.; et al. Hemostatic powder TC-325 treatment of malignancy-related upper gastrointestinal bleeds: International registry outcomes. *J. Gastroenterol. Hepatol.* **2021**, *36*, 3027–3032. [CrossRef]
44. Kwek, B.E.A.; Ang, T.L.; Ong, P.L.J.; Tan, Y.L.J.; Ang, S.W.D.; Law, N.M.; Thurairajah, P.H.; Fock, K.M. TC-325 versus the conventional combined technique for endoscopic treatment of peptic ulcers with high-risk bleeding stigmata: A randomized pilot study. *J. Dig. Dis.* **2017**, *18*, 323–329. [CrossRef]
45. Vitali, F.; Naegel, A.; Atreya, R.; Zopf, S.; Neufert, C.; Siebler, J.; Neurath, M.F.; Rath, T. Comparison of Hemospray® and EndoclotTM for the treatment of gastrointestinal bleeding. *World J. Gastroenterol.* **2019**, *25*, 1592–1602. [CrossRef] [PubMed]
46. Lau, J.Y.W.; Pittayanon, R.; Kwek, A.; Tang, R.S.; Chan, H.; Rerknimitr, R.; Lee, J.; Ang, T.L.; Suen, B.Y.; Yu, Y.Y.; et al. Comparison of a hemostatic powder and standard treatment in the control of active bleeding from upper nonvariceal lesions: A multicenter, noninferiority, randomized trial. *Ann. Intern. Med.* **2022**, *175*, 171–178. [CrossRef] [PubMed]
47. Sung, J.J.; Moreea, S.; Dhaliwal, H.; Moffatt, D.C.; Ragunath, K.; Ponich, T.; Barkun, A.N.; Kuipers, E.J.; Bailey, R.; Donnellan, F.; et al. Use of topical mineral powder as monotherapy for treatment of active peptic ulcer bleeding. *Gastrointest. Endosc.* **2022**, *96*, 28–35.e1. [CrossRef] [PubMed]
48. Martins, B.C.; Abnader Machado, A.; Scomparin, R.C.; Paulo, G.A.; Safatle-Ribeiro, A.; Naschold Geiger, S.; Lenz, L.; Lima, M.S.; Pennacchi, C.; Ribeiro, U.; et al. TC-325 hemostatic powder in the management of upper gastrointestinal malignant bleeding: A randomized controlled trial. *Endosc. Int. Open.* **2022**, *10*, E1350–E1357. [CrossRef] [PubMed]
49. Beg, S.; Al-Bakir, I.; Bhuva, M.; Patel, J.; Fullard, M.; Leahy, A. Early clinical experience of the safety and efficacy of EndoClot in the management of non-variceal upper gastrointestinal bleeding. *Endosc. Int. Open* **2015**, *03*, E605–E609. [CrossRef]
50. Prei, J.C.; Barmeyer, C.; Bürgel, N.; Daum, S.; Epple, H.J.; Günther, U.; Maul, J.; Siegmund, B.; Schumann, M.; Tröger, H.; et al. EndoClot polysaccharide hemostatic system in nonvariceal gastrointestinal bleeding: Results of a prospective multicenter observational pilot study. *J. Clin. Gastroenterol.* **2016**, *50*, e95–e100. [CrossRef]
51. Kim, Y.J.; Park, J.C.; Kim, E.H.; Shin, S.K.; Kil Lee, S.; Lee, Y.C. Hemostatic powder application for control of acute upper gastrointestinal bleeding in patients with gastric malignancy. *Endosc. Int. Open* **2018**, *06*, E700–E705. [CrossRef]
52. Park, J.C.; Kim, Y.J.; Kim, E.H.; Lee, J.; Yang, H.S.; Kim, E.H.; Hahn, K.Y.; Shin, S.K.; Lee, S.K.; Lee, Y.C. Effectiveness of the polysaccharide hemostatic powder in non-variceal upper gastrointestinal bleeding: Using propensity score matching. *J. Gastroenterol. Hepatol.* **2018**, *33*, 1500–1506. [CrossRef]
53. Hagel, A.F.; Raithel, M.; Hempen, P.; Preclik, G.; Dauth, W.; Neurath, M.F.; Gschossman, J.; Konturek, P.C.; Albrecht, H. Multicenter analysis of endoclot as hemostatic powder in different endoscopic settings of the upper gastrointestinal tract. *J. Physiol. Pharmacol.* **2020**, *71*, 657–664.
54. Kurt, M.; Akdogan, M.; Onal, I.K.; Kekilli, M.; Arhan, M.; Shorbagi, A.; Aksu, S.; Kurt, O.K.; Haznedaroglu, I.C. Endoscopic topical application of Ankaferd Blood Stopper for neoplastic gastrointestinal bleeding: A retrospective analysis. *Dig. Liver Dis.* **2010**, *42*, 196–199. [CrossRef] [PubMed]
55. Karaman, A.; Baskol, M.; Gursoy, S.; Torun, E.; Yurci, A.; Çelikbilek, M.; Guven, K.; Ozbakir, O.; Yucesoy, M. Endoscopic Topical Application of Ankaferd Blood Stopper® in Gastrointestinal Bleeding. *J. Altern. Complement. Med.* **2012**, *18*, 65–68. [CrossRef] [PubMed]
56. Gungor, G.; Goktepe, M.H.; Biyik, M.; Polat, I.; Tuna, T.; Ataseven, H.; Demir, A. Efficacy of ankaferd blood stopper application on non-variceal upper gastrointestinal bleeding. *World, J. Gastrointest. Endosc.* **2012**, *4*, 556–560. [CrossRef]
57. Shin, J.; Cha, B.; Park, J.-S.; Ko, W.; Kwon, K.S.; Lee, J.-W.; Kim, H.K.; Shin, Y.W. Efficacy of a novel hemostatic adhesive powder in patients with upper gastrointestinal tumor bleeding. *BMC Gastroenterol.* **2021**, *21*, 40. [CrossRef]

58. Facciorusso, A.; Takahashi, M.; Postula, C.E.; Buccino, V.R.; Muscatiello, N. Efficacy of hemostatic powders in upper gastrointestinal bleeding: A systematic review and meta-analysis. *Dig. Liver Dis.* **2019**, *51*, 1633–1640. [CrossRef] [PubMed]
59. Mutneja, H.; Bhurwal, A.; Go, A.; Sidhu, G.S.; Arora, S.; Attar, B.M. Efficacy of Hemospray in Upper Gastrointestinal Bleeding: A Systematic Review and Meta-Analysis. *J. Gastrointest. Liver Dis.* **2020**, *29*, 69–76. [CrossRef] [PubMed]
60. Sung, J.J.Y.; Chiu, P.; Chan, F.K.L.; Lau, J.Y.; Goh, K.-L.; Ho, L.H.; Jung, H.-Y.; Sollano, J.D.; Gotoda, T.; Reddy, N.; et al. Asia-Pacific working group consensus on non-variceal upper gastrointestinal bleeding: An update 2018. *Gut* **2018**, *67*, 1757–1768. [CrossRef] [PubMed]
61. Gralnek, I.M.; Stanley, A.J.; Morris, A.J.; Camus, M.; Lau, J.; Lanas, A.; Laursen, S.B.; Radaelli, F.; Papanikolaou, I.S.; Gonçalves, T.C.; et al. Endoscopic diagnosis and management of nonvariceal upper gastrointestinal hemorrhage (NVUGIH): European Society of Gastrointestinal Endoscopy (ESGE) Guideline—Update 2021. *Endoscopy* **2021**, *53*, 300–332. [CrossRef]
62. Sung, J.J.; Barkun, A.; Kuipers, E.J.; Mössner, J.; Jensen, D.M.; Stuart, R.; Lau, J.Y.; Ahlbom, H.; Kilhamn, J.; Lind, T.; et al. Intravenous esomeprazole for prevention of recurrent peptic ulcer bleeding: A randomized trial. *Ann. Intern. Med.* **2009**, *150*, 455–464. [CrossRef]
63. Laine, L.; McQuaid, K.R. Endoscopic Therapy for Bleeding Ulcers: An Evidence-Based Approach Based on Meta-Analyses of Randomized Controlled Trials. *Clin. Gastroenterol. Hepatol.* **2009**, *7*, 33–47. [CrossRef]
64. Roberts, S.E.; Button, L.A.; Williams, J.G. Prognosis following Upper Gastrointestinal Bleeding. *PLoS ONE* **2012**, *7*, e49507. [CrossRef] [PubMed]
65. Akhtar, K.; Byrne, J.P.; Bancewicz, J.; Attwood, S.E. Argon beam plasma coagulation in the management of cancers of the esophagus and stomach. *Surg. Endosc.* **2000**, *14*, 1127–1130. [CrossRef]
66. Ofosu, A.; Ramai, D.; Latson, W.; Adler, D.G. Endoscopic management of bleeding gastrointestinal tumors. *Ann. Gastroenterol.* **2019**, *32*, 346–351. [CrossRef] [PubMed]
67. Karna, R.; Deliwala, S.; Ramgopal, B.; Mohan, B.P.; Kassab, L.; Becq, A.; Dhawan, M.; Adler, D.G. Efficacy of topical hemostatic agents in malignancy-related gastrointestinal bleeding: A systematic review and meta-analysis. *Gastrointest. Endosc.* 2022, in press. [CrossRef]
68. Da Costa Martins, B.; Scomparin, R.C.; Bento, L.H.; Pires, C.B.; Pennacchi, C.; Lenz, L.; Franco, M.C.; Kawaguti, F.S.; Safatle-Ribeiro, A.V.; Ribeiro, U. Preliminary results of a randomized controlled trial comparing hemostatic powder versus optimal clinical treatment in the management of gastro-intestinal bleeding from malignancy. *Gastrointest. Endosc.* **2018**, *87*, AB415–AB416. [CrossRef]
69. Bazarbashi, A.N.; Al Obaid, L.; McCarty, T.R.; Hathorn, K.; Aihara, H.; Thompson, C.C. Endoscopic he-mostatic powder for the treatment of malignancy related gastrointestinal bleeding: A single cen-ter US experience. *Gastrointest. Endosc.* **2020**, *91*, AB48. [CrossRef]
70. Disney, B.; Kurup, A.; Muhammad, H.; Ishaq, S. PTU-031 Hemospray use for the management of acute bleeding from upper gastrointestinal cancer: The russells hall experience. *Gut* **2015**, *64*, A71–A72. [CrossRef]

Disclaimer/Publisher's Note: The statements, opinions and data contained in all publications are solely those of the individual author(s) and contributor(s) and not of MDPI and/or the editor(s). MDPI and/or the editor(s) disclaim responsibility for any injury to people or property resulting from any ideas, methods, instructions or products referred to in the content.

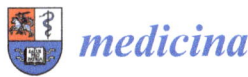

Review

A Comprehensive Review on Bariatric Endoscopy: Where We Are Now and Where We Are Going

Aurelio Mauro [1,*], Francesca Lusetti [1,2], Davide Scalvini [1,2], Marco Bardone [1], Federico De Grazia [1], Stefano Mazza [1], Lodovica Pozzi [1], Valentina Ravetta [1], Laura Rovedatti [1], Carmelo Sgarlata [1], Elena Strada [1], Francesca Torello Viera [1], Letizia Veronese [1], Daniel Enrique Olivo Romero [1,3] and Andrea Anderloni [1]

1. Gastroenterology and Endoscopy Unit, Fondazione IRCCS Policlinico San Matteo, 27100 Pavia, Italy
2. Specialization School of Diseases of Digestive System Pavia, University of Pavia, 27100 Pavia, Italy
3. Digestive Endoscopy Unit, Hospital Nacional Zacamil, San Salvador 01120, El Salvador
* Correspondence: a.mauro@smatteo.pv.it

Abstract: *Background:* Obesity is a chronic disease that impairs quality of life and leads to several comorbidities. When conservative therapies fail, bariatric surgical options such as Roux-en-Y gastric bypass (RYGB) and sleeve gastrectomy (SG) are the most effective therapies to induce persistent weight loss. Over the last two decades, bariatric endoscopy has become a valid alternative to surgery in specific settings. *Primary bariatric endoscopic therapies:* Restrictive gastric procedures, such as intragastric balloons (IGBs) and endoscopic gastroplasty, have been shown to be effective in inducing weight loss compared to diet modifications alone. Endoscopic gastroplasty is usually superior to IGBs in maintaining weight loss in the long-term period, whereas IGBs have an established role as a bridge-to-surgery approach in severely obese patients. IGBs in a minority of patients could be poorly tolerated and require early removal. More recently, novel endoscopic systems have been developed with the combined purpose of inducing weight loss and improving metabolic conditions. Duodenal mucosal resurfacing demonstrated efficacy in this field in its early trials: significant reduction from baseline of HbA1c values and a modest reduction of body weight were observed. Other endoscopic malabsorptive have been developed but need more evidence. For example, a pivotal trial on duodenojejunal bypasses was stopped due to the high rate of severe adverse events (hepatic abscesses). Optimization of these more recent malabsorptive endoscopic procedures could expand the plethora of bariatric patients that could be treated with the intention of improving their metabolic conditions. *Revisional bariatric therapies:* Weight regain may occur in up to one third of patients after bariatric surgery. Different endoscopic procedures are currently performed after both RYGB and SG in order to modulate post-surgical anatomy. The application of argon plasma coagulation associated with endoscopic full-thickness suturing systems (APC-TORe) and Re-EndoSleeve have shown to be the most effective endoscopic treatments after RYGB and SG, respectively. Both procedures are usually well tolerated and have a very low risk of stricture. However, APC-TORe may sometimes require more than one session to obtain adequate final results. The aim of this review is to explore all the currently available primary and revisional endoscopic bariatric therapies focusing on their efficacy and safety and their potential application in clinical practice.

Keywords: endoscopic bariatric therapy; obesity; sleeve gastrectomy; intragastric balloons; endoscopic sleeve gastroplasty; POSE; transoral outlet reduction; duodenal mucosal resurfacing

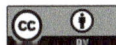

1. Introduction

Obesity is defined as a body mass index (BMI) equal to or higher than 30 kg/m². It is a pandemic disease that affects 650 million people throughout the world with a continuously increasing incidence [1,2].

Genetic predisposition, unbalanced long-term diets, and sedentary habits are the main factors contributing to the multifactorial etiology of this disease. Numerous illnesses result from obesity, mainly type 2 diabetes, arterial hypertension, liver steatosis, and other cardiovascular complications [3]. Moreover, the social implications of this disease significantly hamper everyday activities, contributing to the reduced quality of life of bariatric patients [4].

The first-line treatment is based on diet regimens and modifications of lifestyle habits to increase physical activities. In order to obtain valid results, patients' compliance is essential due to the long-lasting challenging process required [5]. However, these options are frequently insufficient to reach adequate weight loss, and associated treatments are necessary. Pharmacotherapy with medications mainly promoting satiety [3] can be associated with dietary measures, but their efficacy is limited, and their various side effects limit long-term use [6]. Therefore, bariatric surgery has gained relevance in the field, becoming by far the most effective and durable option for obesity treatment. Different types of bariatric surgery have been developed over the years, among which Roux-en-Y gastric bypass (RYGB) and Sleeve gastrectomy (SG) are the most frequently performed [3]. Different from medical and dietary approaches, bariatric surgery allows significant results in terms of weight loss, up to 25–30% from basal weight, even during the long-term period [7,8].

The efficacy and safety of bariatric surgery are currently consolidated by a large number of publications [9,10]. As far as the safety profile is concerned, perioperative mortality has dramatically improved since the early 2000s [10,11]. A recent meta-analysis showed an early (<30 days) major adverse events rate of 0–1.6% with a mortality rate of 0–0.6% [12]. However, since obesity is continuously increasing in prevalence [2] and patients addressed to bariatric surgery are often young and/or fragile with multiple comorbidities, less invasive and safer options are desirable to treat this challenging benign disease.

With this purpose, over the years, bariatric endoscopic procedures have been developed in order to offer less invasive options, with an expected total body weight loss of at least 10–20% [13] when associated with appropriate dietary restrictions [14–16]. They can be classified as primary treatments or revisional procedures after surgery failure.

Primary bariatric endoscopic treatments, which are currently approved by the Food and Drug Administration (FDA) or the European Community (CE), work by reducing gastric volume by means of specific devices. The reduction of gastric volume can be either achieved by placing space-occupying devices or by creating an endoscopic gastroplasty, plicating the stomach walls in order to decrease gastric lumen [14]. In recent years, new endoscopic devices and procedures that reduce the contact between food and the gastrointestinal wall have been developed, with the aim of mimicking surgical malabsorptive procedures [17–19]. One of the main goals of these novel endoscopic treatments is to combine the weight loss effect with an improvement of metabolic complications that are the most common cause of morbidity in obese patients. Revisional bariatric endoscopic procedures have been developed to maximize patients' outcomes after surgical treatments [15]. Indeed, weight regain after bariatric surgery potentially occurs in one third of patients, and re-surgery in this category of patients is characterized by a high rate of complications [20]. After RYGB, dilation of the gastro-jejunal anastomosis and of the gastric pouch may occur, reducing the satiety sensation. Similarly, afterward, SG, dilation of the gastric remnant could lead to weight regain [15]. Endoscopic bariatric revisional procedures are aimed to have a restrictive effect, suturing full-thickness procedures being the most commonly performed after both RYGB and SG. The present review aims to detail the primary bariatric endoscopic procedures currently performed in clinical practice focusing on their mechanisms of action, efficacy, and application in the clinical practice. Revisional bariatric endoscopic procedures are detailed in the review focusing on endoscopic management after RYGB and SG.

2. Primary Bariatric Endoscopic Therapies
2.1. Restrictive Gastric Procedures
2.1.1. Intragastric Balloons

IGBs were the first endoscopic therapeutic option developed for obesity [21]. IGBs carry out their action by occupying space in the stomach, thus reducing its volume, creating a physical impediment to the ingestion of food, and slowing gastric emptying.

Most of the IGBs available today have a round or oval shape made of silicone, limiting gastric mucosal injury (Figure 1).

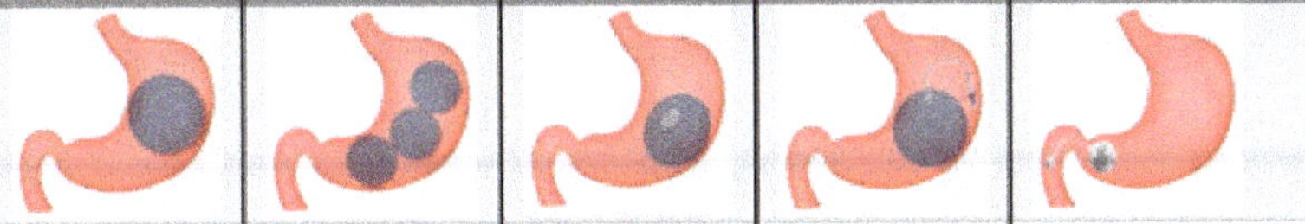

	ORBERA®	OBALON®	ELIPSE™	SPATZ3®	TRANSPYLORIC SHUTTLE®
FILLING CHARACTERISTICS	Single liquid filled	Up to 3 gas-filled	Single liquid filled	Single liquid filled with adjustable volume	Internal coil
POSITIONING	Endoscopic positioning and removal	Swallable; endoscopic removal	Swallable; self-deflating valve	Endoscopic positioning and removal	Endoscopic positioning and removal
TIMING OF REMOVAL	FDA: 6 months CE: 12 months	6 months	4 months	12 months	12 months
FDA/CE APPROVAL	FDA approved CE approved	FDA approved CE approved	CE approved	CE approved FDA approved	FDA approved

Figure 1. Schematic representation and characteristics of commercially available space-occupying devices.

They are usually inflated with a fluid (saline solution, together with methylene blue) or, less frequently, with a gas, to a volume of 500–700 mL. Larger volumes lead to greater total body weight loss (TBWL), but smaller volumes are better tolerated by the patient. IGBs are generally placed endoscopically under sedation; the majority remain implanted for an average of six months and are subsequently removed endoscopically. The presence of gastric, duodenal, and esophageal ulcers, irrespective of the presence of active bleeding, a previous gastric surgery, gastric and esophageal varices, hiatal hernia >5 cm, and anticoagulant use are absolute contraindications to implantation [22].

Although the placement of an IGB is generally well tolerated, some patients may complain of adaptive symptoms or experience adverse events (AEs). The formers, such as persistent nausea, vomiting, generalized abdominal pain and/or discomfort, and reflux symptoms, are related to the space-occupying action in the gastric lumen and usually appear immediately after the insertion of the IGB and are self-limiting. However, the persistence of obstructive symptoms may require early IGB removal, which usually occurs in less than 5% of patients limiting their efficacy [23]. Serious AEs (SAE) include mucosal injury or perforation of the stomach or esophagus, gastrointestinal obstruction due to the migration of the balloon, gastric outflow obstruction, and infections due to bacterial overgrowth in the fluid filling the balloon [23,24]. A meta-analysis by Trang et al. conducted on a total of 938 patients who underwent the positioning of different types of IGBs, showed that nausea and vomiting were very frequent after an IGB positioning (63.3%; 95%CI 61.5–65.2% and 55.3%; 95%CI 53.6–57% respectively) whereas the account rate of SAEs was lower (5.2%; 95% CI 4.8–5.6%) [25].

IGBs are completely reversible, and once removed, the stomach returns to its pre-implantation condition of anatomy and functioning. This kind of reversibility allows for an application in different clinical situations. IGBs could be used as primary therapy in patients who are overweight or have mild to moderate obesity, with a target of TBWL around 10–12% [13]. A meta-analysis of nine RCTs showed that IGB implantation is superior to diet modification alone in achieving BMI loss and EWL loss [26]. However, after IGB removal, compliance with diet in the long-term period is essential in order to prevent weight regain. A recent meta-analysis reported a decrease in %TBWL to 6.9 at 18–24 month follow-up after IGB removal, indicating weight regain [27,28]. Another well-established indication is the implantation of IGB as a bridge to surgery. It is known that surgery could be challenging and associated with increased morbidity in patients with severe and very-severe obesity compared to patients with lower BMI [29,30]. For this reason, bridging therapy has been proposed for weight reduction before bariatric surgery to decrease operative difficulties and achieve better outcomes. IGBs efficacy as a bridge-to-surgery therapy in very-severe obesity patients was shown in a recent meta-analysis that reported a BMI reduction of 6.6 kg/m^2 before surgery [31].

To date, three IGBs have been approved by the FDA in the US, whereas one more device is available only in Europe.

The first balloon designed in accordance with the Tarpon Springs Directives of 1987 [32], which represented the first guidelines regarding IGBs, was the Bioenterics IGB (now available as "Orbera").

Orbera® (Apollo Endosurgery, Austin, TX, USA), commercially available since 1991 and approved by the FDA in 2005 and subsequently by CE, is a single spherical silicone balloon of about 13 cm in maximum diameter. The device is positioned endoscopically. Then the balloon is inflated with saline solution to a volume of 500–700 mL. After the phase of filling, the infusion system is closed, and a self-sealing valve allows the safe release of the filling tube, which is extracted through the mouth. The balloon is inflated in the gastric fundus, and when released, it is free to float in the whole stomach. It remains in place for 6 months, and then it is removed in order to avoid mucosal injuries [33,34]. A systematic review and meta-analysis conducted by the ASGE, including 1683 patients from 17 studies, showed that Orbera® achieved 11.27% of TBWL (95% CI, 8.17–14.36%) at 12 months after implantation and a significant weight loss compared to controls (+26.9% percent excess weight loss (EWL); p, 0.01) [35]. Another large meta-analysis by Kumar et al. [36] showed that the percentage of TBWL was 13.2% (95%CI: 12.3–14.0) at 6 months, with no differences between balloon filling volumes (400 mL vs. 700 mL). The most frequent side effects, similarly to other IGBs, are nausea and vomiting; the aforementioned meta-analysis by Trang reported a nausea and vomiting rate slightly higher than other IGBs (82%;95% CI 77–87 and 72.2; 95% CI 66.7–77.7 respectively) [25].

An Obalon® (Obalon Therapeutics Inc, Carlsbad, CA, USA) balloon is compressed into a gelatinous capsule attached to a thin 2 Fr catheter. Under fluoroscopic guidance, the patient ingests the capsule, and once it reaches the stomach, the balloon is inflated with a gas (mostly nitrogen) to a maximum volume of 250 mL. Finally, the inflation catheter is removed. A maximum of 3 balloons can be placed in the stomach of a patient [37]. After a maximum of 6 months the balloons should be removed endoscopically [14,33,38]. Recently, the FDA approved the Obalon navigation system, that is, a portable console that dynamically tracks the balloon during placement using magnetic resonance and does not require X rays to confirm balloon positioning. The SMART trial, a comparative study of

387 patients between Obalon and the placebo, showed at six months a TBWL of 7.1 ± 5.3 kg in the Obalon group compared to 3.6 ± 5.1 kg in the placebo group ($p < 0.0001$) [39].

An interesting balloon is Elipse™ (Allurion, Natick, MA, USA), a swallowable balloon liquid-filled that has a self-deflating valve mechanism that allows self emptying after 4 months and spontaneous expulsion without the need for an endoscopy [40]. A study conducted on 112 patients showed a total weight loss of 10.9% at 6 months after implantation [41]. Spatz3® (Spatz, Fort Lauderdale, FL, USA) is a balloon filled with 400–700 mL of saline solution that requires endoscopic positioning; its peculiarity is the guaranteed duration of 12 months and the possibility to increase or reduce the volume of the balloon endoscopically in case of low efficacy or intolerance respectively [42]. A recent study by Fittipaldi-Fernandez et al. showed that after Spatz3® placement, mean BMI decreased from 39.5 to 32.8 kg/m^2 ($p < 0.0001$) [43]. Another randomized trial on 288 patients evaluated the efficacy of Spatz3® placement for 8 months compared with diet modification alone. Filling volumes of IGB were modified during the implantation period according to its efficacy or patients' tolerance. TBWL was 15% (95%CI 13.9–16.1) in the IGB group compared to 3.3% (95%CI 2–4.6%) in the control group ($p < 0.0001$). At 6 months from IGB removal, 74% of patients had weight loss maintenance satisfying the endpoint (>50%) [44]. Spatz3® received FDA approval in 2021, whereas Elipse™ is approved only by CE.

ReShape Duo was an approved integrated dual balloon system (ReShape Medical, Inc, San Clemente, CA, USA) that consisted of two liquid-filled silicone spheres joined by a flexible silicone shaft [45]. However, at the end of 2018, ReShape Medical was purchased by Apollo Endosurgery (Apollo Endosurgery, Austin, TX, USA), which decided to stop the production of ReShape Duo and provide Orbera only.

The recent Spanish Intragastric Balloon Consensus provided practical recommendations for IGB implantation. The minimum BMI for balloon implantation is 25 kg/m^2 after failed clinical treatment. Regarding patients with a BMI of 25–30 kg/m^2, a 6-month fluid-filled balloon is preferred, whereas in patients with BMI > 40 kg/m^2, a 12-month fluid-filled balloon is preferred (consensus > 75%). For patients with a BMI of 30–40 kg/m^2, which is the most common indication for IGBs implantation, there is a lower consensus to use a 12-month fluid-filled balloon [23].

2.1.2. Transpyloric Shuttle

Transpyloric shuttle (TPS) (BARONova Inc, San Carlos, CA, USA) is an FDA-approved device since 2019, indicated for obese patients with a body mass index (BMI) of 30 to 40 kg/m^2. It consists of a large spherical bulb attached to a smaller cylindrical bulb through a catheter. TPS is endoscopically released and fully assembled in the stomach, and designed to remain in place for up to 12 months. After the release, peristalsis carries the smaller sphere beyond the pylorus, causing intermittent gastric outlet obstruction and, thus, delaying gastric emptying [46]. To date, few studies have evaluated its safety and effectiveness. In a recent sham-controlled study conducted by Rothstein et al., 270 patients were randomized to a 12-month treatment or sham procedure; the preliminary abstract-based data showed a 30.9% excess weight loss (EWL) in the treatment group vs. 9.8% EWL in controls ($p < 0.0001$). Early device removal was required in 10.3% of patients, and the SAE rate was 2.5% [47].

2.1.3. Endoscopic Gastroplasties

Endoscopic gastroplasty is proposed as the endoluminal equivalent of surgical SG. FDA- and CE-approved dedicated devices (the OverStitch™ by Apollo Endosurgery, Austin, TX and Per-Oral Incisionless Operating Platform– IOP by USGI Medical, San Clemente, CA, USA) are used in order to plicate the gastric wall and to reduce the volume of the stomach inducing an early sensation of fullness. The procedure is performed under general anesthesia.

Endoscopic sleeve gastroplasty (ESG) was first described in 2013 by Abu Dayyeh [48] and is performed with the OverStich™ system. A suturing device is mounted on the tip of a dual-channel endoscope and is equipped with a curved needle guide that allows for either interrupted or continuous sutures. This system also uses an instrument to grasp the tissue called a "tissue helix" that is inserted through one of the channels [49].

On the other hand, primary obesity surgery endoluminal (POSE) is performed with the IOP system. It is a more complex device, equipped with a 54 Fr handle-controlled tube (TransPort®) able to be maneuvered in four directions and with four channels that house specialized instruments for grasping tissue folds (g-Lix™ and g-Prox EZ®) for positioning tissue anchors (g-Cath EZ™), and for lumen visualization with an ultra-slim endoscope [50,51].

The two procedures, as shown in Figure 2, result in two different types of gastroplasty. During ESG, the plication generally starts from the incisura angularis and then rises towards the gastric body along the greater curvature, shortening the distance between the anterior and posterior walls.

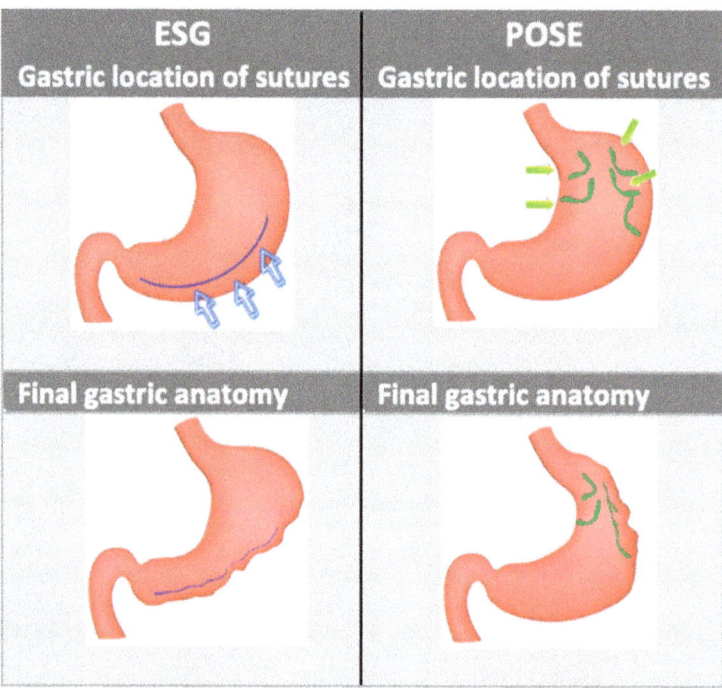

Figure 2. Schematic representation of endoscopic gastroplasties: on the left, an ESG procedure performed with Overstich™, and on the right, a POSE procedure performed with IOP. Blu and green arrows indicate position of endoscopic sutures during ESG and during POSE respectively. ESG, endoscopic sleeve gastroplasty; POSE, primary obesity surgery endoluminal; IOP, Incisionless Operating Platform.

During the POSE procedure, the anchor points are usually positioned in the fundus by creating eight to nine plications; three to four plications are usually placed in the distal body near the mouth of the antrum opposite to the incisura angularis in order to disrupt the gastric antral mill. A meta-analysis conducted by Gys et al., including 2475 patients, compared ESG vs. POSE, showing that both procedures were effective and safe, with only

25 patients experiencing major AEs but without the occurrence of deaths; however, ESG seemed superior in terms of EWL (68.3% vs. 44.9% respectively at 12 months) [52].

An interesting meta-analysis by Mohan et al. [53] compared ESG with surgery, showing that ESG had lower TBWL at 12 months compared to surgery (17% vs. 30.5%, $p = 0.001$) but a significantly lower rate of AEs (2.9% vs. 11.8%, $p = 0.001$).

In their recent systematic review and meta-analyses, Hedjoudje et al. confirmed the promising results of ESG in the long-term period, showing a mean TBWL of 15.1% (95% CI, 14.3–16.0) at six months, of 16.5% (95% CI, 15.2–17.8) at 12 months, and 17.2% (95% CI, 14.6–19.7) at 18–24 months. The procedure was also safe, with a pooled rate of severe AEs of 2.2% (95% CI, 1.6–3.1%), including pain or nausea requiring hospitalization (1.1%), upper gastrointestinal bleeding (0.6%), and peri-gastric leak or fluid collection (0.5%) [54]. A recent RCT comparing ESG with diet modifications alone (MERIT study) in patients with obesity grade 1 and 2 showed significant TBWL (13.6%) at 52 weeks in the ESG group that was maintained at 104 weeks in almost 70% of patients [55]. Few data are also present in the literature about the application of ESG in super obese patients with contraindications to surgery [56] or as a bridge-to-surgery procedure [57].

More recently, different plication technique variants have been proposed by leading centers in order to optimize the efficacy of gastroplasty [58–60]. The group of Lopez-Nava et al. modified the POSE technique performing the plication in the gastric body in order to alter its motility (POSE-2) [58]. Their preliminary data on 73 patients have been encouraging, showing a TBWL of 15.7% at 6 months with no AEs. Further studies are needed in order to confirm the lower rate of AEs and their efficacy compared to other techniques.

Regarding the comparison between endoscopic gastroplasty and IGBs, several studies showed that IGBs are less effective than gastroplasty. A retrospective study showed a significantly lower percentage of TBWL at 6 months (15.0 vs. 19.5%) and 12 months (13.9% vs. 21.3%) and higher AEs rates (17% vs. 5.2%, $p < 0.048$) in IGBs group compared to endoscopic gastroplasty [61]. Interestingly, a higher AEs rate was found in the IGBs group. A recent meta-analysis confirmed that IGB might be inferior to EGS in terms of WL; IGB-related AEs were lower than those of EGS [27].

Endoscopic gastroplasty also appears to have a significant metabolic effect: an observational study by Sharaiha et al. showed that ESG induces favorable changes in metabolism and obesity complications. In this study, patients had a significant reduction in liver enzymes, HbA1c, triglyceride level, and systolic blood pressure at 12-month follow-up following ESG [62]. The MERIT study also showed a significant improvement in metabolic comorbidities in patients who underwent ESG compared to controls [55].

2.2. Aspiration Therapy

Aspiration therapy was a promising technique performed with AspireAssist® System (Aspire Bariatrics, Inc. King of Prussia, PA, USA) for class II-III obesity approved by the FDA. It consists of a customized percutaneous endoscopic gastrostomy tube associated with an external device, which aspirates approximately 30% of the gastric content after a meal. In a multicenter American study, 171 patients were randomized into two groups (aspiration + lifestyle changes vs. lifestyle modification alone) and followed up for 4 years. The average BMI of patients at the beginning of this study was 41.6 ± 4.5 kg/m^2. After 12 months, the average BMI in the aspiration group (82 patients) was 34.1 ± 5.4 kg/m^2 with a %TWL decreased of 18.3 ± 8.0%, and after 48 months, the %TWL in 58 patients was 18.7% [63]. Unfortunately, on February 2022, the AspireAssist system was withdrawn from the market due to financial reasons [64].

3. Endoscopic Malabsorptive Interventions

3.1. Duodenal Mucosal Resurfacing

Duodenal mucosal resurfacing (DMR), better known by the brand name Revita® (Fractyl Health, Lexington, MA USA), is a catheter-based technique that hydrothermally ablates the duodenal mucosa, primarily designed for the treatment of T2DM. The Revita®

DMR is introduced through the mouth into the duodenum and placed distally to the Ampulla of Vater over a guidewire using fluoroscopic guidance; once in place, the gastroscope is re-inserted in order to control the procedure. The 2 cm balloon catheter is designed to isolate the mucosa from the deeper layers of the duodenum by the injection of saline solution and then hydrothermally ablate the mucosa between the Ampulla of Vater and the Treitz ligament [65].

The theoretical basis of this technique derives from the assumption that the duodenal mucosa of T2DM patients is abnormally hypertrophied with a higher concentration of enteroendocrine cells leading to a higher secretion of GIP that produces insulin hypersecretion and insulin resistance.

In the first human study (proof-of-concept) [65], 39 patients with T2DM were treated with DMR, with a baseline HbA1c of 9.6% ± 1.4 and a BMI of 30.8 ± 3.5 kg. HbA1c was reduced by 1.2% at 6 months in the full cohort ($p < 0.001$), with more effects in the long segment cohort, also accompanied by a modest weight reduction of 3.9 ± 0.5 kg at 3 months ($p < 0.001$) and 2.5 ± 0.1 kg at 6 months ($p < 0.05$). In this study, no perforation, gastrointestinal bleeding, or evidence of malabsorption occurred, but three patients developed duodenal stenosis.

A recent randomized, double-blind, sham-controlled trial (REVITA-2) included 56 patients from Europe and Brazil treated with Revita® DMR and 52 with a sham procedure [66]. The primary endpoint was the change of HbA1c, and one of the secondary endpoints was the change of weight at 24 weeks compared to baseline. Statistical analysis of the groups was stratified by region due to the statistical differences between sham groups. In particular, in the European group treated with DMR (N = 39), the median reduction of HbA1c from baseline at 24 weeks was −6.6 mmol/mol (2.8%), compared with −3.3 mmol/mol (2.5%) in the sham procedure group ($p = 0.033$).

Considering the secondary endpoint, in the European DMR group, the median weight reduction at 24 weeks was −2.4 kg, significantly greater than the −1.4 kg observed in the sham group ($p = 0.012$).

The device appeared to be safe: the most common AEs in the first 30 days were transient and mild abdominal pain (17.9%) and hypoglycemia (7.7%). No severe complications occurred in the European group, whereas one jejunal perforation repaired surgically was observed in the Brazilian group. There were no episodes of pancreatitis nor infection in either group, and follow-up endoscopies revealed complete healing of the duodenal mucosa. Revita® is currently for investigational use only.

3.2. Duodenal-Jejunal Bypass

EndoBarrier® (GI Dynamics, Boston, MA USA) is a 60 cm thin and flexible Teflon-coated tube that works as a duodenal-jejunal bypass liner. The device is placed endoscopically and anchored to the duodenal bulb like a self-expanding metal stent for up to 12 months. It is a malabsorptive device that works mimicking RYGB: it brings the food to the proximal jejunum, bypassing the duodenum, preventing contact with the mucosa and the absorption of food. EndoBarrier®, should not interact with the Ampulla of Vater, allowing pancreatic and biliary fluids to flow down outside the tube and meet the chyme at the end of the tube [67]. Different RCTs comparing EndoBarrier® to lifestyle modifications were performed around 2010, showing interesting results in both weight loss and diabetes control [35]. The first systematic review and meta-analyses conducted by Rohde et al., including five RCTs with 235 subjects and ten observational studies with 211 subjects, showed that EndoBarrier® was associated with significant differences in body weight (−5.1 kg; 95% CI −7.3, −3.0) and EWL (12.6%; 95% CI 9.0, 16.2) compared to diet modification alone, even if the reduction of HbA1c and fasting plasma glucose did not reach statistical significance [68]. A subsequent systematic review reported greater reductions in both HbA1c (1.3% or 13.3 mmol/mol) and weight (TBWL 18.9%) [69]. However, the spread of EndoBarrier® into clinical practice was deeply affected by the removal of the CE mark and suspension of FDA approval during the pivotal trial (ENDO trial) [70] owing to the high incidence of liver abscess in the cohort of Endobarrier patients. However, after a review of the relevant safety data, the FDA and Institutional Review Board approved the new STEP-1 pivotal trial (NCT04101669) on Endobarrier in the United States in February 2019, with study closure expected in 2025 [71].

Recently, a multicenter RCT was performed in the UK on 170 adults with obesity and uncontrolled T2DM [72]. The study did not achieve the primary outcome because the reduction of HbA1c $\geq$ 20% at 12 months did not differ in the two groups [DJB 54.6% (n = 30) vs. control 55.2% (n = 32); odds ratio (OR) 0.93, 95% CI 0.44–2.0; p = 0.85]. However, the study demonstrated the superiority of DJB over intensive medical care alone to achieve weight loss at 12 months: 24% (n = 16) of patients achieved $\geq$ 15% weight loss in the DJB group compared to 4% (n = 2) in the control group (OR 8.3, 95% CI: 1.8–39; p = 0.007).

The weakness of these results was confirmed in a recent meta-analysis, where the DJBL group showed superior excess weight loss (+ 11.4% [+ 7.75 to + 15.03%], p < 0.00001), higher decrease in HbA1c compared to the control group (-2.73 ± 0.5 vs. -1.73 ± 0.4, p = 0.0001), and a SAEs rate of 19.7%, criteria that were not sufficient to reach the ASGE threshold for the treatment of obesity (i.e., $\geq$25% excess weight loss (%EWL) compared to the control group and $\leq$5% SAEs) [73].

3.3. Gastroduodenojejunal Bypass

Gastroduodenojejunal Bypass (GDJB) (Endo Bypass System, ValenTx, Maple Grove, MN, USA) is a 120 cm fluoropolymer sleeve anchored in the region of gastroesophageal junction that leads the food into the small bowel with a combined endoscopic/laparoscopic procedure. This liner induces weight loss by mimicking an RYGB for 12 months until removal. In the first study evaluating the safety and efficacy of GDJB, 13 patients (mean BMI 42 kg/m^2) were prospectively enrolled for a 1-year trial [74]. Ten patients concluded the study period, although four patients had a partial cuff detachment. At 12 months, the average EWL was 35.9% and 54% in the fully-attached subgroup. The sleeve was safe and well tolerated, with no esophageal leak, ulceration, or pancreatitis observed during the follow-up period. Five of the six patients that elapsed a period of one year with a fully attached device were followed up, and they had maintained an average EWL of 30% at the 14-month post-explant control (26 months from the beginning of the study). No further studies were performed with this type of device. Endo Bypass System is not yet approved by the FDA and CE for sale.

3.4. The Incisionless Magnetic Anastomotic System

The Incisionless Magnetic Anastomotic System (IMAS) (GI Windows, Westwood, MA, USA) is a novel technique that creates an anastomosis without bowel incision by using simultaneously two octagonal magnets. They are delivered into the proximal jejunum and terminal ileum with a simultaneous enteroscopy and colonoscopy (even if laparoscopic assistance is necessary), creating an anastomosis by causing local tissue necrosis. When the anastomosis is completely created, the magnets usually fall into the stool within 2 weeks. The anastomosis diverts nutrients and bile acids into the ileum, causing malabsorption.

The pilot study enrolled ten patients with an average BMI of 41 kg/m^2 [75]. After 12 months, the average TBWL was 14.6% with an EWL% of 40.2%; moreover, in the subgroup of diabetes patients, IMAS induced a reduction of HbA1c by 1.9% and by 1.0% for prediabetic patients. All patients experienced diarrhea in the following days, and four patients had frequent diarrhea. The anastomosis is not reversible, and no data are available about long-term malabsorption consequences.

4. Revisional Endoscopy after Bariatric Surgery

Primary bariatric surgery, both restrictive and malabsorptive, has a notable efficacy, inducing up to 20–50% of TBWL. However, up to 1/3 of patients undergoing bariatric surgery have subsequent weight regain or insufficient weight loss. In the case of ESG, weight regain could be higher, involving up to 75% of patients [76]. Different definitions of weight regain are available, but the most commonly used definitions in clinical practice and in the literature are (1) BMI ≥ 35 kg/m^2 after successful weight loss; (2) an increase >25% EWL from nadir; (3) an increase >10 kg from nadir; and (4) maintaining <20% of TWL [77]. The causes of weight regain are multifactorial, with the main contributing factors being a lack of lifestyle changes (i.e., sedentary life) and a lack of change in eating habits. Post-surgical anatomical factors also play an important role in weight regain. In the case of RYGB, dilation of the gastro-jejunal anastomosis (GJA) is sometimes observed, which induces a reduction of satiety and contributes to weight regain. Similarly, in ESG, dilation of the gastric remnant can be observed, leading to pre-surgical treatment satiety perception. In the past, lifestyle corrections and re-surgery were the only options available in case of weight regain. However, they carried insufficient results or significant (15–50%) post-surgical comorbidities, respectively [15]. Endoscopic therapies are attractive, as they are more effective than lifestyle modification and are associated with lower AEs rates compared with revision bariatric surgery. Below are detailed all the available endoscopic techniques applied for revision after bariatric surgery.

4.1. Endoscopic Revision after Roux-en-Y Gastric Bypass

Argon plasma coagulation (APC) applied at the level of GJA is a commonly available and easy-to-use treatment in the cases of endoscopic revision after RYGB. The rationale of this type of treatment is that mucosal healing of GJA mucosa after APC application induces an increase of tissue fibrosis and reduction of GJA size, thereby reducing the amount of food passing through the anastomosis [78]. More recently, a similar rationale has been exploited with the cryoablation technique commonly used for Barrett's mucosal eradication. Similarly to APC, a cryoablation balloon is applied at the level of GJA and could also be extended at the gastric pouch leading to a fibrotic stricture and consequently to a reduction of both size of GJA and pouch [79]. APC treatment requires more than one endoscopic session (usually every 2–3 months) in order to reach the target of GJA diameter of 8–10 mm, whereas cryoablation is a one-session technique. One limitation of cryoablation is that the balloon requires a gastric pouch length of at least 4 cm. One retrospective study showed that high-dose APC (70–80 W) compared to low-dose APC (45–55 W) induced higher TBWL (10% vs. 5%) in the long term [80]. A recent RCT demonstrated the efficacy of APC over the standard multidisciplinary diet approach in terms of significant weight loss (9.73 vs. + 1.38) and improvement of quality of life after bariatric surgery [81]. Similar results have been shown for cryoablation in the only available study: significant reduction of the GJA diameter (24 to 17 mm, $p < 0.001$), pouch length (5 to 4 cm, $p < 0.05$), and short-term TBWL (8% at two months). However, it is necessary to highlight that in this study, three severe Aes (13.6%) occurred. One was GJA stenosis requiring endoscopic dilation, and two involved bleeding from the treated area [79].

Another technique aimed at reducing the GJA size is the full-thickness suture, specifically named transoral outlet reduction endoscopically (TORe). The procedure consists of the application of interrupted or purse-string stitches with the OverStich™ system at the level of GJA in order to reduce its size. Several studies have demonstrated the efficacy of TORe, showing a TBWL at one year between 6.6% and 8.6% [15,82,83]. The procedure is usually safe, and the most common AE is stricture which occurs in 3.3–4.8% of patients, whereas only one episode of severe bleeding has been described in a previous study [83]. A modified technique consists of the application of APC at the level of GJA before the execution of the TORe (Figure 3).

A recent meta-analysis showed that APC-TORe is more effective than TORe alone, showing a TBWL at 12 months of 9.5% (5.7–13.2) vs. 5.8% (4.3–7.1) [83].

Older studies described the application of sodium morrhuate at the level of GJA for the treatment of weight regain after bariatric surgery. However, subsequent studies demonstrated its inferiority when compared to other endoscopic procedures (i.e., APC and suturing) [84]. A promising technique is the application of over-the-scope clips on two sides of the GJA, which showed a significant decrease in BMI levels in one study [85].

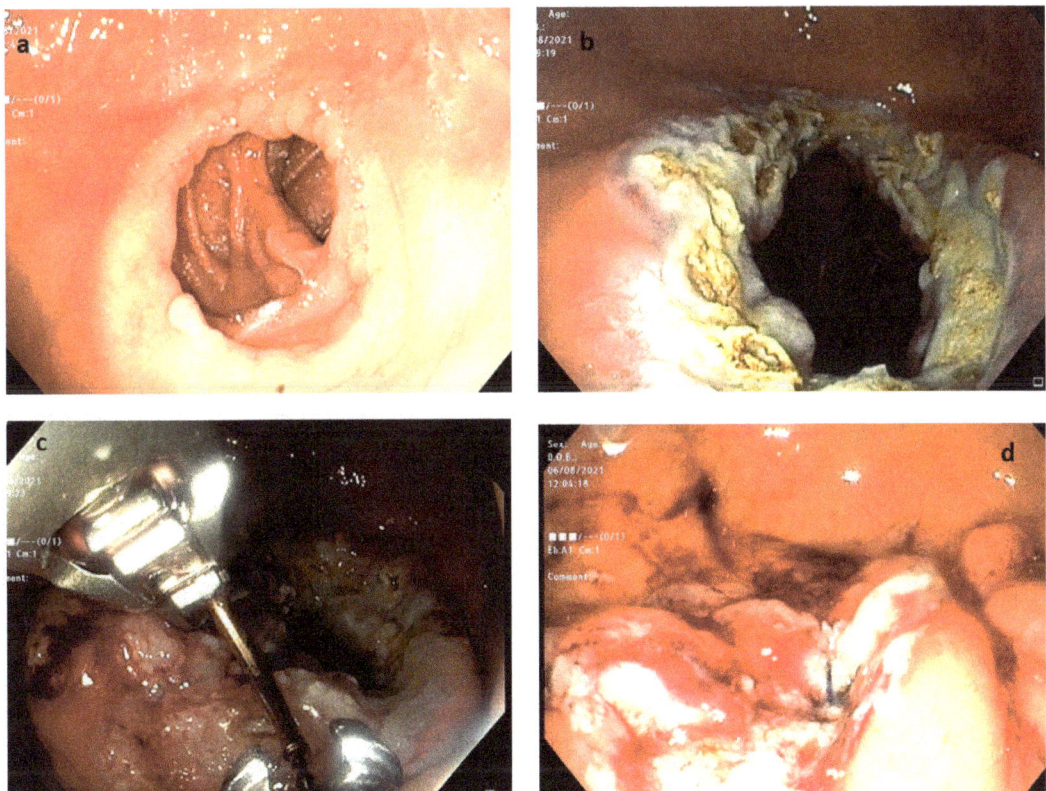

Figure 3. Endoscopic steps of the transoral outlet reduction endoscopic (TORe) procedure: (**a**) visualization of the dilated GJA; (**b**) APC application at the level of GJA; (**c**) suturing performance with OverStich™ system; and (**d**) final GJA at the end of the procedure. GJA, gastrojejunal anastomosis; APC, argon plasma coagulation.

4.2. Endoscopic Revision after Sleeve Gastrectomy

Weight regains after SG is a major challenge considering that it afflicts up to 2/3 of patients. RYGB or repeating SG are the most common surgical solutions for this relevant clinical problem. However, revisional surgery carries a high rate of AEs, described in up to 15% of patients [86]. In 2017 the first series of five patients was published, showing the efficacy of Endosleeve after SG (R-EndoSleeve) [87]. The procedure is analogous to the one performed as a primary intervention: each suture is started at the anterior wall of the sleeve, with subsequent bites progressing along the "greater curvature/staple line" and to the more proximal posterior wall. Approximately 6–10 bites per suture are performed. More recently, the group of de Moura et al. published a larger retrospective series of 34 patients that successfully underwent Endosleeve after SG. The study showed technical success in 100% of cases with a TBWL > 10% at 1 year in 82.4% of patients [76]. The efficacy of R-Endosleeve was confirmed in the recent prospective study by Maselli DB et al. on 82 patients who experienced significant weight regain after SG. The performance of R-endosleeve allowed a TBWL of 15.7% ± 7.6% at 12 months; ≥15% TBWL was achieved in 52.4% of patients at 12 months. The procedure was also safe with only one moderate AE (stricture at the level of the gastroesophageal junction) that was resolved with one session of endoscopic dilation [88].

Table 1 summarizes the results of the most relevant studies present in the literature for all primary and revisional bariatric endoscopic procedures.

Table 1. Summary of the most relevant studies on the efficacy and safety of primary and revisional endoscopic therapies.

			Type of Study	Number of Patients	Comparator Group	Weight Loss Outcome	AEs Outcome
Primary endoscopic therapies	Space occupying devices	Orbera®	Meta-analysis [35]	1638 (17 studies)	None	EWL 25.44 (95% CI, 21.47–29.4) at 1 year	33.7% pain and nausea 1.4% migration 0.1% gastric perforation
		Obalon®	Double-blind RCT with sham group [39]	387	Lifestyle therapy	TBWL 7.1 ± 5.3 vs. 3.6 ± 5.1 kg	0.4% SAEs (one bleeding and one balloon deflation
		Elipse™	Prospective observational [41]	112	None	TBWL 7.9% at 1 year	51% nausea and vomiting 0% SAEs [25] *
		Spatz3®	RCT [44]	288	Lifestyle therapy	TBWL 15.0% vs. 3.3% 32 weeks at 32 wks ($p < 0.0001$)	Seven SAEs (7%). No deaths
		Transpyloric Shuttle®	Observational [46]	20	None	EWL 41% at 6 months	10% early removal for gastric ulceration
	Endoscopic gastroplasties	ESG	Meta-analysis [53]	1815 (8 studies on ESG) 2179 (7 studies on LSG)	Laparoscopic sleeve gastrectomy	TBWL 17.1% vs. 30.5% (ESG vs. LSG) at 1 year	Overall AEs 2.9% (95% CI 1.8–4.4) vs. 11.8% (95% CI 8.4–16.4)
		POSE	Meta-analysis [52]	465 (5 studies on POSE) and 1717 (8 studies on ESG)	ESG	EWL 44.9 ± 2.1% vs. 68.3 ± 3.8% (POSE vs. ESG) at 1 year	4 SAEs for POSE (3 bleeding and 1 hepatic abscess)
	Endoscopic malabsoptive procedures	DMR	RCT [66]	108	Sham procedure	HbA1c reduction from 8.5 ± 0.7% to 7.5 ± 0.8%	None
		EndoBarrier®	RCT [70]	80	Conventional medical therapy	TBWL 9.7% vs. 2.1% at 1 year	19 (39%) SAEs (11 re-intervention)
		Endo Bypass System	Prospective observational [74]	13	None	EWL was 35.9% at 1 year	None
		IMAS	Prospective observational [75]	10	None	TBWL was 14.6%; EWL% 40.2% at 1 year	Diarrhea
Revisional Endoscopic therapies		APC	RCT with sham group [81]	42	Diet	−9.73 kg vs. + 1.38 kg at 6 months	None in 1 year follow-up period
		Cryoablation	Retrospective series [79]	22	None	TBWL 8.1% at 8 weeks	13.6% (one stenosis and 2 bleeding)
		TORe	Meta-analysis [82]	850 (13 studies)	None	TBWL 8.55% at 1 year	Total 11.4% ± 10.11 Severe 0.57% ± 1.35
		TORe + APC	Meta-analysis [83]	1625 (16 studies)	TORe	TBWL at 12 months 9.5% vs. 5.8%	Strictures in 4.8% of patients
		Sodium morrhuate	Prospective comparative [84]	43	TORe	TBWL 2.7% ±5.5 vs. 10.4% ± 2.2	N/A
		OTSC	Observational [85]	94	None	BMI drop from 32.8 (±1.9) to 27.4 (±3.8) at 1 year	Two stenoses requiring endoscopic dilation
		R-Endosleeve	Prospective [88]	82	None	TBWL 15.7% (±7.6%) at 1 year	One moderate adverse event

IGBs, intragastric balloons; ESG, endoscopic sleeve gastroplasty; POSE, primary obesity surgical endoluminal; APC, argon plasma coagulation; TORe, transoral outlet reduction endoscopically; OTSC, over-the-scope clip; LSG, laparoscopic sleeve gastrectomy; TBWL, total body weight loss; EWL, excess of weight loss; AEs, adverse events; SAEs, severe adverse events. * Data extracted from a meta-analysis on two studies with Elipse on 42 patients.

5. Conclusions

Bariatric patients are a complex category that requires a multidisciplinary approach. Different professional figures, such as nutritionists, psychologists, and internal medicine physicians, are involved in the initial evaluation of obese patients and their complications [89]. These figures are essential in order to start the first-line therapeutic approach consisting of dietary regimens and changes in lifestyle habits. However, in severely obese patients and in those not compliant with conservative regimens, more invasive options such as surgery or endoscopy are offered in order to maximize clinical results and improve quality of life [3]. Both types of procedures are offered to obese patients that have failed diet modifications and have no associated psychiatric conditions [90]. Bariatric surgery largely demonstrated efficacy in terms of weight loss in the long-term period [7,10]. In the last decades, several endoscopic options have been developed as a less invasive alternative for the primary treatment of obesity. The availability of different options allows personalized treatment for different clinical situations. IGBs are the most versatile endoscopic procedure that does not alter gastric anatomy. This important feature allows its use both as a primary therapy in patients with mild obesity and also in overweight patients in order to improve metabolic complications [23,28]. Another application is the bridge-to-surgery implantation in severe and very-severe obesity patients in order to reduce intra and post-surgical complications [31]. Different types of IGBs are available in clinical practice. However, there is no evidence of superiority in the efficacy of a brand compared to another one. The general rule is that the higher BMI, the higher volumes and longer times of implantation are required [23].

Endoscopic gastroplasty obtained with both ESG and POSE is a well-established treatment that maximizes efficacy in type 1 and 2 obesity. Endoscopic gastroplasty leads to a lower percentage of TBWL than bariatric surgery but is superior to IGBs in inducing persistent weight loss, and therefore, patients could be offered the option to refuse surgical treatments [54,55,91]. More recently, other endoscopic procedures that have mainly malabsorptive and metabolic-modulating actions have been developed in order to induce weight loss and also to improve glycemic control (Figure 4). Revita® DMR demonstrated encouraging results in pivotal trials, showing a significant reduction of HbA1c compared to controls but associated with a modest weight loss [66]. This type of procedure could be relevant to overweight and mild to moderately obese patients with difficult glycemic control in order to prevent diabetic complications. However, DMR is not yet approved by the bridFDA. An endobarrier is an ideal theoretical device that mimics malabsorptive surgical procedures without altering the anatomy. Initial results were encouraging in terms of weight loss and glycemic control [68]. However, its approval process was troublesome for the occurrence of SAE (i.e., hepatic abscess), which led to the suspension of the pivotal trial [70]. After the review of safety data, a new pivotal trial was started, and data about efficacy and safety will be available in 2–3 years [71]. IMAS and GDJB were both developed with malabsorptive intentions, but evidence of their efficacy is still limited to a few studies [74,75].

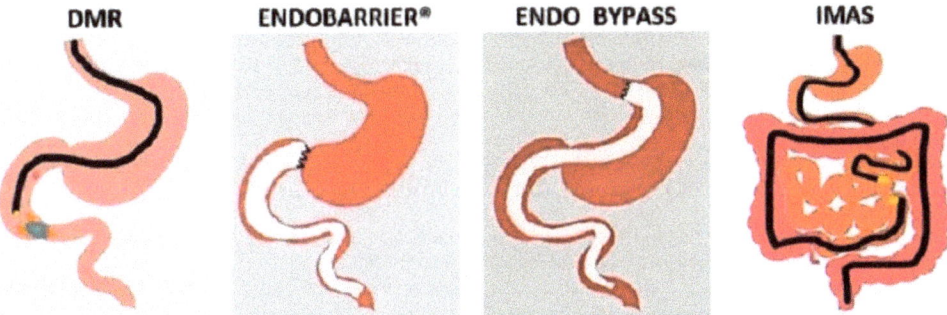

Figure 4. Schematic representation of the endoscopic malabsorptive procedures. IMAS, Incisionless Magnetic Anastomotic System; DMR, duodenal mucosal resurfacing.

The choice between the different endoscopic bariatric procedures and bariatric surgery should be guided according to each specific clinical situation and should therefore be taken according to multidisciplinary decisions aiming to reduce the potentially life-threatening complications of obesity and to improve quality of life and life expectancy of these patients.

Considering patients who have already undergone bariatric surgery, insufficient results are reported in up to one third of cases. Endoscopy has proved efficacy in revisional therapies, allowing for the optimization of surgical results and the avoidance of unacceptable rates of complications of redo-surgery [15]. In the case of RYGB, the application of APC at the GJA in association with TORe has proven the most effective results [83]. Other procedures, such as cryoablation and the application of OTSC at the level of GJA, have shown promising results in recent studies [79,85]. In case of failed SG, bariatric endoscopy could offer the R-EndoSleeve as an optimizing therapy [76,88].

In conclusion, bariatric endoscopy is a valid alternative to surgery for the treatment of obesity, offering different options that can be tailored to the patient guaranteeing good clinical results if associated with adequate diet control. As a minimally invasive technique, bariatric endoscopy may also limit the burden of AEs. The continuous evolution of endoscopic bariatric procedures has also led to the development of techniques that have the potential role of improving metabolic alterations.

Author Contributions: A.M. concept of the study, writing and paper revision; F.L., D.S. and S.M. writing and paper revision; M.B., F.D.G., D.E.O.R., L.P., V.R., L.R., E.S., C.S., F.T.V. and L.V., original draft preparation and editing; A.A. concept of the study, writing and final approval of the manuscript. All authors have read and agreed to the published version of the manuscript.

Funding: This research received no external funding.

Institutional Review Board Statement: Not applicable.

Informed Consent Statement: Not applicable.

Data Availability Statement: Not applicable.

Conflicts of Interest: A.A. consultant for Boston Scientifics and Olympus.

References

1. World Health Organization. Obesity and Overweight. Available online: https://www.who.int/news-room/fact-sheets/detail/obesity-and-overweight (accessed on 22 November 2022).
2. Sturm, R.; Hattori, A. Morbid obesity rates continue to rise rapidly in the United States. *Int. J. Obes.* **2013**, *37*, 889–891. [CrossRef]
3. Heymsfield, S.B.; Wadden, T.A. Mechanisms, Pathophysiology, and Management of Obesity. *N. Engl. J. Med.* **2017**, *376*, 1492. [CrossRef]
4. Berkowitz, R.I.; Fabricatore, A.N. Obesity, psychiatric status, and psychiatric medications. *Psychiatr. Clin. N. Am.* **2011**, *34*, 747–764. [CrossRef] [PubMed]
5. Executive Summary: Guidelines (2013) for the Management of Overweight and Obesity in Adults, a Report of the American College of Cardiology/American Heart Association Task Force on Practice Guidelines and the Obesity Society Published by the Obesity Society and American College of Cardiology/American Heart Association Task Force on Practice Guidelines. Based on a systematic review from the The Obesity Expert Panel, 2013. *Obesity* **2014**, *22* (Suppl. 2), S5–S39.
6. Yanovski, S.Z.; Yanovski, J.A. Long-term drug treatment for obesity, a systematic and clinical review. *JAMA* **2014**, *311*, 74–86. [CrossRef] [PubMed]
7. Sjöström, L.; Narbro, K.; Sjöström, C.D.; Karason, K.; Larsson, B.; Wedel, H.; Lystig, T.; Sullivan, M.; Bouchard, C.; Carlsson, B.; et al. Effects of bariatric surgery on mortality in Swedish obese subjects. *N. Engl. J. Med.* **2007**, *357*, 741–752. [CrossRef] [PubMed]
8. Schauer, P.R.; Mingrone, G.; Ikramuddin, S.; Wolfe, B. Clinical Outcomes of Metabolic Surgery, Efficacy of Glycemic Control, Weight Loss, and Remission of Diabetes. *Diabetes Care* **2016**, *39*, 902–911. [CrossRef]
9. O'Brien, P.E.; Hindle, A.; Brennan, L.; Skinner, S.; Burton, P.; Smith, A.; Crosthwaite, G.; Brown, W. Long-Term Outcomes After Bariatric Surgery, a Systematic Review and Meta-analysis of Weight Loss at 10 or More Years for All Bariatric Procedures and a Single-Centre Review of 20-Year Outcomes After Adjustable Gastric Banding. *Obes. Surg.* **2019**, *29*, 3–14. [CrossRef]
10. Arterburn, D.E.; Telem, D.A.; Kushner, R.F.; Courcoulas, A.P. Benefits and Risks of Bariatric Surgery in Adults: A Review. *JAMA* **2020**, *324*, 879–887. [CrossRef]
11. Flum, D.R.; Belle, S.H.; King, W.C.; Wahed, A.S.; Berk, P.; Chapman, W.; Pories, W.; Courcoulas, A.; McCloskey, C.; Mitchell, J.; et al. Perioperative safety in the longitudinal assessment of bariatric surgery. *N. Engl. J. Med.* **2009**, *361*, 445–454.

12. Chang, S.H.; Freeman, N.L.B.; Lee, J.A.; Stoll, C.R.T.; Calhoun, A.J.; Eagon, J.C.; Colditz, G.A. Early major complications after bariatric surgery in the USA, 2003–2014, a systematic review and meta-analysis. *Obes. Rev.* **2018**, *19*, 529–537. [CrossRef] [PubMed]
13. Mechanick, J.I.; Apovian, C.; Brethauer, S.; Garvey, W.T.; Joffe, A.M.; Kim, J.; Kushner, R.F.; Lindquist, R.; Pessah-Pollack, R.; Seger, J.; et al. Clinical practice guidelines for the perioperative nutrition, metabolic, and nonsurgical support of patients undergoing bariatric procedures—2019 update, cosponsored by american association of clinical endocrinologists/american college of endocrinology, the obesity society, american society for metabolic & bariatric surgery, obesity medicine association, and american society of anesthesiologists—Executive summary. *Endocr. Pract.* **2019**, *25*, 1346–1359.
14. Sullivan, S.; Edmundowicz, S.A.; Thompson, C.C. Endoscopic Bariatric and Metabolic Therapies, New and Emerging Technologies. *Gastroenterology* **2017**, *152*, 1791–1801. [CrossRef] [PubMed]
15. Bulajic, M.; Vadalà di Prampero, S.F.; Boškoski, I.; Costamagna, G. Endoscopic therapy of weight regain after bariatric surgery. *World J. Gastrointest. Surg.* **2021**, *13*, 1584–1596. [CrossRef]
16. Kumbhari, V.; le Roux, C.W.; Cohen, R.V. Endoscopic Evaluation and Management of Late Complications After Bariatric Surgery, a Narrative Review. *Obes. Surg.* **2021**, *31*, 4624–4633. [CrossRef] [PubMed]
17. Karlas, T.; Petroff, D.; Feisthammel, J.; Beer, S.; Blüher, M.; Schütz, T.; Lichtinghagen, R.; Hoffmeister, A.; Wiegand, J. Endoscopic Bariatric Treatment with Duodenal-Jejunal Bypass Liner Improves Non-invasive Markers of Non-alcoholic Steatohepatitis. *Obes. Surg.* **2022**, *32*, 2495–2503. [CrossRef]
18. Na, H.K.; De Moura, D.T.H. Various Novel and Emerging Technologies in Endoscopic Bariatric and Metabolic Treatments. *Clin. Endosc.* **2021**, *54*, 25–31. [CrossRef]
19. van Baar, A.C.G.; Meiring, S.; Smeele, P.; Vriend, T.; Holleman, F.; Barlag, M.; Mostafavi, N.; Tijssen, J.G.P.; Soeters, M.R.; Nieuwdorp, M.; et al. Duodenal mucosal resurfacing combined with glucagon-like peptide-1 receptor agonism to discontinue insulin in type 2 diabetes, a feasibility study. *Gastrointest. Endosc.* **2021**, *94*, 111–120.e3. [CrossRef]
20. Buchwald, H.; Estok, R.; Fahrbach, K.; Banel, D.; Sledge, I. Trends in mortality in bariatric surgery, a systematic review and meta-analysis. *Surgery* **2007**, *142*, 621–632; discussion 32–35. [CrossRef]
21. Nieben, O.G.; Harboe, H. Intragastric balloon as an artificial bezoar for treatment of obesity. *Lancet* **1982**, *1*, 198–199. [CrossRef]
22. Neto, M.G.; Silva, L.B.; Grecco, E.; de Quadros, L.G.; Teixeira, A.; Souza, T.; Scarparo, J.; Parada, A.A.; Dib, R.; Moon, R.; et al. Brazilian Intragastric Balloon Consensus Statement (BIBC), practical guidelines based on experience of over 40,000 cases. *Surg. Obes. Relat. Dis.* **2018**, *14*, 151–159. [CrossRef]
23. Espinet Coll, E.; Del Pozo García, A.J.; Turró Arau, R.; Nebreda Durán, J.; Cortés Rizo, X.; Serrano Jiménez, A.; Escartí Usó, M.; Muñoz Tornero, M.; Carral Martínez, D.; Bernabéu López, J.; et al. Spanish Intragastric Balloon Consensus Statement (SIBC), practical guidelines based on experience of over 20 000 cases. *Rev. Esp. Enferm. Dig.* **2023**, *115*, 22–34.
24. Ribeiro, I.B.; Kotinda, A.; Sánchez-Luna, S.A.; de Moura, D.T.H.; Mancini, F.C.; de Souza, T.F.; Matuguma, S.E.; Sakai, C.M.; Rocha, R.S.P.; Luz, G.O.; et al. Adverse Events and Complications with Intragastric Balloons, a Narrative Review (with Video). *Obes. Surg.* **2021**, *31*, 2743–2752. [CrossRef] [PubMed]
25. Trang, J.; Lee, S.S.; Miller, A.; Cruz Pico, C.X.; Postoev, A.; Ibikunle, I.; Ibikunle, C.A. Incidence of nausea and vomiting after intragastric balloon placement in bariatric patients—A systematic review and meta-analysis. *Int. J. Surg.* **2018**, *57*, 22–29. [CrossRef] [PubMed]
26. Moura, D.; Oliveira, J.; De Moura, E.G.; Bernardo, W.; Galvão Neto, M.; Campos, J.; Popov, V.B.; Thompson, C. Effectiveness of intragastric balloon for obesity, A systematic review and meta-analysis based on randomized control trials. *Surg. Obes. Relat. Dis.* **2016**, *12*, 420–429. [CrossRef]
27. Singh, S.; de Moura, D.T.H.; Khan, A.; Bilal, M.; Chowdhry, M.; Ryan, M.B.; Bazarbashi, A.N.; Thompson, C.C. Intragastric Balloon Versus Endoscopic Sleeve Gastroplasty for the Treatment of Obesity, a Systematic Review and Meta-analysis. *Obes. Surg.* **2020**, *30*, 3010–3029. [CrossRef] [PubMed]
28. Fittipaldi-Fernandez, R.J.; Zotarelli-Filho, I.J.; Diestel, C.F.; Klein, M.; de Santana, M.F.; de Lima, J.H.F.; Bastos, F.S.S.; Dos Santos, N.T. Intragastric Balloon, a Retrospective Evaluation of 5874 Patients on Tolerance, Complications, and Efficacy in Different Degrees of Overweight. *Obes. Surg.* **2020**, *30*, 4892–4898. [CrossRef] [PubMed]
29. Schwartz, M.L.; Drew, R.L.; Chazin-Caldie, M. Factors determining conversion from laparoscopic to open Roux-en-Y gastric bypass. *Obes. Surg.* **2004**, *14*, 1193–1197. [CrossRef] [PubMed]
30. Khan, M.A.; Grinberg, R.; Johnson, S.; Afthinos, J.N.; Gibbs, K.E. Perioperative risk factors for 30-day mortality after bariatric surgery, is functional status important? *Surg. Endosc.* **2013**, *27*, 1772–1777. [CrossRef]
31. Loo, J.H.; Lim, Y.H.; Seah, H.L.; Chong, A.Z.Q.; Tay, K.V. Intragastric Balloon as Bridging Therapy Prior to Bariatric Surgery for Patients with Severe Obesity (BMI $\geq$ 50 kg/m(2)), a Systematic Review and Meta-analysis. *Obes. Surg.* **2022**, *32*, 489–502. [CrossRef]
32. Schapiro, M.; Benjamin, S.; Blackburn, G.; Frank, B.; Heber, D.; Kozarek, R.; Randall, S.; Stern, W. Obesity and the gastric balloon, a comprehensive workshop. *Gastrointest. Endosc.* **1987**, *33*, 323–327. [CrossRef] [PubMed]
33. Stavrou, G.; Shrewsbury, A.; Kotzampassi, K. Six intragastric balloons, Which to choose? *World J. Gastrointest. Endosc.* **2021**, *13*, 238–259. [CrossRef] [PubMed]
34. Wahlen, C.H.; Bastens, B.; Herve, J.; Malmendier, C.; Dallemagne, B.; Jehaes, C.; Markiewicz, S.; Monami, B.; Weerts, J. The BioEnterics Intragastric Balloon (BIB), how to use it. *Obes. Surg.* **2001**, *11*, 524–527. [CrossRef] [PubMed]

35. Abu Dayyeh, B.K.; Kumar, N.; Edmundowicz, S.A.; Jonnalagadda, S.; Larsen, M.; Sullivan, S.; Thompson, C.C.; Banerjee, S. ASGE Bariatric Endoscopy Task Force systematic review and meta-analysis assessing the ASGE PIVI thresholds for adopting endoscopic bariatric therapies. *Gastrointest. Endosc.* **2015**, *82*, 425–438.e5. [CrossRef]
36. Kumar, N.; Bazerbachi, F.; Rustagi, T.; McCarty, T.R.; Thompson, C.C.; Galvao Neto, M.P.; Zundel, N.; Wilson, E.B.; Gostout, C.J.; Abu Dayyeh, B.K. The Influence of the Orbera Intragastric Balloon Filling Volumes on Weight Loss, Tolerability, and Adverse Events, a Systematic Review and Meta-Analysis. *Obes. Surg.* **2017**, *27*, 2272–2278. [CrossRef]
37. Mion, F.; Ibrahim, M.; Marjoux, S.; Ponchon, T.; Dugardeyn, S.; Roman, S.; Deviere, J. Swallowable Obalon® gastric balloons as an aid for weight loss, a pilot feasibility study. *Obes. Surg.* **2013**, *23*, 730–733. [CrossRef]
38. Král, J.; Machytka, E.; Horká, V.; Selucká, J.; Doleček, F.; Špičák, J.; Kovářová, V.; Haluzík, M.; Bužga, M. Endoscopic Treatment of Obesity and Nutritional Aspects of Bariatric Endoscopy. *Nutrients* **2021**, *13*, 4268. [CrossRef]
39. Sullivan, S.; Swain, J.; Woodman, G.; Edmundowicz, S.; Hassanein, T.; Shayani, V.; Fang, J.C.; Noar, M.; Eid, G.; English, W.J.; et al. Randomized sham-controlled trial of the 6-month swallowable gas-filled intragastric balloon system for weight loss. *Surg. Obes. Relat. Dis.* **2018**, *14*, 1876–1889. [CrossRef]
40. Machytka, E.; Gaur, S.; Chuttani, R.; Bojkova, M.; Kupka, T.; Buzga, M.; Giannakou, A.; Ioannis, K.; Mathus-Vliegen, E.; Levy, S.; et al. Elipse, the first procedureless gastric balloon for weight loss, a prospective, observational, open-label, multicenter study. *Endoscopy* **2017**, *49*, 154–160. [CrossRef]
41. Jamal, M.H.; Almutairi, R.; Elabd, R.; AlSabah, S.K.; Alqattan, H.; Altaweel, T. The Safety and Efficacy of Procedureless Gastric Balloon, a Study Examining the Effect of Elipse Intragastric Balloon Safety, Short and Medium Term Effects on Weight Loss with 1-Year Follow-Up Post-removal. *Obes. Surg.* **2019**, *29*, 1236–1241. [CrossRef]
42. Machytka, E.; Klvana, P.; Kornbluth, A.; Peikin, S.; Mathus-Vliegen, L.E.; Gostout, C.; Lopez-Nava, G.; Shikora, S.; Brooks, J. Adjustable intragastric balloons, a 12-month pilot trial in endoscopic weight loss management. *Obes. Surg.* **2011**, *21*, 1499–1507. [CrossRef] [PubMed]
43. Fittipaldi-Fernandez, R.J.; Zotarelli-Filho, I.J.; Diestel, C.F.; Klein, M.; de Santana, M.F.; de Lima, J.H.F.; Bastos, F.S.S.; Dos Santos, N.T. Randomized Prospective Clinical Study of Spatz3® Adjustable Intragastric Balloon Treatment with a Control Group, a Large-Scale Brazilian Experiment. *Obes. Surg.* **2021**, *31*, 787–796. [CrossRef]
44. Abu Dayyeh, B.K.; Maselli, D.B.; Rapaka, B.; Lavin, T.; Noar, M.; Hussan, H.; Chapman, C.G.; Popov, V.; Jirapinyo, P.; Acosta, A.; et al. Adjustable intragastric balloon for treatment of obesity, a multicentre, open-label, randomised clinical trial. *Lancet* **2021**, *398*, 1965–1973. [CrossRef]
45. Ponce, J.; Quebbemann, B.B.; Patterson, E.J. Prospective, randomized, multicenter study evaluating safety and efficacy of intragastric dual-balloon in obesity. *Surg. Obes. Relat. Dis.* **2013**, *9*, 290–295. [CrossRef] [PubMed]
46. Marinos, G.; Eliades, C.; Raman Muthusamy, V.; Greenway, F. Weight loss and improved quality of life with a nonsurgical endoscopic treatment for obesity, clinical results from a 3- and 6-month study. *Surg. Obes. Relat. Dis.* **2014**, *10*, 929–934. [CrossRef]
47. Rothstein, R.; Woodman, G.; Swain, J. Weight Reduction in Patients with Obesity Using the Transpyloric Shuttle®, ENDObesity® II Study. In Proceedings of the Obesity Week 2018, Nashville, TN, USA, 11–15 November 2018.
48. Abu Dayyeh, B.K.; Rajan, E.; Gostout, C.J. Endoscopic sleeve gastroplasty, a potential endoscopic alternative to surgical sleeve gastrectomy for treatment of obesity. *Gastrointest. Endosc.* **2013**, *78*, 530–535. [CrossRef]
49. Lopez-Nava, G.; Galvão, M.P.; Bautista-Castaño, I.; Jimenez-Baños, A.; Fernandez-Corbelle, J.P. Endoscopic Sleeve Gastroplasty, How I Do It? *Obes. Surg.* **2015**, *25*, 1534–1538. [CrossRef] [PubMed]
50. Espinós, J.C.; Turró, R.; Mata, A.; Cruz, M.; da Costa, M.; Villa, V.; Buchwald, J.N.; Turró, J. Early experience with the Incisionless Operating Platform™ (IOP) for the treatment of obesity, the Primary Obesity Surgery Endolumenal (POSE) procedure. *Obes. Surg.* **2013**, *23*, 1375–1383. [CrossRef]
51. Telese, A.; Sehgal, V.; Magee, C.G.; Naik, S.; Alqahtani, S.A.; Lovat, L.B.; Haidry, R.J. Bariatric and Metabolic Endoscopy, A New Paradigm. *Clin. Transl. Gastroenterol.* **2021**, *12*, e00364. [CrossRef]
52. Gys, B.; Plaeke, P.; Lamme, B.; Lafullarde, T.; Komen, N.; Beunis, A.; Hubens, G. Endoscopic Gastric Plication for Morbid Obesity, a Systematic Review and Meta-analysis of Published Data over Time. *Obes. Surg.* **2019**, *29*, 3021–3029. [CrossRef]
53. Mohan, B.P.; Asokkumar, R.; Khan, S.R.; Kotagiri, R.; Sridharan, G.K.; Chandan, S.; Ravikumar, N.P.; Ponnada, S.; Jayaraj, M.; Adler, D.G. Outcomes of endoscopic sleeve gastroplasty, how does it compare to laparoscopic sleeve gastrectomy? A systematic review and meta-analysis. *Endosc. Int. Open* **2020**, *8*, E558–E565. [CrossRef]
54. Hedjoudje, A.; Abu Dayyeh, B.K.; Cheskin, L.J.; Adam, A.; Neto, M.G.; Badurdeen, D.; Morales, J.G.; Sartoretto, A.; Nava, G.L.; Vargas, E.; et al. Efficacy and Safety of Endoscopic Sleeve Gastroplasty, A Systematic Review and Meta-Analysis. *Clin. Gastroenterol. Hepatol.* **2020**, *18*, 1043–1053.e4. [CrossRef] [PubMed]
55. Abu Dayyeh, B.K.; Bazerbachi, F.; Vargas, E.J.; Sharaiha, R.Z.; Thompson, C.C.; Thaemert, B.C.; Teixeira, A.F.; Chapman, C.G.; Kumbhari, V.; Ujiki, M.B.; et al. Endoscopic sleeve gastroplasty for treatment of class 1 and 2 obesity (MERIT), a prospective, multicentre, randomised trial. *Lancet* **2022**, *400*, 441–451. [CrossRef] [PubMed]
56. Li, R.; Veltzke-Schlieker, W.; Adler, A.; Specht, M.; Eskander, W.; Ismail, M.; Badakhshi, H.; Galvao, M.P.; Zorron, R. Endoscopic Sleeve Gastroplasty (ESG) for High-Risk Patients, High Body Mass Index (> 50 kg/m(2)) Patients, and Contraindication to Abdominal Surgery. *Obes. Surg.* **2021**, *31*, 3400–3409. [CrossRef] [PubMed]

57. Zorron, R.; Veltzke-Schlieker, W.; Adler, A.; Denecke, C.; Dziodzio, T.; Pratschke, J.; Benzing, C. Endoscopic sleeve gastroplasty using Apollo Overstitch as a bridging procedure for superobese and high risk patients. *Endoscopy* **2018**, *50*, 81–83. [CrossRef] [PubMed]
58. Lopez-Nava, G.; Asokkumar, R.; Turró Arau, R.; Neto, M.G.; Dayyeh, B.A. Modified primary obesity surgery endoluminal (POSE-2) procedure for the treatment of obesity. *VideoGIE* **2020**, *5*, 91–93. [CrossRef]
59. Jirapinyo, P.; Thompson, C.C. Endoscopic gastric body plication for the treatment of obesity, technical success and safety of a novel technique (with video). *Gastrointest. Endosc.* **2020**, *91*, 1388–1394. [CrossRef]
60. Graus Morales, J.; Crespo Pérez, L.; Marques, A.; Marín Arribas, B.; Bravo Arribas, R.; Ramo, E.; Escalada, C.; Arribas, C.; Himpens, J. Modified endoscopic gastroplasty for the treatment of obesity. *Surg. Endosc.* **2018**, *32*, 3936–3942. [CrossRef]
61. Fayad, L.; Adam, A.; Schweitzer, M.; Cheskin, L.J.; Ajayi, T.; Dunlap, M.; Badurdeen, D.S.; Hill, C.; Paranji, N.; Lalezari, S.; et al. Endoscopic sleeve gastroplasty versus laparoscopic sleeve gastrectomy, a case-matched study. *Gastrointest. Endosc.* **2019**, *89*, 782–788. [CrossRef]
62. Sharaiha, R.Z.; Kumta, N.A.; Saumoy, M.; Desai, A.P.; Sarkisian, A.M.; Benevenuto, A.; Tyberg, A.; Kumar, R.; Igel, L.; Verna, E.C.; et al. Endoscopic Sleeve Gastroplasty Significantly Reduces Body Mass Index and Metabolic Complications in Obese Patients. *Clin. Gastroenterol. Hepatol.* **2017**, *15*, 504–510. [CrossRef]
63. Thompson, C.C.; Abu Dayyeh, B.K.; Kushner, R.; Sullivan, S.; Schorr, A.B.; Amaro, A.; Apovian, C.M.; Fullum, T.; Zarrinpar, A.; Jensen, M.D.; et al. Percutaneous Gastrostomy Device for the Treatment of Class II and Class III Obesity, Results of a Randomized Controlled Trial. *Am. J. Gastroenterol.* **2017**, *112*, 447–457. [CrossRef] [PubMed]
64. Crothall, K. 2022. Available online: https://www.aspirebariatrics.com/ (accessed on 25 November 2022).
65. Rajagopalan, H.; Cherrington, A.D.; Thompson, C.C.; Kaplan, L.M.; Rubino, F.; Mingrone, G.; Becerra, P.; Rodriguez, P.; Vignolo, P.; Caplan, J.; et al. Endoscopic Duodenal Mucosal Resurfacing for the Treatment of Type 2 Diabetes, 6-Month Interim Analysis From the First-in-Human Proof-of-Concept Study. *Diabetes Care* **2016**, *39*, 2254–2261. [CrossRef] [PubMed]
66. Mingrone, G.; van Baar, A.C.; Devière, J.; Hopkins, D.; Moura, E.; Cercato, C.; Rajagopalan, H.; Lopez-Talavera, J.C.; White, K.; Bhambhani, V.; et al. Safety and efficacy of hydrothermal duodenal mucosal resurfacing in patients with type 2 diabetes, the randomised, double-blind, sham-controlled, multicentre REVITA-2 feasibility trial. *Gut* **2022**, *71*, 254–264. [CrossRef] [PubMed]
67. Rodriguez-Grunert, L.; Galvao Neto, M.P.; Alamo, M.; Ramos, A.C.; Baez, P.B.; Tarnoff, M. First human experience with endoscopically delivered and retrieved duodenal-jejunal bypass sleeve. *Surg. Obes. Relat. Dis.* **2008**, *4*, 55–59. [CrossRef]
68. Rohde, U.; Hedbäck, N.; Gluud, L.L.; Vilsbøll, T.; Knop, F.K. Effect of the EndoBarrier Gastrointestinal Liner on obesity and type 2 diabetes, a systematic review and meta-analysis. *Diabetes Obes. Metab.* **2016**, *18*, 300–305. [CrossRef] [PubMed]
69. Jirapinyo, P.; Haas, A.V.; Thompson, C.C. Effect of the Duodenal-Jejunal Bypass Liner on Glycemic Control in Patients With Type 2 Diabetes With Obesity, A Meta-analysis With Secondary Analysis on Weight Loss and Hormonal Changes. *Diabetes Care* **2018**, *41*, 1106–1115. [CrossRef]
70. Caiazzo, R.; Branche, J.; Raverdy, V.; Czernichow, S.; Carette, C.; Robert, M.; Disse, E.; Barthet, M.; Cariou, B.; Msika, S.; et al. Efficacy and Safety of the Duodeno-Jejunal Bypass Liner in Patients With Metabolic Syndrome, A Multicenter Randomized Controlled Trial (ENDOMETAB). *Ann. Surg.* **2020**, *272*, 696–702. [CrossRef]
71. ClinicalTrials. Available online: https://clinicaltrials.gov/ct2/show/NCT04101669 (accessed on 1 March 2023).
72. Ruban, A.; Miras, A.D.; Glaysher, M.A.; Goldstone, A.P.; Prechtl, C.G.; Johnson, N.; Chhina, N.; Al-Najim, W.; Aldhwayan, M.; Klimowska-Nassar, N.; et al. Duodenal-Jejunal Bypass Liner for the management of Type 2 Diabetes Mellitus and Obesity, A Multicenter Randomized Controlled Trial. *Ann. Surg.* **2022**, *275*, 440–447. [CrossRef]
73. Yvamoto, E.Y.; de Moura, D.T.H.; Proença, I.M.; do Monte Junior, E.S.; Ribeiro, I.B.; Ribas, P.; Hemerly, M.C.; de Oliveira, V.L.; Sánchez-Luna, S.A.; Bernardo, W.M.; et al. The Effectiveness and Safety of the Duodenal-Jejunal Bypass Liner (DJBL) for the Management of Obesity and Glycaemic Control, a Systematic Review and Meta-Analysis of Randomized Controlled Trials. *Obes. Surg.* **2023**, *33*, 585–599. [CrossRef]
74. Sandler, B.J.; Rumbaut, R.; Swain, C.P.; Torres, G.; Morales, L.; Gonzales, L.; Schultz, J.; Talamini, M.A.; Jacobsen, G.R.; Horgan, S. One-year human experience with a novel endoluminal, endoscopic gastric bypass sleeve for morbid obesity. *Surg. Endosc.* **2015**, *29*, 3298–3303. [CrossRef]
75. Machytka, E.; Bužga, M.; Zonca, P.; Lautz, D.B.; Ryou, M.; Simonson, D.C.; Thompson, C.C. Partial jejunal diversion using an incisionless magnetic anastomosis system, 1-year interim results in patients with obesity and diabetes. *Gastrointest. Endosc.* **2017**, *86*, 904–912. [CrossRef]
76. De Moura, D.T.H.; Barrichello, S., Jr.; de Moura, E.G.H.; de Souza, T.F.; Dos Passos Galvão Neto, M.; Grecco, E.; Sander, B.; Hoff, A.C.; Matz, F.; Ramos, F.; et al. Endoscopic sleeve gastroplasty in the management of weight regain after sleeve gastrectomy. *Endoscopy* **2020**, *52*, 202–210.
77. Cambi, M.P.C.; Baretta, G.A.P.; Magro, D.O.; Boguszewski, C.L.; Ribeiro, I.B.; Jirapinyo, P.; de Moura, D.T.H. Multidisciplinary Approach for Weight Regain-how to Manage this Challenging Condition, an Expert Review. *Obes. Surg.* **2021**, *31*, 1290–1303. [CrossRef]
78. Brunaldi, V.O.; Jirapinyo, P.; de Moura, D.T.H.; Okazaki, O.; Bernardo, W.M.; Galvão Neto, M.; Campos, J.M.; Santo, M.A.; de Moura, E.G.H. Endoscopic Treatment of Weight Regain Following Roux-en-Y Gastric Bypass, a Systematic Review and Meta-analysis. *Obes. Surg.* **2018**, *28*, 266–276. [CrossRef] [PubMed]

79. Fayad, L.; Trindade, A.J.; Benias, P.C.; Simsek, C.; Raad, M.; Badurdeen, D.; Hill, C.; Brewer Gutierrez, O.I.; Fayad, G.; Dunlap, M.; et al. Cryoballoon ablation for gastric pouch and/or outlet reduction in patients with weight regain post Roux-en-Y gastric bypass. *Endoscopy* **2020**, *52*, 227–230. [CrossRef]
80. Jirapinyo, P.; de Moura, D.T.H.; Dong, W.Y.; Farias, G.; Thompson, C.C. Dose response for argon plasma coagulation in the treatment of weight regain after Roux-en-Y gastric bypass. *Gastrointest. Endosc.* **2020**, *91*, 1078–1084. [CrossRef]
81. de Quadros, L.G.; Neto, M.G.; Marchesini, J.C.; Teixeira, A.; Grecco, E.; Junior, R.L.K.; Zundel, N.; Filho, I.J.Z.; de Souza, T.F.; Filho, A.C.; et al. Endoscopic Argon Plasma Coagulation vs. Multidisciplinary Evaluation in the Management of Weight Regain After Gastric Bypass Surgery, a Randomized Controlled Trial with SHAM Group. *Obes. Surg.* **2020**, *30*, 1904–1916. [CrossRef] [PubMed]
82. Dhindsa, B.S.; Saghir, S.M.; Naga, Y.; Dhaliwal, A.; Ramai, D.; Cross, C.; Singh, S.; Bhat, I.; Adler, D.G. Efficacy of transoral outlet reduction in Roux-en-Y gastric bypass patients to promote weight loss, a systematic review and meta-analysis. *Endosc. Int. Open* **2020**, *8*, E1332–E1340. [CrossRef] [PubMed]
83. Jaruvongvanich, V.; Vantanasiri, K.; Laoveeravat, P.; Matar, R.H.; Vargas, E.J.; Maselli, D.B.; Alkhatry, M.; Fayad, L.; Kumbhari, V.; Fittipaldi-Fernandez, R.J. Endoscopic full-thickness suturing plus argon plasma mucosal coagulation versus argon plasma mucosal coagulation alone for weight regain after gastric bypass, a systematic review and meta-analysis. *Gastrointest. Endosc.* **2020**, *92*, 1164–1175.e6. [CrossRef]
84. Jirapinyo, P.; Dayyeh, B.K.; Thompson, C.C. Gastrojejunal anastomotic reduction for weight regain in roux-en-y gastric bypass patients, physiological, behavioral, and anatomical effects of endoscopic suturing and sclerotherapy. *Surg. Obes. Relat. Dis.* **2016**, *12*, 1810–1816. [CrossRef]
85. Heylen, A.M.; Jacobs, A.; Lybeer, M.; Prosst, R.L. The OTSC®-clip in revisional endoscopy against weight gain after bariatric gastric bypass surgery. *Obes. Surg.* **2011**, *21*, 1629–1633. [CrossRef] [PubMed]
86. Lee, Y.; Ellenbogen, Y.; Doumouras, A.G.; Gmora, S.; Anvari, M.; Hong, D. Single- or double-anastomosis duodenal switch versus Roux-en-Y gastric bypass as a revisional procedure for sleeve gastrectomy, A systematic review and meta-analysis. *Surg. Obes. Relat. Dis.* **2019**, *15*, 556–566. [CrossRef]
87. Eid, G. Sleeve gastrectomy revision by endoluminal sleeve plication gastroplasty, a small pilot case series. *Surg. Endosc.* **2017**, *31*, 4252–4255. [CrossRef]
88. Maselli, D.B.; Alqahtani, A.R.; Abu Dayyeh, B.K.; Elahmedi, M.; Storm, A.C.; Matar, R.; Nieto, J.; Teixeira, A.; Al Khatry, M.; Neto, M.G. Revisional endoscopic sleeve gastroplasty of laparoscopic sleeve gastrectomy, an international, multicenter study. *Gastrointest. Endosc.* **2021**, *93*, 122–130. [CrossRef] [PubMed]
89. Kushner, R.F.; Ryan, D.H. Assessment and lifestyle management of patients with obesity, clinical recommendations from systematic reviews. *JAMA* **2014**, *312*, 943–952. [CrossRef] [PubMed]
90. Acosta, A.; Streett, S.; Kroh, M.D.; Cheskin, L.J.; Saunders, K.H.; Kurian, M.; Schofield, M.; Barlow, S.E.; Aronne, L. White Paper AGA, POWER—Practice Guide on Obesity and Weight Management, Education, and Resources. *Clin. Gastroenterol. Hepatol.* **2017**, *15*, 631–649.e10. [CrossRef] [PubMed]
91. Lopez Nava, G.; Arau, R.T.; Asokkumar, R.; Maselli, D.B.; Rapaka, B.; Matar, R.; Bautista, I.; Espinos Perez, J.C.; Bilbao, A.M.; Jaruvongvanich, V.; et al. Prospective Multicenter Study of the Primary Obesity Surgery Endoluminal (POSE 2.0) Procedure for Treatment of Obesity. *Clin. Gastroenterol. Hepatol.* **2023**, *21*, 81–89.e4. [CrossRef]

Disclaimer/Publisher's Note: The statements, opinions and data contained in all publications are solely those of the individual author(s) and contributor(s) and not of MDPI and/or the editor(s). MDPI and/or the editor(s) disclaim responsibility for any injury to people or property resulting from any ideas, methods, instructions or products referred to in the content.

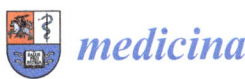

Case Report

Accidental Sewing Pin Ingestion by a Tailor: A Case Report and Literature Review

Stefan Stojkovic [1,*], Milica Bjelakovic [2], Milica Stojkovic Lalosevic [1,3], Milos Stulic [1,3], Nina Pejic [1], Nemanja Radivojevic [3,4], Nemanja Stojkovic [5], Jelena Martinov Nestorov [1,3] and Djordje Culafic [1,3]

1. Clinic for Gastroenterology and Hepatology, University Clinical Center of Serbia, 11000 Belgrade, Serbia
2. Clinic for Gastroenterology and Hepatology, University Clinical Center of Nis, 18000 Nis, Serbia
3. Faculty of Medicine, University of Belgrade, 11000 Belgrade, Serbia
4. Clinic for Otorhinolaryngology and Maxillofacial Surgery, University Clinical Center of Serbia, 11000 Belgrade, Serbia
5. Department of Cardiology, University Clinical Hospital Center "Dr. Dragisa Misovic-Dedinje", 11000 Belgrade, Serbia
* Correspondence: stefanstojkovic@ymail.com

Abstract: Foreign body ingestion is a frequently encountered emergency in healthcare institutions. It mostly affects pediatric populations, although it can also affect adults with developmental delays, those with psychiatric diseases, drug abusers, and prisoners. Endoscopy is a diagnostic and treatment method for suspected foreign body ingestion. In this article, we discuss a 45-year-old tailor who swallowed a sewing pin while at work. The abdominal X-ray showed a needle-shaped metal shadow in the stomach region. During an upper endoscopy, it was discovered that a sewing pin with a sharp edge was stuck in the pylorus. The sewing pin was extracted endoscopically, and the patient was discharged the same day in good condition. Since the estimated risk of complications of foreign body ingestion in the adult population is about 35%, and the most common complications include impaction, laceration, bleeding, or perforation of the gastrointestinal wall, endoscopic or surgical removal is necessary. This also emphasizes the importance of a careful endoscopic evaluation of some at-risk occupations for foreign body ingestion with or without gastrointestinal complaints.

Keywords: foreign body ingestion; sewing pin; stomach; endoscopy; tailor

1. Introduction

Foreign body (FB) ingestion is a frequently encountered emergency in healthcare institutions. Although the majority of patients with FB ingestions are found in the pediatric population, these emergencies also affect adults. In particular, impaction with meat or fish bones while eating is the most common cause of FB ingestion in adults. Patients with developmental delays, psychiatric diseases, abusers of illicit drugs or alcohol, and prisoners are recognized as high-risk groups for accidental or intentional ingestion of FB [1]. While most of the FB pass spontaneously through the gastrointestinal tract, in 10% to 20% of patients, endoscopic extraction is necessary, and in less than 1% of patients, surgical intervention is required [2]. Swallowed objects, especially sharp ones, may cause serious complications during their passage through the digestive tube [3,4]. Symptoms may vary depending on the type of FB ingested and the time interval until diagnosis.

Swallowed sharp foreign objects cause 15–35% of intestinal perforations and should be removed, especially if found in the esophagus or stomach [5]. Endoscopy is a well-known diagnostic and treatment modality for suspected FB ingestion since it reduces the need for surgery and makes it possible to diagnose other diseases at the same time [6,7].

Here we report a case of accidental sewing pin ingestion by a tailor.

2. Case Presentation

A 45-year-old female tailor was admitted to the emergency department due to the possible swallowing of a sewing pin. She reported that she had been holding several sewing pins with her lips during work the day before when she accidentally coughed. She did not know if she had swallowed a pin because she could not remember the exact number of pins she was holding. Later that day, she felt slight discomfort in her upper abdominal parts. Past medical and surgical history was not specific. Abdominal palpation revealed a slight pain in the epigastrium. Other physical and laboratory findings were unremarkable. The patient was immediately referred to a plain abdominal X-ray, which showed a needle-shaped metal shadow, approximately 4 cm long, in the stomach region (shown in Figure 1). Thereafter, an urgent upper endoscopy was performed, and a needle was seen in the pyloric part of the stomach. The sharp point of the pin was stuck in the pylorus with surrounding tissue reaction, while the blunt, rounded, purple-colored pinhead was in the duodenal bulb (shown in Figure 2a). Alligator jaw forceps were used, and the pin was gripped near its center, between the pinhead and the tip. Firstly, a gentle push was applied towards the bulbus to disengage the pin from the pylorus. After that, the pin was slowly pulled through the pylorus in the antrum. In the antrum grasp of alligator forceps was relocated from the pin's center towards the tip (shown in Figure 2b). After a firm grip was obtained, the pin was gently extracted with the tip of the forceps about a centimeter away from the endoscope tip to provide direct visualization during extubation. Protective overtubes were not used because of the endoscopist's certainty of the forceps grip, direct visualization at all times, and the fact that the pinhead was rounded and not supposed to damage the tissues by contact (shown in Figure 3). After the procedure, a control endoscopy was performed, and since there was no mucosal laceration on the esophagus or stomach, the patient was discharged in good condition.

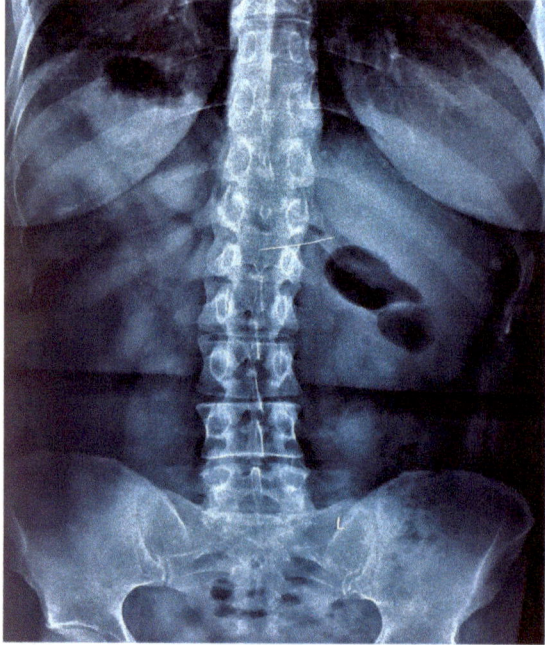

Figure 1. A metal shadow in the stomach region shown in a plain abdominal X-ray image.

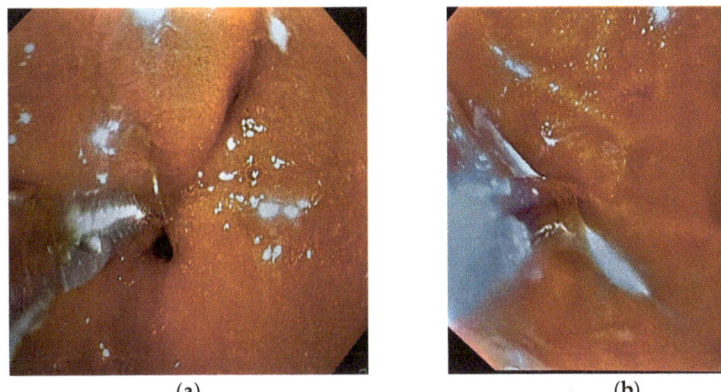

Figure 2. Upper endoscopy findings. (**a**) A sewing pin stuck in the pylorus with surrounding tissue reaction. (**b**) An alligator jaw forceps holding the sewing pin in the stomach.

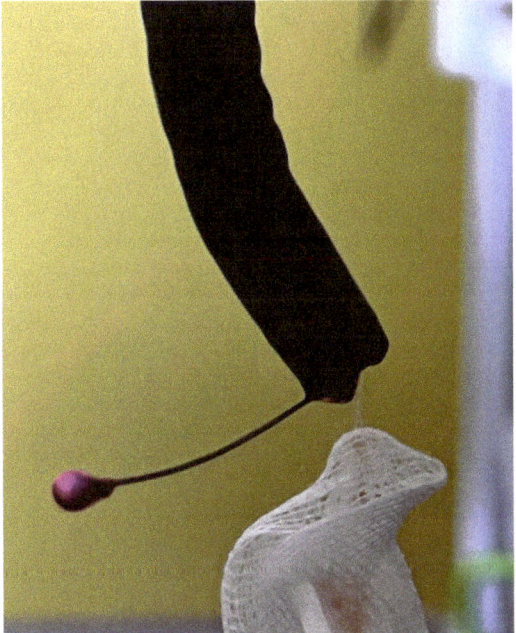

Figure 3. An extracted sewing pin.

3. Discussion

The management of patients with FB ingestion requires different diagnostic and therapeutic approaches due to the specificity of each individual case. The lack of specific complaints that are clearly related to the localization of the FB and the need for timely identification, as well as the treatment of complications, require the coordinated work of radiologists, endoscopists, and surgeons [4,8].

In patients presenting with FB ingestion, symptoms may vary from asymptomatic or mildly uncomfortable to dramatic and life-threatening. Most patients have symptoms, and they vary depending on the type and location of the FB [9]. Usually, patients after FB ingestion present with sensations of FB, dysphagia, chest or abdominal pain, nausea, or vomiting [10]. In symptomatic patients, FB are more likely to be located in the esophagus and pharynx. By contrast, in asymptomatic patients, FBs are more frequently located in the stomach or duodenum [9,11]. Moreover, sharp objects are more likely to cause symptoms than blunt FBs. Furthermore, the absence of symptoms leads to a late diagnosis and the development of complications [12]. Therefore, all patients suspected of FB ingestion should undergo radiologic and/or laryngological examination to exclude oropharyngeal location [10]. Since our patient had very mild symptoms and was not sure that she had swallowed a needle, the decision to perform an X-ray and endoscopy proved to be very useful. Endoscopic treatment can be challenging because the estimated risk of complications is as high as 35%, especially if the FB is not removed at the right time [13]. The success rate of endoscopic FB removal is 95%, while adverse events are rare and include mucosal laceration, bleeding, infection, perforation, or aspiration [9,14]. According to the European Society of Gastrointestinal Endoscopy, emergency upper endoscopy is recommended within 6 h in cases of esophageal obstruction or sharp objects in the esophagus and within 24 h in cases of other FBs. An endoscopic examination is also recommended after removing the FB [3]. A study by Liu et al. showed that a time interval of 6 h can reduce all complications, while a time interval between 6 and 24 h can reduce major complications but not all of them [15].

Complications of sharp object ingestion include impaction, laceration, bleeding, or perforation of the gastrointestinal wall, especially in the anatomically narrow parts of the gastrointestinal tract, such as the upper and lower esophageal sphincters, the pylorus, the ileocecal valve, and, in rare cases, the appendiceal lumen [4]. In our case, the needle was impacted in the pylorus, so the risk of serious complications was high. Thus, endoscopic treatment was performed immediately with great caution to avoid injury to the gastrointestinal wall and potential aspiration. Endoscopic management of sharp FB extraction includes various techniques and instruments. These techniques involve using an overtube or a transparent cup, or fashioning a protective hood [4]. Shishido et al. [16] described the successful extraction of a sewing needle that was grasped by biopsy forceps and withdrawn together with the endoscope through a flexible overtube placed in the duodenum. Instead, in our case, we were able to remove the pin safely only by grasping the tip of the needle using endoscopic forceps, whereas a smooth pinhead should not be able to cause complications. Similarly, Costa et al. [17] successfully removed thirteen needles from the gastric body and one from the duodenum by grasping the sharp end of the needle with continuous suction into the working channel of the endoscope. Thus, endoscopic extraction of such objects is easier than that of objects with two pointed sides because there is low risk of injury to the contralateral wall. Therefore, a detailed description of the swallowed FB and an X-ray are necessary [18]. The possibility of spontaneous passage is affected by several factors, including the size, shape, and composition of the ingested FB. The duration of ingestion and the age of the patient also play a significant role in the management of these patients [1].

Objects less than 2.5 cm in diameter can pass spontaneously [19], but cases of later complications due to their migration have been described by some authors. Sharp objects may reach the liver or pancreas in 1% of cases by penetrating the small intestine or stomach wall. Considering the high possibility of unhindered passage through the gastrointestinal tract, some authors still advocate conservative treatment in the case of sharp or pointed FB, regardless of the potential risk. As a result, Bazabih and Getu [5] only used follow-up and serial radiological exams to successfully treat a 23-year-old male who ingested a metal nail. In contrast, Dal et al. [20] described an accidentally swallowed sewing needle in a 23-year-old female that was revealed starting from the posterior of the small curvature of the stomach and reaching the head and body of the pancreas. This patient required laparoscopic surgery for the removal of the FB. In the literature, the most commonly reported complications of an unextracted FB are intestinal perforation, abscess formation, fistulae, and appendicitis [21,22]. In order to prevent complications, it is recommended that sharp FBs be extracted whenever possible, and in the event of unsuccessful extraction, clinical follow-up and daily radiographs are necessary. If it is observed that the FB does not progress within three days after ingestion, surgical intervention should be considered [3].

Several observational studies have shown that up to 80% of patients who ingest FBs are children [21]. In adults, most FB ingestion or food bolus impaction occurs accidentally during eating. It is important to emphasize that underlying esophageal pathology, such as stricture or malignancy, is found in more than 75% of patients with food bolus impaction [23,24]. The rest of the patients marked as having a high risk of FB ingestion are the geriatric population, adults with psychiatric illnesses, and individuals under the influence of drugs or alcohol. A special group consists of patients who benefit from FB ingestion, such as prisoners or drug couriers [3]. The most frequently found ingestions of sharp FBs include meat bones, toothpicks, needles, safety pins, and dental appliances [25]. The type of FB that is swallowed is influenced by various factors, including dietary habits, behavior, and religion. For example, several studies have shown that the accidental ingestion of date pits while eating is very common in China, while ingestion of hijab pins is common among Muslim women [26,27]. Hijab pins provide a tiny but significant risk of catastrophic sequelae, especially in cases of needle impaction lasting longer than a few months, according to a large cohort study by Yogev et al. that included 208 patients who swallowed a hijab needle. [28] A CT scan should be done on patients who have ingested a needle in the last several weeks or months to rule out infectious or mechanical issues [29]. However, there is little information in the literature about the ingestion of FB in specific professions.

We performed a literature search in the PubMed database (Medline) using the keywords "foreign body ingestion", "sewing pin", and "tailor" and identified only two related publications. Ha et al. [30] reported the case of a 34-year-old tailor who swallowed a sewing needle and, after an unsuccessful colonoscopy, underwent a laparoscopic appendectomy. Another publication by Espin et al. [31] describes the case of a tailor who was diagnosed with colonic perforation after swallowing a needle and was treated surgically with a laparoscopic approach. To our knowledge, this is the first case report found in the literature of an endoscopic retraction of a sewing pin in a patient who is at occupational risk for ingestion—a tailor. This further emphasizes that patients with specific occupations should be noted as high-risk groups for FB ingestion.

4. Conclusions

An ingested sharp FB may cause serious complications in the gastrointestinal tract, such as perforation or migration into other organs. An endoscopy ought to be performed even when FB ingestion is suspected. The presence of a sharp FB requires endoscopic or surgical removal. This therapeutic method must be performed with extreme caution to avoid injury to the gastrointestinal wall and aspiration. A CT scan should be done if the patient presents later than two to three weeks after ingesting. Even seasoned tailors who hold pins with their lips while working, though this is a widespread technique throughout the world, run the risk of ingesting them.

Author Contributions: S.S., M.S. and N.P. diagnosed and treated the patient, and participated in the design of the manuscript. M.B., N.R. and N.S. reviewed the literature and participated in the writing. M.S.L., J.M.N. and D.C. critically revised the report for intellectual input and gave final approval of the version to be published. All authors have read and agreed to the published version of the manuscript.

Funding: This research received no external funding.

Institutional Review Board Statement: This case report did not require IRB approval. The patient provided verbal and written consent for the publication of this report.

Informed Consent Statement: Written informed consent has been obtained from the patient to publish this paper.

Data Availability Statement: All information is publicly available, and data regarding this particular patient can be obtained from the corresponding author upon request.

Conflicts of Interest: The authors declare no conflict of interest.

References

1. Wang, X.; Su, S.; Chen, Y.; Wang, Z.; Li, Y.; Hou, J.; Zhong, W.; Wang, Y.; Wang, B. The removal of foreign body ingestion in the upper gastrointestinal tract: A retrospective study of 1182 adult cases. *Ann. Transl. Med.* **2021**, *9*, 502. [CrossRef] [PubMed]
2. Feng, S.; Peng, H.; Xie, H.; Bai, Y.; Yin, J. Management of Sharp-Pointed Esophageal Foreign-Body Impaction With Rigid Endoscopy: A Retrospective Study of 130 Adult Patients. *Ear Nose Throat J.* **2020**, *99*, 251–258. [CrossRef] [PubMed]
3. Birk, M.; Bauerfeind, P.; Deprez, P.H.; Häfner, M.; Hartmann, D.; Hassan, C.; Hucl, T.; Lesur, G.; Aabakken, L.; Meining, A. Removal of foreign bodies in the upper gastrointestinal tract in adults: European Society of Gastrointestinal Endoscopy (ESGE) Clinical Guideline. *Endoscopy* **2016**, *48*, 489–496. [CrossRef]
4. Fung, B.M.; Sweetser, S.; Wong Kee Song, L.M.; Tabibian, J.H. Foreign object ingestion and esophageal food impaction: An update and review on endoscopic management. *World J. Gastrointest. Endosc.* **2019**, *11*, 174–192. [CrossRef]
5. Bezabih, Y.S.; Getu, M.E. Spontaneous passage of accidentally ingested metallic nail in an adult: A case report. *Int. J. Surg. Case Rep.* **2022**, *92*, 106865. [CrossRef]
6. Li, Z.S.; Sun, Z.X.; Zou, D.W.; Xu, G.M.; Wu, R.P.; Liao, Z. Endoscopic management of foreign bodies in the upper-GI tract: Experience with 1088 cases in China. *Gastrointest. Endosc.* **2006**, *64*, 485–492. [CrossRef] [PubMed]
7. Chen, Q.; Chu, H.; Tong, T.; Tao, Y.; Zhou, L.; Chen, J.; Liu, Y.; Peng, L. Predictive factors for complications associated with penetrated fish bones outside the upper gastrointestinal tract. *Eur. Arch. Otorhinolaryngol.* **2019**, *276*, 185–191. [CrossRef] [PubMed]
8. Chen, B.; Cyr, D.G.; Hales, B.F. Role of apoptosis in mediating phosphoramide mustard-induced rat embryo malformations in vitro. *Teratology* **1994**, *50*, 1–12. [CrossRef] [PubMed]
9. Geng, C.; Li, X.; Luo, R.; Cai, L.; Lei, X.; Wang, C. Endoscopic management of foreign bodies in the upper gastrointestinal tract: A retrospective study of 1294 cases. *Scand J. Gastroenterol.* **2017**, *52*, 1286–1291. [CrossRef]
10. Boo, S.J.; Kim, H.U. Esophageal Foreign Body: Treatment and Complications. *Korean J. Gastroenterol.* **2018**, *72*, 1–5. [CrossRef] [PubMed]
11. Jaan, A.; Mulita, F. *Gastrointestinal Foreign Body*; StatPearls Publishing LLC: Treasure Island, FL, USA, 2023.
12. Zhang, S.; Cui, Y.; Gong, X.; Gu, F.; Chen, M.; Zhong, B. Endoscopic management of foreign bodies in the upper gastrointestinal tract in South China: A retrospective study of 561 cases. *Dig. Dis. Sci.* **2010**, *55*, 1305–1312. [CrossRef]
13. Yoo, D.R.; Im, C.B.; Jun, B.G.; Seo, H.I.; Park, J.K.; Lee, S.J.; Han, K.H.; Kim, Y.D.; Jeong, W.J.; Cheon, G.J.; et al. Clinical outcomes of endoscopic removal of foreign bodies from the upper gastrointestinal tract. *BMC Gastroenterol.* **2021**, *21*, 385. [CrossRef]
14. Boumarah, D.N.; Binkhamis, L.S.; AlDuhileb, M. Foreign body ingestion: Is intervention always a necessity? *Ann. Med. Surg.* **2022**, *84*, 104944. [CrossRef]
15. Mosca, S.; Manes, G.; Martino, R.; Amitrano, L.; Bottino, V.; Bove, A.; Camera, A.; De Nucci, C.; Di Costanzo, G.; Guardascione, M.; et al. Endoscopic management of foreign bodies in the upper gastrointestinal tract: Report on a series of 414 adult patients. *Endoscopy* **2001**, *33*, 692–696. [CrossRef]
16. Shishido, T.; Oka, S.; Tanaka, S.; Aoyama, T.; Watari, I.; Imagawa, H.; Yoshida, S.; Hiyama, T.; Chayama, K. Removal of a sewing needle penetrating the wall of the third portion of the duodenum by double-balloon endoscopy. *Clin. J. Gastroenterol.* **2012**, *5*, 79–81. [CrossRef] [PubMed]
17. Costa, S.; Gonçalves, R.; Rolanda, C. Endoscopic removal of multiple sharp gastro-duodenal foreign bodies. *Rev. Esp. Enferm. Dig.* **2017**, *109*, 144–145. [PubMed]
18. Liu, Q.; Liu, F.; Xie, H.; Dong, J.; Chen, H.; Yao, L. Emergency Removal of Ingested Foreign Bodies in 586 Adults at a Single Hospital in China According to the European Society of Gastrointestinal Endoscopy (ESGE) Recommendations: A 10-Year Retrospective Study. *Med. Sci. Monit.* **2022**, *28*, e936463. [CrossRef]
19. Yu, M.; Li, K.; Zhou, S.; Wang, H.; Le, M.; Li, C.; Liu, D.; Tan, Y. Endoscopic Removal of Sharp-Pointed Foreign Bodies with Both Sides Embedded into the Duodenal Wall in Adults: A Retrospective Cohort Study. *Int. J. Gen. Med.* **2021**, *14*, 9361–9369. [CrossRef]
20. Dal, F.; Hatipoğlu, E.; Teksöz, S.; Ertem, M. Foreign body: A sewing needle migrating from the gastrointestinal tract to pancreas. *Turk. J. Surg.* **2018**, *34*, 256–258. [CrossRef] [PubMed]
21. Bekkerman, M.; Sachdev, A.H.; Andrade, J.; Twersky, Y.; Iqbal, S. Endoscopic Management of Foreign Bodies in the Gastrointestinal Tract: A Review of the Literature. *Gastroenterol. Res. Pract.* **2016**, *2016*, 8520767. [CrossRef]
22. Cheng He, R.; Nobel, T.; Greenstein, A.J. A case report of foreign body appendicitis caused by tongue piercing ingestion. *Int. J. Surg. Case Rep.* **2021**, *81*, 105808. [CrossRef] [PubMed]
23. Jutte, E.; Cense, H. Liver abscess due to sewing needle perforation. *Sci. World J.* **2010**, *10*, 1532–1534. [CrossRef] [PubMed]
24. Ikenberry, S.O.; Jue, T.L.; Anderson, M.A.; Appalaneni, V.; Banerjee, S.; Ben-Menachem, T.; Decker, G.A.; Fanelli, R.D.; Fisher, L.R.; Fukami, N.; et al. Management of ingested foreign bodies and food impactions. *Gastrointest. Endosc.* **2011**, *73*, 1085–1091. [CrossRef] [PubMed]
25. Wu, W.T.; Chiu, C.T.; Kuo, C.J.; Lin, C.J.; Chu, Y.Y.; Tsou, Y.K.; Su, M.Y. Endoscopic management of suspected esophageal foreign body in adults. *Dis. Esophagus.* **2011**, *24*, 131–137. [CrossRef]
26. Sugawa, C.; Ono, H.; Taleb, M.; Lucas, C.E. Endoscopic management of foreign bodies in the upper gastrointestinal tract: A review. *World J. Gastrointest. Endosc.* **2014**, *6*, 475–481. [CrossRef]
27. Siti Soraya, A.R. Ingested pins—A potential hazard for hijabis: A case report. *Med. J. Malays.* **2020**, *75*, 78–79.

28. Yogev, D.; Mahameed, F.; Gileles-Hillel, A.; Millman, P.; Davidovics, Z.; Hashavya, S.; Rekhtman, D.; Wilschanski, M.; Berkun, Y.; Slae, M. Hijab Pin Ingestions. *Pediatrics* **2020**, *145*, e20193472. [CrossRef]
29. Zong, Y.; Zhao, H.; Sun, C.; Ji, M.; Wu, Y.; Zhang, S.; Wang, Y. Differences between intentional and accidental ingestion of foreign body in China. *BMC Gastroenterol.* **2020**, *20*, 90. [CrossRef]
30. Ha, N.R.; Lee, H.L.; Yoon, J.H.; Jo, S.C.; Lee, K.N.; Shim, S.G.; Lee, O.Y.; Yoon, B.C.; Choi, H.S.; Hahm, J.S.; et al. A case of an ingested sewing needle in the appendix. *Gastrointest. Endosc.* **2009**, *70*, 1244–1245. [CrossRef]
31. Espin, D.S.; Tufiño, J.F.; Cevallos, J.M.; Zumárraga, F.; Orozco, V.E.; Proaño, E.J.; Molina, G.A. A needle in the colon, the risk of ingested foreign objects: A case report. *J. Surg. Case Rep.* **2021**, *2021*, rjab455. [CrossRef]

Disclaimer/Publisher's Note: The statements, opinions and data contained in all publications are solely those of the individual author(s) and contributor(s) and not of MDPI and/or the editor(s). MDPI and/or the editor(s) disclaim responsibility for any injury to people or property resulting from any ideas, methods, instructions or products referred to in the content.

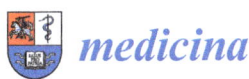

Review

Endoscopic Management of Postoperative Esophageal and Upper GI Defects—A Narrative Review

Cecilia Binda [1,*], Carlo Felix Maria Jung [1], Stefano Fabbri [1], Paolo Giuffrida [2], Monica Sbrancia [1], Chiara Coluccio [1], Giulia Gibiino [1] and Carlo Fabbri [1]

[1] Gastroenterology and Digestive Endoscopy Unit, Forlì—Cesena Hospitals, AUSL Romagna, 47121 Forlì Cesena, Italy
[2] Department of Health Promotion, Mother and Child Care, Internal Medicine and Medical Specialties, PROMISE, University of Palermo, 90127 Palermo, Italy
* Correspondence: cecilia.binda@gmail.com

Abstract: Anastomotic defects are deleterious complications after either oncologic or bariatric surgery, leading to high morbidity and mortality. Besides surgical revision in early stages or instable patients, endoscopic treatment has become the mainstay. To date, many options for endoscopic treatment in this setting exist, including fully covered metal stent placement, endoscopic vacuum therapy (EVT), endoscopic internal drainage with pigtail placement (EID), leak closure with through the scope or over the scope clips, endoluminal suturing, fibrin glue sealing and a combination of all these techniques. Current evidence is mostly based on retrospective single and multicenter studies. No guidelines exist in this important field. Treatment options have to be chosen upon each case individually, taking into account clinical and anatomic criteria, such as timing, size, infectious wound complications and hemodynamic stability. Local expertise and availability of treatment devices need to be taken into account whenever choosing a treatment strategy. This review aimed to present current treatment options in terms of effectiveness, advantages and disadvantages in order to guide the clinician for his decision making. Additionally, we aimed to provide a treatment algorithm.

Keywords: endoscopic treatment of anastomotic defects; esophageal fistula; perforation; esophageal leakage

1. Introduction

Leaks, fistulas and anastomotic defects after either oncologic or bariatric surgery are feared complications. They occur in up to 13.1% of cases after esophagectomy [1,2] and in up to 7.5% after gastrectomy in large patient cohorts [3,4]. Leakage sites may be intrathoracic or intra-abdominal in these patients.

Patients undergoing bariatric surgery including sleeve gastrectomy and Roux en Y bypass may also be subject to postoperative anastomotic defects, leakages or fistulas. After gastric sleeve, they are reported in 1–3.9% [5–7] and after Roux en Y bypass, in 0.6–5.25% [8–10]. Leak site after sleeve gastrectomy typically is situated at the stapler line whereas after bypass surgery the leak most commonly (in up to 50%) is situated at the gastrojejunal anastomosis followed by the gastric pouch [11,12].

Classifications try to systemize clinical appearance and treatment decisions. According to the ECCG (esophagectomy complications consensus group), postoperative defects after esophageal surgery are defined as full thickness GI defects involving the esophagus, anastomosis, staple line or conduit. They are subclassified into three groups: type I local defect requiring no change in therapy; type II localized defect requiring interventional but not surgical therapy and type III localized defect requiring surgical therapy [13]. Defects can also be classified by timing of occurrence, for which either surgical reintervention or endoscopic management might be the treatment of choice. Here, a general accepted subdivision at least for esophageal and post-gastrectomy defects is proposed by Bludau et al.

"Early leaks "are considered to occur within 72 h after operation, "classic leaks are observed in a period from 4–10 days after operation and late leaks occur after postoperative day 10 [14].

Besides conservative treatment, septic conditions frequently require surgical re-intervention or application of endoscopic therapies.

For anastomotic defects after oncologic upper GI surgery (Ivor Lewis and gastrectomy), early surgical reintervention in these conditions is favored during the first postoperative days. Endoscopic therapies remain treatment of choice after the third postoperative days [14–17].

After bariatric operations: surgical reintervention will normally be performed in early leaks (<5 days postop) whereas non-surgical treatment is favored in patients with chronic leaks [18].

Many options for the endoscopic treatment for any kind of anastomotic defect exist, including fully covered metal stent placement, endoscopic vacuum therapy (EVT), endoscopic internal drainage with pigtail placement (EID), leak closure with through the scope or over the scope clips, endoluminal suturing, fibrin glue sealing and a combination. Table 1 summarizes the main features of endoscopic closure techniques of upper GI fistula, leaks and perforations.

Table 1. Comparison of endoscopic closure techniques of upper GI fistula, leaks and perforations.

	Device	Main Indication	Pros	Cons	AEs
STENT	SEPS FCSEMS PCSEMS BDs	Leaks Fistula Perforation > 2 cm	Easy placement High technical and clinical success Avoid stenosis Combined approach with clips	Expensive High migration rate Possible multiple sessions Need of percutaneous drainage of collection	Migration Food impaction Mucosal erosions Bleeding Perforation Stent ruptures Drooling, foreign body sensation
CLIP	TTSc	Leaks or perforations < 1 cm Acute perforations	Large availability Different shapes and sizes available Integration with other techniques	Limited efficacy Need of multiple interventions No full-thickness closure Need of percutaneous drainage of collection	Failure Migration
	OTSc	Leaks or perforations up to 2–3 cm Acute and chronic perforations	Full-thickness closure Single-step procedure	Need of percutaneous drainage of collection	Misdeployment
ENDOSUTURING	Overstitch Overstitch SX	Early defects > 2 cm	Full thickness closure High clinical and technical success	Expensive Need of high expertise Challenging use in angulated GI regions Need of percutaneous drainage of collection	Bleeding Strictures

Table 1. Cont.

Device		Main Indication	Pros	Cons	AEs
ENDOSCOPIC VACUUM THERAPY (EVT)	Esosponge Suprasorb	Leaks, fistula, perforation with associated cavity	High clinical and technical success rate Simultaneous drainage of collection	Patient discomfort due to external tube drainage Need of multiple sessions	Bleeding Sponge ingrowth Strictures
ENDOSCOPIC INTERNAL DRAINAGE (EID)		Perforation and leaks with associated cavity	High clinical and technical success rate Low cost Oral feeding feasible	Need odultiple session	Bleeding Migration Splenic Hematoma

SEPS: self-expandable plastic stents; FCSEMS: fully covered self-expandable metallic stents; PCSEMS: partially covered self-expandable metallic stents; BDs: biodegradable stents; TTSc: through the scope clip; OTSc: over the scope clip.

Until now, no guidelines for endoscopic treatment for defects in the upper GI after oncologic or bariatric surgery are available. Current ESGE guidelines only comprise treatment suggestions for intestinal perforations (for any cause) [19]. Large quantitative or qualitative data which could serve for guidelines are still scarce. The data published mostly consist of retrospective single and multicenter studies. Most definitely, due to ethical aspects, randomized controlled trials will hardly exist.

No leak/fistula or defect is anatomically the same and needs individual treatment approaches, which might be changed during the course of treatment. Time of detection, anatomy, size, presence of a wound cavity including presence of a drainage need to be taken into account in order to choose the right endoscopic armamentarium.

In this narrative review, we look at the current literature comprising endoscopic techniques for the management of upper GI anastomotic defects, their indications, contraindications, technical aspects, treatment algorithms and complications.

2. Endoscopic Techniques

2.1. Stenting

Endoluminal stent placement has been proven to be a safe and effective treatment option for upper GI leaks and fistula. Once released under fluoroscopic or endoscopic control or both, the meshes expand radially to its maximal diameter and the stent adheres to the mucosal wall. The rationale of stent deployment is to seal the breach and divert luminal content, allowing the closure of wall defect. Diversion therapy offers the advantages of early oral intake and early discharge. In addition, stent placement prevents the onset of gastric stenosis in patients affected by sleeve gastrectomy leak [20].

In two recent published guidelines, ESGE recommends that temporary stent placement can be considered for the treatment of leaks, fistulas and perforations >2 cm in size, but no specific type of stent can be recommended [19,21]. Indeed, different types of stents are commercially available: self-expandable plastic stents (SEPS), self-expandable metal stents (SEMS), both fully covered (FCSEMS) or partially covered (PCSEMS) and biodegradable stents.

The most used self-expandable plastic stent (SEPS) is Polyflex (Boston Scientific, Natick, MA, USA), made of polyester, completely covered with silicon. SEPSs guarantee an easy removal and a low cost, but their use is burdened by a high rate of migration [22].

Self-expandable metal stents (SEMSs) are composed of various metal alloys, which confer them a higher radial force compared to SEPSs. FCSEMSs have a plastic or silicone rubber coating along its full length. PCSEMSs has uncovered distal and proximal ends. These help for the optimal fitting and prevention of migration. On the other hand, uncovered parts of the stent are exposed to mucosal in-growth. This could lead to increased risk of bleeding, mucosal stripping and perforation during stent removal. A recent multicenter retrospective study showed that FCSEMSs were more successfully removed than self-expandable plastic stents and PCSEMSs. However, esophageal stent removal in the setting of benign disease was affected by a low rate of adverse events (2.1%) [23].

The results of three systematic reviews on the use of PCSEMSs, FCSEMSs, and SEPSs reported a clinical success rate of esophageal stent placement of 81%–87%, with similar efficacy between the different stents (SEPS 84%; FCSEMS 85%; PCSEMS 86%; $p = 0.97$) [24–26]. SEMSs are reported to perform better than SEPSs in leaks and perforations, with higher technical success (95% vs. 91%; $p = 0.03$), and reduced risk of migration (16% vs. 24%; $p = 0.001$) and stent repositioning (3% vs. 11%; $p < 0.001$) [26].

Freeman et al. identified four factors associated with failure of stenting therapy for esophageal wall defects, such as location of the defect at the proximal cervical esophagus, stent traversing the gastroesophageal junction, esophageal injury longer than 6 cm and an anastomotic leak associated with a more distal conduit leak [27]. The presence of fluid collection is another unfavorable factor in successful treatment with stents, especially when the fluid collection is >5 cm, thus appropriate drainage of any pre-existing or concurrent extra-luminal collection is mandatory [28].

The most frequently reported adverse event is stent migration, which is higher for FCSEMSs (26%) and SEPSs (31%) compared with PCSEMSs (12%), as might be expected [24]. Migration risk can be reduced by fixating the proximal flange of the stent to the esophageal wall with TTSC, OTSC or endosuturing devices. Ngamruengphong et al. found no statistically significant difference in stent migration rate between PCSEMS and FCSEMS fixed with the OverStitch suturing device (Apollo Endosurgery, Austin, TX, United States) [29]. Moreover, fixation of FCSEMSs with a novel dedicated over-the-scope clip device, Stentfix OTSC® (Ovesco Endoscopy, Tubingen, Germany) significantly reduced migration rate compared with unfixed stents [30].

Other stent-related adverse events include stricture development, stent rupture, food impaction, mucosal erosion with perforation or massive bleeding due to erosion into the major vessel [24–26,31].

According to the ESGE guidelines, the timing of stent retrieval is still subject to debate [21]. Stents are usually removed 6–8 weeks after insertion [24–26], but some authors report success with only 2 weeks of deployment [32]. In order to avoid complications, Van Heel et al. suggests stent indwelling within 6 weeks after insertion [33]. A survey questionnaire, distributed among international expert interventional endoscopists, reported the tendency to reduce the stent dwell time to 4–5 weeks in clinical practice [34].

Biodegradable stents (BDs) such as SX-Ella (Milady Horakrove, Hradc Kralove, Czech Republic) are made of polydioxanone, an absorbable polymer which degrades after 3 to 4 months in a low ambient pH. Therefore, it is a potentially ideal solution for temporary use in benign indications because BDs do not need to be removed, but data regarding their use in clinical practice are still limited. Promising results were published by Cerna et al [35] who reported a case series of five patients with esophageal perforation or anastomotic leak treated with covered biodegradable stents. Technical success was achieved in 100% of patients and clinical success was achieved in four out of five patients (80%), but stent migration occurred in three patients (60%). Although biodegradable stents eliminate complications involved in stent removal, they are more expensive. Additional side effects reported in the literature include drooling, retrosternal pain, "foreign body"—sensation and aversion to water for up to 2 months [36].

Customized SEMS have been recently designed for the treatment of leaks after bariatric surgery, especially for sleeve gastrectomy leaks (SGL). Customized bariatric stents (CBS) include Niti-S Mega [37,38] and Niti-S Beta [39,40] (TaeWoong Medical Industries, Seoul, Republic of Korea), Hanaro GastroSeal [41] and Hanaro ECBB [42] (M.I. Tech, Seoul, Republic of Korea). These stents have common characteristics: CBS are fully covered SEMSs with a longer length (18–24 cm) that ensures the complete coverage of the leak area and to bypass the wide gastric lumen. A large diameter ensures a complete seal and reduces the risk of migration. Significant flexibility allows to conform to the tortuous bariatric surgery anatomy. Moreover, every CBS is equipped with a specific anti-migration system.

Hamid et al. has recently published a systematic review and meta-analysis aiming to evaluate the cumulative efficacy and safety of CBS and to compare them with the conventional esophageal stents (CES) [43]. In total, 12 studies (141 patients) used CBS and 11 studies (167 patients) used CES. Treatment with CBS was associated with a similar technical success rate, fewer stent insertions and endoscopic interventions, and shorter time to leak closure compared to CES. Non-Niti-S Mega stents had a higher clinical success rate (89%) than Niti-S Mega stents (66%), and a similar clinical success rate to CES (93%). Of note, in the Niti-S Mega group, 11% of patients had combined sleeve leakage and stenosis, which were reported to be associated with lower clinical success [7]. On the other hand, non-Niti-S Mega stents had the highest migration rate (41%) compared to other types of stents, including CES and Niti-S Mega stents (15–24%). Anyway, the overall quality of evidence was very low and further studies, including randomized trials, are warranted.

2.2. Endoscopic Clip Placement (TTSC and OTSC)

Through-the-scope clips (TTSC) are available in different sizes and opening lengths. TTSC are inserted and deployed through the operative channel. Multiple clips can be applied in a parallel manner.

A recent updated ESGE position paper suggests the use of TTSC for upper GI leaks or perforations <1 cm in size, in general due to small clip size and low tissue compression force [19]. Their application is also limited by location of the defect and endoscopist experience [44,45].

Clip application might be difficult and lead to suboptimal closure if the tissue surrounding the defect is inflamed, necrotic or fibrotic.

A pooled analysis performed by Qadeer et al. demonstrated that TTSC can be effective for closing both acute and chronic esophageal defects; however, there is a statistically significant correlation between the duration of a perforation and the time of healing, which is longer for chronic perforations than for acute perforations [46].

A retrospective study including 20 patients with anastomotic leak after gastric surgery, published by Lee et al., reported a 95% technical and 100% clinical success rate after TTS clip deployment [47].

Other than the TTSC, over-the-scope clips have demonstrated several advantages in closing GI defects, including as the ability to capture larger area of tissue and applying higher compression force. OTS clip can achieve full-thickness closure of GI defects up to 2–3 cm. In the recent published ESGE Position Paper, the use of OTSC is suggested for upper GI leaks or perforations larger than 1 cm in size [19].

The first developed and most used OTS clip is the OTSC® (Ovesco Endoscopy AG, Tübingen, Germany). The OTSC® has a bear-trap shape design made of Nitinol, a biocompatible, super-elastic, shape-memory material which firmly anchors the tissue and can remain in the body as a long-term implant.

The edges of the wall defect can be approximated and pulled inside the application cap mounted at the tip of the endoscope by simply applying suction. Otherwise, the edges can be pulled actively into the cap using additional devices (twin grasper/tissue anchor).

Once the whole leak is engulfed into the cap, the clip is deployed by turning an handwheel located in the endoscope handle, similar to a variceal band ligator. OTSC® are available in different sizes and with different dental shapes (atraumatic/traumatic).

The traumatic Ovesco OTSC, equipped with spiked teeth, is the most used to close fistula and perforations.

In a recent systematic review analyzing 381 patients with anastomotic leak, the overall technical and clinical success rate for OTSCs closure was 86.7 and 72.6%, respectively [48]. A large single center case series included in this review reported long-term clinical resolution in 83% patients affected by post-operative leaks in the upper GI-tract [49].

In 2021, Rogalski et al. published a systematic review and meta-analysis of 13 studies including a total of 85 cases of leaks and fistulas after bariatric surgery [50]. Overall, successful closure of a leak/fistula with the OTSC system was achieved in 57 of 85 patients (67.1%). Only two studies reported complications related to the OTSC system including clip migration (1 patient), mediogastric stenosis (1 patient) and one case of anchor blocked within the clip during the deployment.

Another advantage of OTS over TTS clips is the ability to close long-term leakages and fistulas even if the surrounding tissue is inflamed or fibrotic. Several studies suggest to de-epithelialize the edges of the fistula with Argon Plasma Coagulation or with a cytology brush before OTS clip placement in order to promote granulation tissue and obtain a stronger grip of the tissues [20].

A large multicenter retrospective study was published in 2014 by Haito-Chavez et al. including 188 patients undergoing OTSC placement for closure of GI defects, of which 62.8% were in the upper GI tract. The rate for the successful closure of perforations (90%) and leaks (73.3%) was significantly higher than that of the fistulae (42.9%) ($p < 0.05$). Long-term clinical success did not differ between all three defect types but was significantly higher when OTSCs were applied as primary therapy as compared with rescue therapy (69.1% vs. 46.9%, respectively; $p = 0.004$) [51].

If the fistula is in communication with an abscess cavity, OTSC is significantly more efficient in the case of patients having a prior endoluminal drainage (88.2% healing in this subgroup vs. 53.8%, $p = 0.049$) [52].

In conclusion, the use of OTS clips is suggested in the case of early detection, perforation diameter ranging from 10 to 20 mm and the absence of fluid collections [45].

A new OTSC device, the Padlock Clip (Aponos Medical, Kingston, NH, United States), has been introduced [53]. It differs from Ovesco in the hexagonal shape and in the deployment system. Clinical data are currently limited, but several case reports describe the successful treatment of tracheoesophageal fistula [54], gastrocutaneous fistula [55] and iatrogenic duodenal perforation [56].

2.3. Endoscopic Suturing

Recent development of endoscopic suturing techniques has allowed for the full-thickness closure of large GI luminal defects. The OverStitch system (Apollo Endosurgery, TX, USA) was first developed in 2009 and is currently the most common endoscopic suturing device [57]. The original OverStitch is a single operator, disposable platform that requires a double-channel therapeutic endoscope. Instead, the newly introduced OverStitch SX (Apollo Endosurgery, TX, United States) can be mounted on every single channel endoscope commercially available. The device is composed of a handle attached to the endoscope controls, a metallic needle on the tip of the endoscope, devices for tissue retraction and a specially designed non absorbable suture.

Endoscopic suturing is a complex technique, requiring specific training and a high level of expertise, limiting its use to tertiary centers only. Due to its size and reduced maneuverability, endoscopic suturing may be challenging in narrow or angulated GI locations, such as the gastric fundus, duodenum or sigmoid colon. Similar to TTS clips, suturing requires robust and healthy mucosa to hold the sutures when tissues are approximated and is therefore adapted for early leakages in the absence of an associated wound cavity.

In a large multicenter retrospective study, including 122 patients undergoing endoscopic suturing, clinical success was 91.4% in stent anchorage, 93% in perforations, 80% in fistulas, but only 27% in anastomotic leak closure [58]. Long-term clinical success was more likely if the leak was closed within days of diagnosis, indicating its usefulness in mainly treating acute and early leaks.

Chon et al. performed a retrospective, single-center study of 13 patients affected by leaks in the upper gastrointestinal tract treated with OverStitch [59]. The mean size of the leak was 22.31 ± 22.6 mm. Interventional success was achieved in all endoscopic attempts ($n = 16$, 100%) with a mean closure time of 28.0 ± 12.36 min per patient. Clinical success was achieved in 8 of the 13 patients (61.5%). These eight patients had not received prior treatment for the leak.

A recently published systematic review and meta-analysis showed a pooled technical success for any GI defect treated with Apollo OverStitch of 92.7% (95% [84.4–96.8]), clinical success was 67.9% [59.2–75.5], and adverse events occurred in 6.9% [3.8–12.5] [60]. The pooled clinical success for perforations was higher when compared to fistulae/leaks (respectively 89.5% [73.8–96.3] vs. 60.4% [50.1–69.9]).

Endoscopic suturing can also be used for esophageal stent fixation in order to prevent migration [29]. In this regard, Granata et al. reported a recent case series of 20 patients with post-operative leaks [61]. The therapeutic approach was stratified in three groups according to the clinical scenario and structural condition of the wall defect layers: Pure endoscopic direct suture (group A: healthy tissue and feasible suture), combined therapy with endoscopic direct suture + FC-SEMS placement + anchoring (group B: unhealthy tissue and feasible sutures) and FC-SEMS placement + anchoring (group C: unhealthy tissue and suture not feasible). The overall long-term clinical success was 80%. The clinical success rate for each group was 77% (7/9) in group A, 85% (6/7) in group B and 75% (3/4) in group C. No evidence of migration was detected.

Endoscopic suturing is a well-accepted treatment option for long-term complications after bariatric surgery such as dilation of the gastrojejunal anastomosis (TORE procedure) [62]. There are few studies explicitly examining the effectiveness of endoscopic suturing of anastomotic malformations and stapler line leaks after bariatric surgery. Therefore, no conclusions or recommendations can be drawn for this indication.

2.4. Endoscopic Vacuum Therapy (EVT)

Endoscopic vacuum therapy has been applied for the treatment of various types of defects in the gastrointestinal tract. First applied for anastomotic leakage after colonic surgery with promising results, it was successfully used for the treatment of anastomotic defects after upper GI oncologic surgery [63–66].

So far, EVT has mostly been used for defects (leaks, fistulas, but also perforations) in the upper GI after oncologic surgery. Recent systematic reviews confirm high defect closure rates (81.6–85%) for these indications [67,68]. Less frequently EVT has also been proposed for the treatment of defects/leaks after bariatric surgery (staple line defects after laparoscopic sleeve gastrectomy and anastomotic defects after Roux en Y bypass) showing high healing rates up to 90% [69–72].

EVT consists of an open pore polyurethane sponge attached to a suction tube to which negative pressure of −125 mmHg is applied (for example Eso-Sponge® Braun B Melsungen Germany); see also Figure 1. The sponge and suction tube are inserted endoscopically via an overtube, externalized transnasally and attached to a suction device which generates negative pressure. EVT works through at least five different mechanisms: 1. wound adaption; 2. cavitary collapse; 3. induction of angiogenesis; 4. wound granulation; and 5. bacterial clearance.

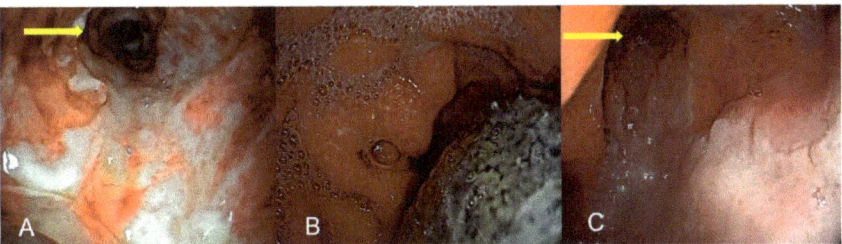

Figure 1. (**A–C**) partial closure of anastomotic esophageal defect after Ivor Lewis esophagectomy: (**A**) pleural drainage channel (yellow arrow); (**B**) EVT removal; (**C**) partial defect closure after EVT.

Animal experiments showed the highest efficiency of negative pressure therapy for inducing granulation, wound adaption and induction of angiogenesis at around −125 mmHg [73]. Studies with negative pressure inferior to −125 mmHg exist but are scarce. Here, EVT is considered to act by diverting possibly toxic fluids (bile, pancreatic enzymes, gastric acid) away from the anastomosis, and less through wound adaption/cavity collapse and aspiration of bacterial fluids. Nevertheless, administration of low negative pressure around −50 mmHg still proved to be efficient [74]. Loske et al. recently described postoperative pre-emptive active drainage of reflux using negative pressure with a 25 cm open pore film drainage esosponge device after Ivor Lewis esophagectomy to be effective for anastomoses at risk with focal necrosis [75]. No randomized controlled trials investigating the effect on different negative pressures exist.

Lately, a new form of EVT using an open pore film wrapped around the drainage tube (Suprasorb CNP, Drainage Film; Lohmann & Rauscher International GmbH & Co. KG, Rengsdorf, Germany) has been proposed by Loske et al. Its advantage lies in its capability of being applied to cavities behind small defects (4–6 mm), where a classic polyurethan sponge cannot be placed due to its diameter (1.5–3.2 cm) [76].

EVT can be applied either intracavitarily or intraluminally and is adapted for different sizes of defects. When defects measure <10 mm, EVT is generally placed intraluminally outside of the wound cavity. In defects >10 mm, EVT can be placed intracavitarily. In patients with complete anastomotic dehiscence after for example Ivor Lewis operation, EVT can still be placed, although it may not represent the ideal indication [15]. Defects with a size of less than 10 mm can sometimes be dilated in order to fit in the Eso-Sponge® system. In patients with large defects, EVT can be initiated intracavitarily and finished intraluminally. In case of two different defects, simultaneous intraluminal and intracavitary application can be performed [77].

EVT can come with complications. In the literature, procedure-related bleeding, sponge ingrowth and stricture development are described.

Minor bleeding can be addressed endoscopically, in general when it occurs directly associated with the sponge change. Only a few bleedings associated with sponge change have been described that led to fatal consequences. Laukoetter et al. described a case of aortic rupture into the esophagus not manageable by endoscopic means [17].

Strictures associated with therapy are rare (ca. 7.6%) and can be managed by endoscopic pneumatic dilation [17,78]. Recently, stricture incidences up to 35% have been presented in a smaller Korean study. This result must be interpreted carefully due to the small cohort size [79].

Sponge ingrowth poses a serious issue when the sponge is left in place for over 4 days [80]. Then, difficulties in removing may occur resulting in detachment of the sponge and the suction tube. Then, careful endoscopic resection of the ingrown sponge part is necessary.

Timing of EVT after Upper GI Surgery

This subject has not been addressed in major studies or meta-analysis so far. It is not clear whether late onset of therapy after diagnosis leads to longer treatment duration. Risk factors for long treatment so far are patients with neoadjuvant treatment and larger defect sizes >2 cm [79]. Another recent retrospective multicenter study by Hyun Jung et al. investigates factors associated with treatment failure in patients with leaks and perforations. Here, neoadjuvant treatment and interestingly, the intraluminal method, are independent risk factors for treatment failure [81].

According to our own experience, it is important to initiate therapy early after defect diagnosis. At this point, mucosal injury has not turned into fistulous or fibrotic tissue which generally makes it more difficult for EVT to induce wound granulation. Otherwise, risk of longer treatment duration is high. According to Bludau et al., EVT can generally be initiated 3 days after defect diagnosis. Prior to this point, early surgical revision is recommended [14].

Instead, some studies have looked into the prophylactic use of EVT in patients with at-risk anastomoses during upper GI surgery for those with high-risk comorbidities or anastomosis ischemia [82,83]. In the study by Laukoetter et al., high "protection" rates with a low incidence of defect development in anastomotic ischemia were observed (75% of patients). When defects occurred (25% of patients treated pre-emptively), EVT was continued until closure.

So far, no consensus was found to define the failing of EVT treatment. Treatment failure is still a clinical decision comprising leak persistence and ongoing purulent secretion.

Whether SEMS placement or EVT should be preferred for patients with upper GI defects after oncologic surgery is not clear.

By now there are no randomized controlled trials available comparing EVT treatment to SEMS placement. Only retrospective studies on this subject exist. Two recent review and metanalysis studies address this important comparison as these two therapies are most frequently used for the treatment of upper GI defects [84,85]. Here, EVT seems to be superior to SEMS therapy in terms of defect closure, mortality, hospital stay and adverse events. A first phase 2 trial (ESOLEAK-Trial) by Tachezy et al. will try to shed some light on this matter although the primary endpoint is "quality of life". Group sizes in this protocol will not contain more than 20 patients per group (EVT vs. SEMS) [86].

Additionally, patients with defects after bariatric surgery (in case of staple line leaks) seem to profit from EVT compared to SEMS placement. In a study by Archid et al. in 24 patients either treated with EVT or SEMS for staple line leakage after sleeve gastrectomy, EVT was shown to be superior in terms of defect closure, reducing adverse events, hospital stay and duration of endoscopic treatment [87].

More studies using EVT for defects after bariatric surgery are needed.

2.5. Endoscopic Internal Drainage (EID)

Endoscopic internal drainage proves to be a valuable alternative to SEMS—and EVT placement in the treatment of anastomotic defects. First introduced by Pequignot et al. in 2012 and later by Donatelli et al., it was used for defects after bariatric and oncologic esophageal surgery showing promising results [88–92]. From there, many other single center studies showed that EID provides high healing rates up to 78–95% for defects after either upper GI oncologic interventions or bariatric operations [92–96]. The largest single center study by Donatelli et al. describes an experience of 617 EID cases for defects following bariatric surgery demonstrating a cumulative efficacy of 84.7% [97].

Endoscopic internal drainage consists of endoscopically placing one or multiple double pigtail plastic stents into the anastomotic defect and its associated cavity (see Figure 2). When suspecting anastomotic defects, the local situation is being examined by normal gastroscopy. Via fluoroscopy, the cavitary size behind the defect is evaluated. Then, defects are intubated with a straight catheter and a guidewire over which pigtail are inserted (normal pigtail size: 7–10 Fr, 3–5 cm).

EID works by at least two mechanisms. One is the passive drainage of purulent material accumulated in the cavity behind the anastomotic defect, and the second is by continuously irrigating the fistulous tract inducing wound granulation. In the studies demonstrated so far, EID is changed every 3 weeks with no need for hospitalization during treatment. Oral alimentation is generally possible during treatment. Whenever pigtail exchange is performed, local wound situations are examined, and treatment modalities can be adapted when necessary. So far, no clear treatment algorithms exist but it seems obvious that EID most sufficiently might be working in patients with anastomotic defects up to 2 cm of size. In defects greater than 2 cm, also when placing multiple stents, pigtails can easily dislocate and therefore not induce wound granulation and clearance of purulent fluids. Therefore, EID has no indication in patients with complete anastomotic dehiscence. More studies investigating the success rates including complication rate of EID treatment are necessary. Especially, direct comparative studies between SEMS placement and EID or EVT and EID are needed to confirm treatment effects and define optimal treatment indications.

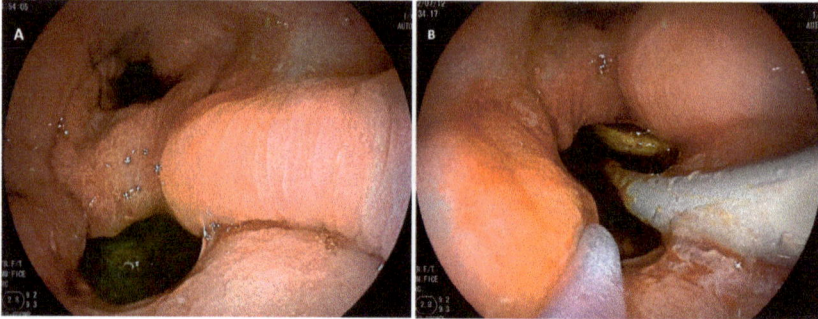

Figure 2. (**A**,**B**): Stapler line dehiscence after sleeve gastrectomy: (**A**) orifice and gastric inlet, (**B**) pigtail placement through the defect into the associated cavity.

A study by Lorenzo et al. compared the effect of EID vs. direct clip closure of defects after sleeve gastrectomy in a cohort of 100 patients. Primary success rates of EID were 86% whereas clip closure had an efficacy of only 63% [28].

A recent review and meta-analysis by Laopemathong et al. compared the effectiveness of EVT and EID: EVT had slightly inferior healing success rates with 85.2% compared to EID with 91.6% when used as first line treatment in patients with post-bariatric leaks [98].

A study by Hallit et al. compared effectiveness of endoscopic treatment with either EID or SEMS placement in patients with oncologic upper GI surgery. Here, in 68 patients with either prior Ivor Lewis esophagectomy, tr-incisional esophagectomy or total gastrectomy, the healing success rate for patients with defects treated by SEMS placement was 77%, whereas the healing success rate in EID was 95% [94].

A study by Jung et al. Comparing EID vs. EVT in defects after oncologic surgery confirmed high healing success after EID with 100% vs. 85.2% after EVT [99].

Only a few complications with EID treatment are described. The most common are ulcerations, upper gastrointestinal symptoms, splenic hematoma, stenosis, bleeding, stent migration (into the spleen or peritoneum) and pneumoperitoneum [89,95,97].

Still, larger studies are needed to confirm the effect, advantages, disadvantages and possible contraindications for EID treatment.

3. New Concepts

One of the new treatment concepts is the sponge over stent method, combining wound fluid suction and defect coverage. It enables draining wound secretions of cavities connected to anastomotic defects, whilst covering the defect itself and enabling liquid/food oral intake.

Technically, either a specially conceived device (Vac Stent GI Microtech^{TM} Endoscopy, Micro-Tech Europe GmbH) or a manually constructed device can be used [100,101].

The MicroTech Vac Stent can be used in defects up to 30 mm and consists of a nitinol stent covered with a silicone membrane and a 10 mm thick sponge system fixed to the outer layer of the stent. Either way, a sponge will be attached to a fully covered metal stent and placed over the anastomotic defect and associated cavity.

Only limited data for this method are available so far. In the study by Valli et al., a total of 12 patients with upper GI wall defects were treated with the stent over sponge method, in 7 patients as a first line treatment with a success rate of 71.4% and in 5 patients as a second line treatment with a success rate of 80%. No severe adverse events were observed [101].

In a preliminary study using the Microtech stent by Lange et al., a total of three patients with different types of defects were treated: one patient presenting a leak after subtotal esophagectomy, one patient with acute Boerhaave syndrome and one patient with a full thickness defect caused by an anti-reflux device. In all patients, successful defect closure was obtained.

An interesting feature of the SOS device is the necessity of changing the stent only every 5 days as sponge ingrowth does not seem to occur as frequently as compared to classic EVT.

A very promising new technique is described by Nachira/Boskoski et al. for leaks that have failed prior classic endoscopic treatment or which may not be treated either endoscopically or surgically for various reasons (e.g., anatomical difficulties). This new innovative method was tested in five patients (two with upper and three with distal esophageal fistulas). The method consists of the submucosal injection/delivery of the stromal vascular fraction obtained by the mechanical emulsification of autologous adipose tissue. The fluid comprises mesenchymal stem cells and fragments of the extracellular matrix obtained by centrifugation of subcutaneous fat of the patient itself. The injection is performed submucosally in each quadrant around the defect until obliteration of the defect. Fistula closure was obtained in all five cases after 7 days of injection. Long-term follow-up after a median of 8 months showed persistent defect closure [102]. These data should be confirmed in larger prospective studies.

4. Treatment Logarithm Proposal

A flowchart for treatment choices according to the clinical situation is illustrated in Figure 3 (modified after Loske et al. and Di Leo et al. [15,103]).

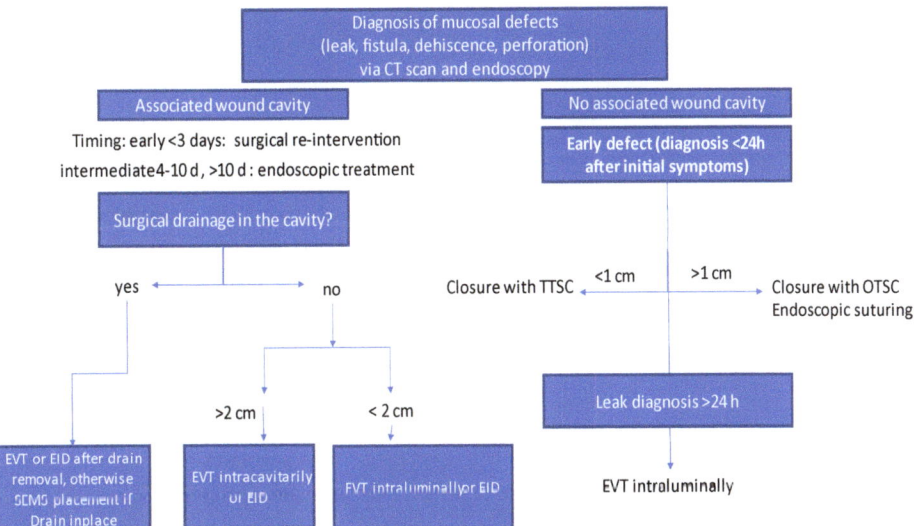

Figure 3. Flowchart treatment of mucosal defects in the upper GI tract, modified after Loschke and Di Leo et al. [15,103].

There are several main parameters that need to be considered when choosing the right treatment for defects after upper GI surgery (either after oncologic or bariatric surgery). This includes timing, anatomical site, presence of an associated wound cavity and hemodynamic stability of the patient.

First, the timing of diagnosis is of crucial interest. Timing of defect detection is divided in "early" <3 d, "classic/intermediate" 4–10 d and "late" >10 d after either bariatric or oncologic surgery [14,104]. Some authors consider early defects in patients after oncologic and bariatric surgery a classic indication for surgical re-intervention [5,14]. Otherwise, the presence of an associated wound cavity is of crucial interest.

In case of an associated wound cavity and intermediate or late diagnosis, it depends whether a surgical drain is still present in the wound cavity. If so, drain removal can be performed enabling treatment with an endoscopic draining method (EVT/EID). Otherwise, SEMS placement can be performed whilst leaving the drainage in place. When no drain is in place, EVT can be placed intracavitarily when the defect size is equal or larger than 2 cm, otherwise the defect can be artificially amplified by dilation; 2 cm is normally the minimal size allowing for EVT—overtube insertion into the defect associated cavity. If the defect is smaller than 2 cm, either EVT can be placed intraluminally or EID placement can be performed.

In patients where the defect has no associated wound cavity and defect diagnosis is made in an early stage, direct defect closure either with TTSC (defect size up to 1 cm) or OTSC (defect size between 1–2 cm) can be performed. The sizes and recommendations for clip use are referred to in the latest ESGE recommendations for endoscopic treatment in gastrointestinal perforations [19]. In selected cases with intact mucosal tissue, endoscopic suturing could be an option for defect closure. If the defect is not amenable to clipping or endoscopic suturing, intraluminal EVT can be performed. TTSC/OTSC placement or endoscopic suturing should not be performed if local wound infection is suspected and no drainages are in place.

Complete anastomotic dehiscence usually cannot be treated with EID. In these cases, when diagnosed >3 days after surgery, a trial with SEMS placement or EVT can be performed. If no wound granulation is observed, surgical reintervention might be necessary.

In general, EVT needs to be changed every 3–4 days. For EID, no clear change intervals are defined. In most publications, EID exchange is performed every 3 weeks. SEMS are generally exchanged every 4 weeks.

5. Discussion

SEMS, EVT and EID are the main treatment options for upper GI defect closure. In 2013, Schniewind et al. retrospectively compared mortality in patients treated with surgical revision, EVT and SEMS placement for defects after upper GI oncologic surgery. Once adjusted for APACHE II score, patients treated with surgical revision and SEMS patients showed significantly higher mortality than patients treated with EVT [105]. This study did not mention closure rates nor documents the postoperative timepoint of treatment after defect diagnosis. Nevertheless, it shows a paradigm shift concerning treatment of postoperative defects towards endoscopic approaches.

For a long time, SEMS placement was the mainstay of endoscopic treatment. With the invention of EVT and clinical data showing slightly higher defect closure rates in single center studies, a shift in first line treatment towards EVT was observed. Do Monte Junior and Scognamiglio et al. addressed this important topic in their meta-analysis for treatment efficacy between SEMS and EVT therapy. They included five studies retrospectively comparing the efficacy of SEMS and EVT in patients with upper GI defects. They found a significant 21% increase in successful defect closure in patients treated with EVT compared to SEMS. Other observations were a significant 12% reduction in mortality for patients treated with EVT compared to SEMS, an average reduction of treatment duration by 14.22 days with EVT vs. SEMS and a 24% reduction in adverse events in patients treated with EVT vs. SEMS [84,85]. Obviously, EVT therapy was associated with higher number of endoscopic interventional sessions.

EID treatment seems to be a valid and less expensive alternative to EVT, needing fewer interventions, leading to high closure rates. Comparative analyses for EVT and EID are extremely scarce. Our literature research has evidenced one study comparing EVT vs. EID in defects after oncologic upper GI surgery with higher treatment success rates in EID treatment (100% overall treatment success in EID vs. 85.2% in EVT, $p = 0.03$) [99]. EID also seems to be superior to EVT for defect closure after bariatric surgery, as outlined in the meta-analysis be Laopemathong et al. (91.6% EID vs. 85.2% EVT) [98]. One recent multicenter retrospective analysis compared the treatment success of SEMS vs. EID in upper GI defects after oncologic surgery, concluding in favor of a higher treatment success after EID (95% EID vs. 77% SEMS, $p = 0.06$) [94].

The scarcity of data makes it difficult to draw final conclusions whether supporting SEMS, EVT or EID as the first line treatment for defect closure either after upper GI oncologic or bariatric surgery. Nevertheless, data published so far seem to favor EVT and EID over SEMS placement as first line therapy. Nonetheless, whenever one treatment technique does not show sufficient defect closure, treatment reevaluation needs to be performed, not excluding device changes. One point not being addressed in studies is local availability of treatment methods and the clinical experience of the endoscopist. Our recommendation is to treat patients with defects in tertiary clinical centers or where sufficient clinical endoscopic expertise in all main closure techniques and intensive care are provided.

Larger prospective, comparative multicenter studies are clearly needed in order to guide clinicians in their decision making. Upper GI defects remain very difficult to treat, not only due to individual anatomic properties of the defect but also due to individual patient comorbidities.

6. Conclusions

Upper GI anastomotic defects after either oncologic or bariatric surgery come along with high morbidity and mortality. Multiple endoscopic treatment modalities exist and they have to be applied looking at each case individually and upon multidisciplinary agreement. The mainstay of therapy has been SEMS placement for over a decade leading to healing success in up to 87% in these scenarios. Indications for SEMS placement range from defects under 1 cm up to complete anastomotic dehiscence. If purulent wound cavities are associated with defects, external drainage besides SEMS placement is necessary. TTSC and OTSC placement can be performed in defects from 5 mm up to ca. 2 cm in early diagnosed defects without wound cavities or as a final closure device when cavities behind defects have been cleaned. Endoscopic vacuum therapy provides high healing rates >90% and can be placed either intraluminally or intracavitarily. Defect size can range from 5 mm to complete anastomotic dehiscence. Endoscopic internal drainage shows high healing success rates up to 95% associated with low costs and few endoscopic interventions and can be placed in defects ranging from 5 mm up to about 2 cm, even in association with wound cavities and when internal drainage of purulent cavities is needed. EID has no rule in complete anastomotic dehiscence as double pigtails cannot be anchored.

Suturing techniques should only be applied by expert hands and in patients with fresh defects and aseptic wound conditions. New devices and methods such as the stent over sponge method or submucosal mesenchymal stem cell injections are on the way but larger clinical trials are needed in order to confirm the preliminary data.

Large-scale cohort studies comparing various treatment techniques for different defect sizes are missing and endoscopic guidelines are not available yet. Optimal treatment strategies according to defect type, size, anatomic characteristics and the presence of wound cavities need to be developed.

Author Contributions: C.B., C.F.M.J. and S.F. were responsible for conceptualization, literature acquisition and preparation of the manuscript. C.C., P.G., G.G., M.S. and C.F. critically revised the manuscript. All authors have read and agreed to the published version of the manuscript.

Funding: This research received no external funding.

Informed Consent Statement: No informed consent was necessary for this review.

Data Availability Statement: All articles listed in this review are listed in PubMed.

Conflicts of Interest: The authors declare no conflict of interest.

Abbreviations

BDS	biodegradable stent
CBS	customized bariatric stents
CES	conventional esophageal stents
EID	endoscopic internal drainage
EVT	endoscopic vacuum therapy
ESGE	European Society of Gastrointestinal Endoscopy
FCSEMS	fully covered self-expandable metallic stents
OTSC	over the scope clip
PCSEMSs	partially covered self-expandable metallic stents
SEMS	self-expandable metal stent
SEPS	self-expandable plastic stents
SOS	stent over sponge
TTSC	through the scope clip

References

1. Kuppusamy, M.K.; Low, D.E.; International Esodata Study Group. Evaluation of International Contemporary Operative Outcomes and Management Trends Associated with Esophagectomy: A 4-Year Study of >6000 Patients Using ECCG Definitions and the Online Esodata Database. *Ann. Surg.* **2020**, *275*, 515–525. [CrossRef]
2. Aiolfi, A.; Asti, E.; Rausa, E.; Bonavina, G.; Bonitta, G.; Bonavina, L. Use of C-reactive protein for the early prediction of anastomotic leak after esophagectomy: Systematic review and Bayesian meta-analysis. *PLoS ONE* **2018**, *13*, e0209272. [CrossRef]
3. Lang, H.; Piso, P.; Stukenborg, C.; Raab, R.; Jahne, J. Management and results of proximal anastomotic leaks in a series of 1114 total gastrectomies for gastric carcinoma. *Eur. J. Surg. Oncol.* **2000**, *26*, 168–171. [CrossRef] [PubMed]
4. Watanabe, M.; Miyata, H.; Gotoh, M.; Baba, H.; Kimura, W.; Tomita, N.; Nakagoe, T.; Shimada, M.; Kitagawa, Y.; Sugihara, K.; et al. Total gastrectomy risk model: Data from 20,011 Japanese patients in a nationwide internet-based database. *Ann. Surg.* **2014**, *260*, 1034–1039. [CrossRef] [PubMed]
5. Abou Rached, A.; Basile, M.; El Masri, H. Gastric leaks post sleeve gastrectomy: Review of its prevention and management. *World J. Gastroenterol.* **2014**, *20*, 13904–13910. [CrossRef]
6. Rosenthal, R.J.; International Sleeve Gastrectomy Expert, P.; Diaz, A.A.; Arvidsson, D.; Baker, R.S.; Basso, N.; Bellanger, D.; Boza, C.; El Mourad, H.; France, M.; et al. International Sleeve Gastrectomy Expert Panel Consensus Statement: Best practice guidelines based on experience of >12,000 cases. *Surg. Obes. Relat. Dis.* **2012**, *8*, 8–19. [CrossRef]
7. Bashah, M.; Khidir, N.; El-Matbouly, M. Management of leak after sleeve gastrectomy: Outcomes of 73 cases, treatment algorithm and predictors of resolution. *Obes. Surg.* **2020**, *30*, 515–520. [CrossRef]
8. Marshall, J.S.; Srivastava, A.; Gupta, S.K.; Rossi, T.R.; DeBord, J.R. Roux-en-Y gastric bypass leak complications. *Arch. Surg.* **2003**, *138*, 520–523; discussion 523. [CrossRef]
9. Jacobsen, H.J.; Nergard, B.J.; Leifsson, B.G.; Frederiksen, S.G.; Agajahni, E.; Ekelund, M.; Hedenbro, J.; Gislason, H. Management of suspected anastomotic leak after bariatric laparoscopic Roux-en-y gastric bypass. *Br. J. Surg.* **2014**, *101*, 417–423. [CrossRef] [PubMed]
10. Vidarsson, B.; Sundbom, M.; Edholm, D. Incidence and treatment of leak at the gastrojejunostomy in Roux-en-Y gastric bypass: A cohort study of 40,844 patients. *Surg. Obes. Relat. Dis.* **2019**, *15*, 1075–1079. [CrossRef]
11. Csendes, A.; Burgos, A.M.; Braghetto, I. Classification and management of leaks after gastric bypass for patients with morbid obesity: A prospective study of 60 patients. *Obes. Surg.* **2012**, *22*, 855–862. [CrossRef] [PubMed]
12. Burgos, A.M.; Braghetto, I.; Csendes, A.; Maluenda, F.; Korn, O.; Yarmuch, J.; Gutierrez, L. Gastric leak after laparoscopic-sleeve gastrectomy for obesity. *Obes. Surg.* **2009**, *19*, 1672–1677. [CrossRef] [PubMed]
13. Low, D.E.; Alderson, D.; Cecconello, I.; Chang, A.C.; Darling, G.E.; D'Journo, X.B.; Griffin, S.M.; Holscher, A.H.; Hofstetter, W.L.; Jobe, B.A.; et al. International Consensus on Standardization of Data Collection for Complications Associated With Esophagectomy: Esophagectomy Complications Consensus Group (ECCG). *Ann. Surg.* **2015**, *262*, 286–294. [CrossRef]
14. Bludau, M.; Fuchs, H.F.; Herbold, T.; Maus, M.K.H.; Alakus, H.; Popp, F.; Leers, J.M.; Bruns, C.J.; Holscher, A.H.; Schroder, W.; et al. Results of endoscopic vacuum-assisted closure device for treatment of upper GI leaks. *Surg. Endosc.* **2018**, *32*, 1906–1914. [CrossRef] [PubMed]
15. Loske, G.; Muller, C.T. Tips and tricks for endoscopic negative pressure therapy. *Chirurg* **2019**, *90*, 7–14. [CrossRef]
16. Schorsch, T.; Muller, C.; Loske, G. Endoscopic vacuum therapy of anastomotic leakage and iatrogenic perforation in the esophagus. *Surg. Endosc.* **2013**, *27*, 2040–2045. [CrossRef]
17. Laukoetter, M.G.; Mennigen, R.; Neumann, P.A.; Dhayat, S.; Horst, G.; Palmes, D.; Senninger, N.; Vowinkel, T. Successful closure of defects in the upper gastrointestinal tract by endoscopic vacuum therapy (EVT): A prospective cohort study. *Surg. Endosc.* **2017**, *31*, 2687–2696. [CrossRef]

18. Kim, J.; Azagury, D.; Eisenberg, D.; DeMaria, E.; Campos, G.M.; American Society for Metabolic and Bariatric Surgery Clinical Issues Committee. ASMBS position statement on prevention, detection, and treatment of gastrointestinal leak after gastric bypass and sleeve gastrectomy, including the roles of imaging, surgical exploration, and nonoperative management. *Surg. Obes. Relat. Dis.* **2015**, *11*, 739–748. [CrossRef]
19. Paspatis, G.A.; Arvanitakis, M.; Dumonceau, J.M.; Barthet, M.; Saunders, B.; Turino, S.Y.; Dhillon, A.; Fragaki, M.; Gonzalez, J.M.; Repici, A.; et al. Diagnosis and management of iatrogenic endoscopic perforations: European Society of Gastrointestinal Endoscopy (ESGE) Position Statement-Update 2020. *Endoscopy* **2020**, *52*, 792–810. [CrossRef]
20. Souto-Rodriguez, R.; Alvarez-Sanchez, M.V. Endoluminal solutions to bariatric surgery complications: A review with a focus on technical aspects and results. *World J. Gastrointest. Endosc.* **2017**, *9*, 105–126. [CrossRef]
21. Spaander, M.C.; Baron, T.H.; Siersema, P.D.; Fuccio, L.; Schumacher, B.; Escorsell, À.; Garcia-Pagán, J.C.; Dumonceau, J.M.; Conio, M. Esophageal stenting for benign and malignant disease: European Society of Gastrointestinal Endoscopy (ESGE) Clinical Guideline. *Endoscopy* **2016**, *48*, 939–948. [CrossRef]
22. Moyes, L.H.; Mackay, C.K.; Forshaw, M.J. The use of self-expanding plastic stents in the management of oesophageal leaks and spontaneous oesophageal perforations. *Diagn. Ther. Endosc.* **2011**, *2011*, 418103. [CrossRef]
23. van Halsema, E.E.; Wong Kee Song, L.M.; Baron, T.H.; Siersema, P.D.; Vleggaar, F.P.; Ginsberg, G.G.; Shah, P.M.; Fleischer, D.E.; Ratuapli, S.K.; Fockens, P.; et al. Safety of endoscopic removal of self-expandable stents after treatment of benign esophageal diseases. *Gastrointest. Endosc.* **2013**, *77*, 18–28. [CrossRef]
24. van Boeckel, P.G.; Sijbring, A.; Vleggaar, F.P.; Siersema, P.D. Systematic review: Temporary stent placement for benign rupture or anastomotic leak of the oesophagus. *Aliment. Pharmacol. Ther.* **2011**, *33*, 1292–1301. [CrossRef]
25. Dasari, B.V.; Neely, D.; Kennedy, A.; Spence, G.; Rice, P.; Mackle, E.; Epanomeritakis, E. The role of esophageal stents in the management of esophageal anastomotic leaks and benign esophageal perforations. *Ann. Surg.* **2014**, *259*, 852–860. [CrossRef]
26. Kamarajah, S.K.; Bundred, J.; Spence, G.; Kennedy, A.; Dasari, B.V.M.; Griffiths, E.A. Critical Appraisal of the Impact of Oesophageal Stents in the Management of Oesophageal Anastomotic Leaks and Benign Oesophageal Perforations: An Updated Systematic Review. *World J. Surg.* **2020**, *44*, 1173–1189. [CrossRef] [PubMed]
27. Freeman, R.K.; Ascioti, A.J.; Giannini, T.; Mahidhara, R.J. Analysis of unsuccessful esophageal stent placements for esophageal perforation, fistula, or anastomotic leak. *Ann. Thorac. Surg.* **2012**, *94*, 959–964, discussion 964–955. [CrossRef] [PubMed]
28. Lorenzo, D.; Guilbaud, T.; Gonzalez, J.M.; Benezech, A.; Dutour, A.; Boullu, S.; Berdah, S.; Bege, T.; Barthet, M. Endoscopic treatment of fistulas after sleeve gastrectomy: A comparison of internal drainage versus closure. *Gastrointest. Endosc.* **2018**, *87*, 429–437. [CrossRef] [PubMed]
29. Ngamruengphong, S.; Sharaiha, R.; Sethi, A.; Siddiqui, A.; DiMaio, C.J.; Gonzalez, S.; Rogart, J.; Jagroop, S.; Widmer, J.; Im, J.; et al. Fully-covered metal stents with endoscopic suturing vs. partially-covered metal stents for benign upper gastrointestinal diseases: A comparative study. *Endosc. Int. Open* **2018**, *6*, E217–E223. [CrossRef]
30. Schiemer, M.; Bettinger, D.; Mueller, J.; Schultheiss, M.; Schwacha, H.; Hasselblatt, P.; Thimme, R.; Schmidt, A.; Kuellmer, A. Reduction of esophageal stent migration rate with a novel over-the-scope fixation device (with video). *Gastrointest. Endosc.* **2022**, *96*, 1–8. [CrossRef] [PubMed]
31. Fugazza, A.; Lamonaca, L.; Mercante, G.; Civilini, E.; Pradella, A.; Anderloni, A.; Repici, A. The worst adverse event for an endoscopist after esophageal stent placement: An aortoesophageal fistula. *Endoscopy* **2022**, *54*, E44–E45. [CrossRef] [PubMed]
32. Freeman, R.K.; Ascioti, A.J.; Dake, M.; Mahidhara, R.S. An Assessment of the Optimal Time for Removal of Esophageal Stents Used in the Treatment of an Esophageal Anastomotic Leak or Perforation. *Ann. Thorac. Surg.* **2015**, *100*, 422–428. [CrossRef] [PubMed]
33. van Heel, N.C.; Haringsma, J.; Spaander, M.C.; Bruno, M.J.; Kuipers, E.J. Short-term esophageal stenting in the management of benign perforations. *Am. J. Gastroenterol.* **2010**, *105*, 1515–1520. [CrossRef] [PubMed]
34. Rodrigues-Pinto, E.; Repici, A.; Donatelli, G.; Macedo, G.; Deviere, J.; van Hooft, J.E.; Campos, J.M.; Galvao Neto, M.; Silva, M.; Eisendrath, P.; et al. International multicenter expert survey on endoscopic treatment of upper gastrointestinal anastomotic leaks. *Endosc. Int. Open* **2019**, *7*, E1671–E1682. [CrossRef] [PubMed]
35. Cerna, M.; Kocher, M.; Valek, V.; Aujesky, R.; Neoral, C.; Andrasina, T.; Panek, J.; Mahathmakanthi, S. Covered biodegradable stent: New therapeutic option for the management of esophageal perforation or anastomotic leak. *Cardiovasc. Interv. Radiol.* **2011**, *34*, 1267–1271. [CrossRef]
36. Kones, O.; Oran, E. Self-Expanding Biodegradable Stents for Postoperative Upper Gastrointestinal Issues. *JSLS* **2018**, *22*, e2018.00011. [CrossRef]
37. Shehab, H.M.; Hakky, S.M.; Gawdat, K.A. An Endoscopic Strategy Combining Mega Stents and Over-The-Scope Clips for the Management of Post-Bariatric Surgery Leaks and Fistulas (with video). *Obes. Surg.* **2016**, *26*, 941–948. [CrossRef] [PubMed]
38. Shehab, H.; Abdallah, E.; Gawdat, K.; Elattar, I. Large Bariatric-Specific Stents and Over-the-Scope Clips in the Management of Post-Bariatric Surgery Leaks. *Obes. Surg.* **2018**, *28*, 15–24. [CrossRef]
39. Tringali, A.; Bove, V.; Perri, V.; Landi, R.; Familiari, P.; Boskoski, I.; Costamagna, G. Endoscopic treatment of post-laparoscopic sleeve gastrectomy leaks using a specifically designed metal stent. *Endoscopy* **2017**, *49*, 64–68. [CrossRef]
40. Boerlage, T.C.C.; Houben, G.P.M.; Groenen, M.J.M.; van der Linde, K.; van de Laar, A.; Emous, M.; Fockens, P.; Voermans, R.P. A novel fully covered double-bump stent for staple line leaks after bariatric surgery: A retrospective analysis. *Surg. Endosc.* **2018**, *32*, 3174–3180. [CrossRef]

41. Shehab, H.; Mikhail, H. Gastroseal: A Novel Stent Design for the Management of Post-Bariatric Surgery Leaks. *ACG Case Rep. J.* **2018**, *5*, e85. [CrossRef]
42. van Wezenbeek, M.R.; de Milliano, M.M.; Nienhuijs, S.W.; Friederich, P.; Gilissen, L.P. A Specifically Designed Stent for Anastomotic Leaks after Bariatric Surgery: Experiences in a Tertiary Referral Hospital. *Obes. Surg.* **2016**, *26*, 1875–1880. [CrossRef] [PubMed]
43. Hamid, H.K.S.; Emile, S.H.; Saber, A.A.; Dincer, M.; de Moura, D.T.H.; Gilissen, L.P.L.; Almadi, M.A.; Montuori, M.; Vix, M.; Perisse, L.G.S.; et al. Customized bariatric stents for sleeve gastrectomy leak: Are they superior to conventional esophageal stents? A systematic review and proportion meta-analysis. *Surg. Endosc.* **2021**, *35*, 1025–1038. [CrossRef]
44. Ritter, L.A.; Wang, A.Y.; Sauer, B.G.; Kleiner, D.E. Healing of complicated gastric leaks in bariatric patients using endoscopic clips. *JSLS* **2013**, *17*, 481–483. [CrossRef] [PubMed]
45. Yilmaz, B.; Unlu, O.; Roach, E.C.; Can, G.; Efe, C.; Korkmaz, U.; Kurt, M. Endoscopic clips for the closure of acute iatrogenic perforations: Where do we stand? *Dig. Endosc.* **2015**, *27*, 641–648. [CrossRef] [PubMed]
46. Qadeer, M.A.; Dumot, J.A.; Vargo, J.J.; Lopez, A.R.; Rice, T.W. Endoscopic clips for closing esophageal perforations: Case report and pooled analysis. *Gastrointest. Endosc.* **2007**, *66*, 605–611. [CrossRef]
47. Lee, S.; Ahn, J.Y.; Jung, H.Y.; Lee, J.H.; Choi, K.S.; Kim, D.H.; Choi, K.D.; Song, H.J.; Lee, G.H.; Kim, J.H.; et al. Clinical outcomes of endoscopic and surgical management for postoperative upper gastrointestinal leakage. *Surg. Endosc.* **2013**, *27*, 4232–4240. [CrossRef]
48. Bartell, N.; Bittner, K.; Kaul, V.; Kothari, T.H.; Kothari, S. Clinical efficacy of the over-the-scope clip device: A systematic review. *World J. Gastroenterol.* **2020**, *26*, 3495–3516. [CrossRef] [PubMed]
49. Manta, R.; Manno, M.; Bertani, H.; Barbera, C.; Pigo, F.; Mirante, V.; Longinotti, E.; Bassotti, G.; Conigliaro, R. Endoscopic treatment of gastrointestinal fistulas using an over-the-scope clip (OTSC) device: Case series from a tertiary referral center. *Endoscopy* **2011**, *43*, 545–548. [CrossRef]
50. Rogalski, P.; Swidnicka-Siergiejko, A.; Wasielica-Berger, J.; Zienkiewicz, D.; Wieckowska, B.; Wroblewski, E.; Baniukiewicz, A.; Rogalska-Plonska, M.; Siergiejko, G.; Dabrowski, A.; et al. Endoscopic management of leaks and fistulas after bariatric surgery: A systematic review and meta-analysis. *Surg. Endosc.* **2021**, *35*, 1067–1087. [CrossRef]
51. Haito-Chavez, Y.; Law, J.K.; Kratt, T.; Arezzo, A.; Verra, M.; Morino, M.; Sharaiha, R.Z.; Poley, J.W.; Kahaleh, M.; Thompson, C.C.; et al. International multicenter experience with an over-the-scope clipping device for endoscopic management of GI defects (with video). *Gastrointest. Endosc.* **2014**, *80*, 610–622. [CrossRef]
52. Mercky, P.; Gonzalez, J.M.; Aimore Bonin, E.; Emungania, O.; Brunet, J.; Grimaud, J.C.; Barthet, M. Usefulness of over-the-scope clipping system for closing digestive fistulas. *Dig. Endosc.* **2015**, *27*, 18–24. [CrossRef]
53. Dinelli, M.; Omazzi, B.; Andreozzi, P.; Zucchini, N.; Redaelli, A.; Manes, G. First clinical experiences with a novel endoscopic over-the-scope clip system. *Endosc. Int. Open* **2017**, *5*, E151–E156. [CrossRef] [PubMed]
54. Armellini, E.; Crino, S.F.; Orsello, M.; Ballare, M.; Tari, R.; Saettone, S.; Montino, F.; Occhipinti, P. Novel endoscopic over-the-scope clip system. *World J. Gastroenterol.* **2015**, *21*, 13587–13592. [CrossRef] [PubMed]
55. Abraham, A.; Vasant, D.H.; McLaughlin, J.; Paine, P.A. Endoscopic closure of a refractory gastrocutaneous fistula using a novel over-the-scope Padlock clip following de-epithelialisation of the fistula tract. *BMJ Case Rep.* **2015**, *2015*, bcr2015211242. [CrossRef]
56. Anderloni, A.; Bianchetti, M.; Mangiavillano, B.; Fugazza, A.; Di Leo, M.; Carrara, S.; Repici, A. Successful endoscopic closure of iatrogenic duodenal perforation with the new Padlock Clip. *Endoscopy* **2017**, *49*, E58–E59. [CrossRef]
57. Moran, E.A.; Gostout, C.J.; Bingener, J. Preliminary performance of a flexible cap and catheter-based endoscopic suturing system. *Gastrointest. Endosc.* **2009**, *69*, 1375–1383. [CrossRef] [PubMed]
58. Sharaiha, R.Z.; Kumta, N.A.; DeFilippis, E.M.; Dimaio, C.J.; Gonzalez, S.; Gonda, T.; Rogart, J.; Siddiqui, A.; Berg, P.S.; Samuels, P.; et al. A Large Multicenter Experience With Endoscopic Suturing for Management of Gastrointestinal Defects and Stent Anchorage in 122 Patients: A Retrospective Review. *J. Clin. Gastroenterol.* **2016**, *50*, 388–392. [CrossRef] [PubMed]
59. Chon, S.H.; Toex, U.; Plum, P.S.; Kleinert, R.; Bruns, C.J.; Goeser, T.; Berlth, F. Efficacy and feasibility of OverStitch suturing of leaks in the upper gastrointestinal tract. *Surg. Endosc.* **2020**, *34*, 3861–3869. [CrossRef] [PubMed]
60. Mohan, B.; Khan, S.R.; Madhu, D.; Kassab, L.; Jonnadula, S.; Chandan, S.; Facciorusso, A.; Adler, D. Clinical Outcomes of Endoscopic Suturing in Gastrointestinal Fistulas, Leaks, Perforations and Mucosal Defects: A Systematic Review and Meta-Analysis. *Am. J. Gastroenterol.* **2021**, *116*, S470–S471. [CrossRef]
61. Granata, A.; Amata, M.; Ligresti, D.; Martino, A.; Tarantino, I.; Barresi, L.; Traina, M. Endoscopic management of post-surgical GI wall defects with the overstitch endosuturing system: A single-center experience. *Surg. Endosc.* **2020**, *34*, 3805–3817. [CrossRef] [PubMed]
62. Jirapinyo, P.; Kumar, N.; AlSamman, M.A.; Thompson, C.C. Five-year outcomes of transoral outlet reduction for the treatment of weight regain after Roux-en-Y gastric bypass. *Gastrointest. Endosc.* **2020**, *91*, 1067–1073. [CrossRef]
63. Weidenhagen, R.; Gruetzner, K.U.; Wiecken, T.; Spelsberg, F.; Jauch, K.W. Endoscopic vacuum-assisted closure of anastomotic leakage following anterior resection of the rectum: A new method. *Surg. Endosc.* **2008**, *22*, 1818–1825. [CrossRef] [PubMed]
64. Wedemeyer, J.; Schneider, A.; Manns, M.P.; Jackobs, S. Endoscopic vacuum-assisted closure of upper intestinal anastomotic leaks. *Gastrointest. Endosc.* **2008**, *67*, 708–711. [CrossRef]
65. Loske, G.; Muller, C. Vacuum therapy of an esophageal anastomotic leakage—A case report. *Zentralbl. Chir.* **2009**, *134*, 267–270. [CrossRef]

66. Loske, G.; Muller, C. Endoscopic vacuum-assisted closure of upper intestinal anastomotic leaks. *Gastrointest. Endosc.* **2009**, *69*, 601–602, author reply 602. [CrossRef]
67. Jung, D.H.; Yun, H.R.; Lee, S.J.; Kim, N.W.; Huh, C.W. Endoscopic Vacuum Therapy in Patients with Transmural Defects of the Upper Gastrointestinal Tract: A Systematic Review with Meta-Analysis. *J. Clin. Med.* **2021**, *10*, 2346. [CrossRef] [PubMed]
68. Tavares, G.; Tustumi, F.; Tristao, L.S.; Bernardo, W.M. Endoscopic vacuum therapy for anastomotic leak in esophagectomy and total gastrectomy: A systematic review and meta-analysis. *Dis. Esophagus.* **2021**, *34*, doaa132. [CrossRef]
69. Schmidt, F.; Mennigen, R.; Vowinkel, T.; Neumann, P.A.; Senninger, N.; Palmes, D.; Laukoetter, M.G. Endoscopic Vacuum Therapy (EVT)-a New Concept for Complication Management in Bariatric Surgery. *Obes. Surg.* **2017**, *27*, 2499–2505. [CrossRef] [PubMed]
70. Morell, B.; Murray, F.; Vetter, D.; Bueter, M.; Gubler, C. Endoscopic vacuum therapy (EVT) for early infradiaphragmal leakage after bariatric surgery-outcomes of six consecutive cases in a single institution. *Langenbecks Arch. Surg.* **2019**, *404*, 115–121. [CrossRef]
71. Markus, A.; Henrik, B.J.; Benedikt, R.; Alexander, H.; Thomas, B.; Clemens, S.; Jan-Hendrik, E. Endoscopic vacuum therapy in salvage and standalone treatment of gastric leaks after bariatric surgery. *Langenbecks Arch. Surg.* **2021**, *407*, 1039–1046. [CrossRef]
72. Leeds, S.G.; Burdick, J.S. Management of gastric leaks after sleeve gastrectomy with endoluminal vacuum (E-Vac) therapy. *Surg. Obes. Relat. Dis.* **2016**, *12*, 1278–1285. [CrossRef]
73. Argenta, L.C.; Morykwas, M.J. Vacuum-assisted closure: A new method for wound control and treatment: Clinical experience. *Ann. Plast Surg.* **1997**, *38*, 563–576, discussion 577. [CrossRef] [PubMed]
74. Jung, C.F.M.; Muller-Dornieden, A.; Gaedcke, J.; Kunsch, S.; Gromski, M.A.; Biggemann, L.; Seif Amir Hosseini, A.; Ghadimi, M.; Ellenrieder, V.; Wedi, E. Impact of Endoscopic Vacuum Therapy with Low Negative Pressure for Esophageal Perforations and Postoperative Anastomotic Esophageal Leaks. *Digestion* **2021**, *102*, 469–479. [CrossRef]
75. Loske, G.; Müller, J.; Schulze, W.; Riefel, B.; Müller, C.T. Pre-emptive active drainage of reflux (PARD) in Ivor-Lewis oesophagectomy with negative pressure and simultaneous enteral nutrition using a double-lumen open-pore film drain (dOFD). *Surg. Endosc.* **2022**, *36*, 2208–2216. [CrossRef] [PubMed]
76. Loske, G.; Schorsch, T.; Rucktaeschel, F.; Schulze, W.; Riefel, B.; van Ackeren, V.; Mueller, C.T. Open-pore film drainage (OFD): A new multipurpose tool for endoscopic negative pressure therapy (ENPT). *Endosc. Int. Open* **2018**, *6*, E865–E871. [CrossRef] [PubMed]
77. Wedi, E.; Schuler, P.; Kunsch, S.; Ghadimi, B.M.; Seif Amir Hosseini, A.; Ellenrieder, V.; Jung, C. Individual endoscopic management of anastomotic insufficiency after esophagectomy for esophageal squamous cell carcinoma and creation of a neostomach. *Endoscopy* **2018**, *50*, E69–E71. [CrossRef]
78. Brangewitz, M.; Voigtlander, T.; Helfritz, F.A.; Lankisch, T.O.; Winkler, M.; Klempnauer, J.; Manns, M.P.; Schneider, A.S.; Wedemeyer, J. Endoscopic closure of esophageal intrathoracic leaks: Stent versus endoscopic vacuum-assisted closure, a retrospective analysis. *Endoscopy* **2013**, *45*, 433–438. [CrossRef]
79. Min, Y.W.; Kim, T.; Lee, H.; Min, B.H.; Kim, H.K.; Choi, Y.S.; Lee, J.H.; Rhee, P.L.; Kim, J.J.; Zo, J.I.; et al. Endoscopic vacuum therapy for postoperative esophageal leak. *BMC Surg.* **2019**, *19*, 37. [CrossRef]
80. Schniewind, B.; Schafmayer, C.; Both, M.; Arlt, A.; Fritscher-Ravens, A.; Hampe, J. Ingrowth and device disintegration in an intralobar abscess cavity during endosponge therapy for esophageal anastomotic leakage. *Endoscopy* **2011**, *43* (Suppl. 2), E64–E65. [CrossRef]
81. Jung, D.H.; Huh, C.W.; Min, Y.W.; Park, J.C. Endoscopic vacuum therapy for the management of upper GI leaks and perforations: A multicenter retrospective study of factors associated with treatment failure (with video). *Gastrointest. Endosc.* **2022**, *95*, 281–290. [CrossRef] [PubMed]
82. Gubler, C.; Vetter, D.; Schmidt, H.M.; Muller, P.C.; Morell, B.; Raptis, D.; Gutschow, C.A. Preemptive endoluminal vacuum therapy to reduce anastomotic leakage after esophagectomy: A game-changing approach? *Dis. Esophagus* **2019**, *32*, doy126. [CrossRef]
83. Neumann, P.A.; Mennigen, R.; Palmes, D.; Senninger, N.; Vowinkel, T.; Laukoetter, M.G. Pre-emptive endoscopic vacuum therapy for treatment of anastomotic ischemia after esophageal resections. *Endoscopy* **2017**, *49*, 498–503. [CrossRef]
84. Scognamiglio, P.; Reeh, M.; Karstens, K.; Bellon, E.; Kantowski, M.; Schon, G.; Zapf, A.; Chon, S.H.; Izbicki, J.R.; Tachezy, M. Endoscopic vacuum therapy versus stenting for postoperative esophago-enteric anastomotic leakage: Systematic review and meta-analysis. *Endoscopy* **2020**, *52*, 632–642. [CrossRef]
85. do Monte Junior, E.S.; de Moura, D.T.H.; Ribeiro, I.B.; Hathorn, K.E.; Farias, G.F.A.; Turiani, C.V.; Medeiros, F.S.; Bernardo, W.M.; de Moura, E.G.H. Endoscopic vacuum therapy versus endoscopic stenting for upper gastrointestinal transmural defects: Systematic review and meta-analysis. *Dig. Endosc.* **2021**, *33*, 892–902. [CrossRef] [PubMed]
86. Tachezy, M.; Chon, S.H.; Rieck, I.; Kantowski, M.; Christ, H.; Karstens, K.; Gebauer, F.; Goeser, T.; Rosch, T.; Izbicki, J.R.; et al. Endoscopic vacuum therapy versus stent treatment of esophageal anastomotic leaks (ESOLEAK): Study protocol for a prospective randomized phase 2 trial. *Trials* **2021**, *22*, 377. [CrossRef] [PubMed]
87. Archid, R.; Bazerbachi, F.; Abu Dayyeh, B.K.; Hones, F.; Ahmad, S.J.S.; Thiel, K.; Nadiradze, G.; Konigsrainer, A.; Wichmann, D. Endoscopic Negative Pressure Therapy (ENPT) Is Superior to Stent Therapy for Staple Line Leak After Sleeve Gastrectomy: A Single-Center Cohort Study. *Obes. Surg.* **2021**, *31*, 2511–2519. [CrossRef]
88. Pequignot, A.; Fuks, D.; Verhaeghe, P.; Dhahri, A.; Brehant, O.; Bartoli, E.; Delcenserie, R.; Yzet, T.; Regimbeau, J.M. Is there a place for pigtail drains in the management of gastric leaks after laparoscopic sleeve gastrectomy? *Obes. Surg.* **2012**, *22*, 712–720. [CrossRef]

89. Donatelli, G.; Dumont, J.L.; Cereatti, F.; Ferretti, S.; Vergeau, B.M.; Tuszynski, T.; Pourcher, G.; Tranchart, H.; Mariani, P.; Meduri, A.; et al. Treatment of Leaks Following Sleeve Gastrectomy by Endoscopic Internal Drainage (EID). *Obes. Surg.* **2015**, *25*, 1293–1301. [CrossRef]
90. Donatelli, G.; Ferretti, S.; Vergeau, B.M.; Dhumane, P.; Dumont, J.L.; Derhy, S.; Tuszynski, T.; Dritsas, S.; Carloni, A.; Catheline, J.M.; et al. Endoscopic Internal Drainage with Enteral Nutrition (EDEN) for treatment of leaks following sleeve gastrectomy. *Obes. Surg.* **2014**, *24*, 1400–1407. [CrossRef]
91. Donatelli, G.; Dumont, J.L.; Cereatti, F.; Dhumane, P.; Tuszynski, T.; Vergeau, B.M.; Meduri, B. Endoscopic internal drainage as first-line treatment for fistula following gastrointestinal surgery: A case series. *Endosc. Int. Open* **2016**, *4*, E647–E651. [CrossRef]
92. Gonzalez, J.M.; Lorenzo, D.; Guilbaud, T.; Bege, T.; Barthet, M. Internal endoscopic drainage as first line or second line treatment in case of postsleeve gastrectomy fistulas. *Endosc. Int. Open* **2018**, *6*, E745–E750. [CrossRef]
93. Siddique, I.; Alazmi, W.; Al-Sabah, S.K. Endoscopic internal drainage by double pigtail stents in the management of laparoscopic sleeve gastrectomy leaks. *Surg. Obes. Relat. Dis.* **2020**, *16*, 831–838. [CrossRef]
94. Hallit, R.; Calmels, M.; Chaput, U.; Lorenzo, D.; Becq, A.; Camus, M.; Dray, X.; Gonzalez, J.M.; Barthet, M.; Jacques, J.; et al. Endoscopic management of anastomotic leak after esophageal or gastric resection for malignancy: A multicenter experience. *Ther. Adv. Gastroenterol.* **2021**, *14*, 17562848211032823. [CrossRef]
95. Bouchard, S.; Eisendrath, P.; Toussaint, E.; Le Moine, O.; Lemmers, A.; Arvanitakis, M.; Deviere, J. Trans-fistulary endoscopic drainage for post-bariatric abdominal collections communicating with the upper gastrointestinal tract. *Endoscopy* **2016**, *48*, 809–816. [CrossRef]
96. Toh, B.C.; Chong, J.; Yeung, B.P.M.; Lim, C.H.; Lim, E.K.W.; Chan, W.H.; Tan, J.T.H. Endoscopic Internal Drainage with Double Pigtail Stents for Upper Gastrointestinal Anastomotic Leaks: Suitable for All Cases? *Korean J. Gastrointest. Endosc.* **2022**, *55*, 401–407. [CrossRef] [PubMed]
97. Donatelli, G.; Spota, A.; Cereatti, F.; Granieri, S.; Dagher, I.; Chiche, R.; Catheline, J.M.; Pourcher, G.; Rebibo, L.; Calabrese, D.; et al. Endoscopic internal drainage for the management of leak, fistula, and collection after sleeve gastrectomy: Our experience in 617 consecutive patients. *Surg. Obes. Relat. Dis.* **2021**, *17*, 1432–1439. [CrossRef] [PubMed]
98. Laopeamthong, I.; Akethanin, T.; Kasetsermwiriya, W.; Techapongsatorn, S.; Tansawet, A. Vacuum Therapy and Internal Drainage as the First-Line Endoscopic Treatment for Post-Bariatric Leaks: A Systematic Review and Meta-Analysis. *Visc. Med.* **2021**, *38*, 63–71. [CrossRef]
99. Jung, C.F.M.; Hallit, R.; Muller-Dornieden, A.; Calmels, M.; Goere, D.; Chaput, U.; Camus, M.; Gonzalez, J.M.; Barthet, M.; Jacques, J.; et al. Endoscopic internal drainage and low negative-pressure endoscopic vacuum therapy for anastomotic leaks after oncologic upper gastrointestinal surgery. *Endoscopy* **2022**, *54*, 71–74. [CrossRef] [PubMed]
100. Lange, J.; Dormann, A.; Bulian, D.R.; Hugle, U.; Eisenberger, C.F.; Heiss, M.M. VACStent: Combining the benefits of endoscopic vacuum therapy and covered stents for upper gastrointestinal tract leakage. *Endosc. Int. Open* **2021**, *9*, E971–E976. [CrossRef]
101. Valli, P.V.; Mertens, J.C.; Kroger, A.; Gubler, C.; Gutschow, C.; Schneider, P.M.; Bauerfeind, P. Stent-over-sponge (SOS): A novel technique complementing endosponge therapy for foregut leaks and perforations. *Endoscopy* **2018**, *50*, 148–153. [CrossRef] [PubMed]
102. Nachira, D.; Trivisonno, A.; Costamagna, G.; Toietta, G.; Margaritora, S.; Pontecorvi, V.; Punzo, G.; Porziella, V.; Boskoski, I. Successful Therapy of Esophageal Fistulas by Endoscopic Injection of Emulsified Adipose Tissue Stromal Vascular Fraction. *Gastroenterology* **2021**, *160*, 1026–1028. [CrossRef] [PubMed]
103. Di Leo, M.; Maselli, R.; Ferrara, E.C.; Poliani, L.; Al Awadhi, S.; Repici, A. Endoscopic Management of Benign Esophageal Ruptures and Leaks. *Curr. Treat. Options Gastroenterol.* **2017**, *15*, 268–284. [CrossRef]
104. Csendes, A.; Burdiles, P.; Burgos, A.M.; Maluenda, F.; Diaz, J.C. Conservative management of anastomotic leaks after 557 open gastric bypasses. *Obes. Surg.* **2005**, *15*, 1252–1256. [CrossRef]
105. Schniewind, B.; Schafmayer, C.; Voehrs, G.; Egberts, J.; von Schoenfels, W.; Rose, T.; Kurdow, R.; Arlt, A.; Ellrichmann, M.; Jurgensen, C.; et al. Endoscopic endoluminal vacuum therapy is superior to other regimens in managing anastomotic leakage after esophagectomy: A comparative retrospective study. *Surg. Endosc.* **2013**, *27*, 3883–3890. [CrossRef] [PubMed]

Disclaimer/Publisher's Note: The statements, opinions and data contained in all publications are solely those of the individual author(s) and contributor(s) and not of MDPI and/or the editor(s). MDPI and/or the editor(s) disclaim responsibility for any injury to people or property resulting from any ideas, methods, instructions or products referred to in the content.

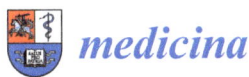

Case Report

Detection of Neuroendocrine Tumours by Enteroscopy: A Case Report

Adriana Ortega Larrode *, Sergio Farrais Villalba, Claudia Guerrero Muñoz, Leonardo Blas Jhon, Maria Jesus Martin Relloso, Paloma Sanchez-Fayos Calabuig, Daniel Calero Baron, Andres Varela Silva and Juan Carlos Porres Cubero

Department of Gastroenterology, Fundación Jiménez Díaz University Hospital, 28040 Madrid, Spain; sfarraisv@quironsalud.es (S.F.V.); claudia.guerrero@quironsalud.es (C.G.M.); lblasjh@fjd.es (L.B.J.); mjmartin@fjd.es (M.J.M.R.); psanchez@quironsalud.es (P.S.-F.C.); dcalerob@fjd.es (D.C.B.); alvarela@quironsalud.es (A.V.S.); jcporres@fjd.es (J.C.P.C.)
* Correspondence: adriana.ortega@quironsalud.es

Abstract: We present the case of a 62-year-old patient who developed melenas and in whom conventional endoscopic tests could not detect any bleeding lesion. In our case, capsule endoscopy and enteroscopy were the pivotal elements in establishing the diagnosis of a neuroendocrine tumour with an atypical location. As a result, it was possible to surgically remove the lesions at an early stage of the malignancy without metastatic disease and without the need for adjuvant therapy. Our case demonstrates the need for these new techniques in tumours of atypical location and aggressive course. Otherwise, this malignancy may be underdiagnosed until an advanced stage.

Keywords: NET; capsule endoscopy; enteroscopy; case report

Citation: Ortega Larrode, A.; Farrais Villalba, S.; Guerrero Muñoz, C.; Blas Jhon, L.; Martin Relloso, M.J.; Sanchez-Fayos Calabuig, P.; Calero Baron, D.; Varela Silva, A.; Porres Cubero, J.C. Detection of Neuroendocrine Tumours by Enteroscopy: A Case Report. *Medicina* 2023, 59, 1469. https://doi.org/10.3390/medicina59081469

Academic Editor: Žilvinas Dambrauskas

Received: 27 July 2023
Revised: 9 August 2023
Accepted: 14 August 2023
Published: 16 August 2023

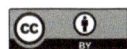

Copyright: © 2023 by the authors. Licensee MDPI, Basel, Switzerland. This article is an open access article distributed under the terms and conditions of the Creative Commons Attribution (CC BY) license (https://creativecommons.org/licenses/by/4.0/).

1. Introduction

Gastrointestinal (GI) neuroendocrine tumours (NET) are rare neoplasms that arise from specialized neuroendocrine cells. Generally, this malignancy can be found anywhere along the gastrointestinal tract and has a poor outcome. They represent a diverse group of neoplasms closely related to the presence of autoimmune atrophic gastritis [1,2]. These tumours represent a therapeutic challenge where endoscopic studies are a fundamental element for their diagnosis [1]. NETs have gained increasing recognition and attention in recent years due to their unique characteristics, complex classification, and diverse clinical presentations. Due to their atypical location, lesions located in the small intestine and colon are usually identified at a late stage, when the disease is at an advanced stage and with widespread dissemination [3]. The development of video capsule endoscopy (VCE) and enteroscopy has facilitated the visualisation of otherwise inaccessible lesions [4]. Our case is a sample of this challenging scenario in which a 62-year-old patient with no previous pathologies developed melenas and in whom previous conventional endoscopic tests did not show any bleeding lesion. Enteroscopy was the decisive and final technique to reach diagnosis.

2. Case Presentation

A 62-year-old male with no past medical history was admitted to hospital two months prior to the current episode with obscure gastrointestinal bleeding (OGIB) in the form of melena. The patient had been taking non-steroidal anti-inflammatory drugs for several days without taking proton pump inhibitors. On arrival at the center of origin, the patient had a hemoglobin of 100 g/L with a mean corpuscular volume of 67 fl.

An upper endoscopy was performed to rule out the presence of gastric lesions, showing the presence of bulbitis with no other findings. Therefore, a colonoscopy was performed, in which only sigmoid diverticula were visualised, showing the presence of hematic debris from the small intestine. No bleeding point was found in the colon.

However, having a strong suspicion that a bleeding lesion in the small intestine was causing the melena, a VCE was performed, which showed a subepithelial lesion in the middle jejunum of about 6–7 mm in size with no hematic debris. Upon remission of the bleeding, the patient was discharged with treatment with oral iron and proton pump inhibitors. After outpatient management with oral iron, hemoglobin improved to 115 g/L one month later. In addition, an abdominal computed tomography scan was performed, which failed to identify signs of active intestinal bleeding but showed mild changes related to acute diverticulitis at the descending colon–sigmoid junction. For a more accurate diagnosis, he was referred to our center for further study.

On arrival at our hospital, the patient showed normal hemoglobin levels of 130 g/L with intense iron deficiency with a 2% iron saturation index, elevated transferrin of 413 mg/dL and ferritin of 14 ng/mL. Elevated circulating Chromogranin Alevels of 277.1 ng/mL were found. With the patient's report and the previous results, it was decided to optimize the diagnosis by performing an enteroscopy.

From proximal to distal ileum (respecting the last cm) around 10 umbilicated, yellowish, submucosal nodular lesions of 3–12 mm, with superficial neovascularization, suggestive of neuroendocrine tumours, were visualized (Figure 1).

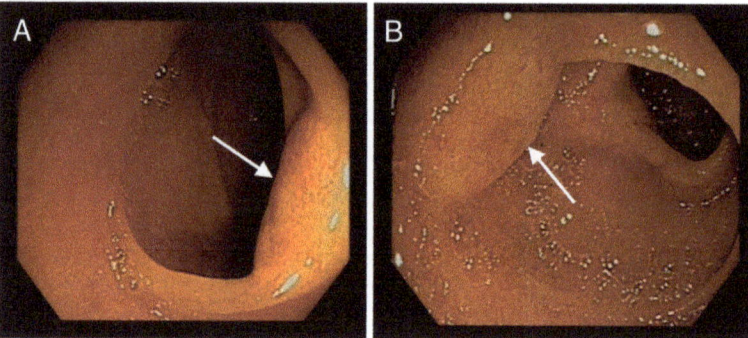

Figure 1. (**A**,**B**): Endoscopic images of jejunum showing nodular, submucosal, umbilicated, yellowish lesions with superficial neovascularization (denoted by arrows).

Multiple biopsies were taken, and the proximal (oral) edge of the first lesion was marked with activated charcoal (Figure 2).

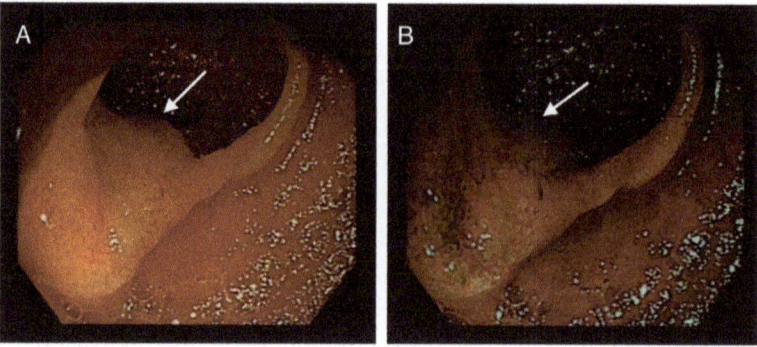

Figure 2. (**A**): arrow pointing at another lesion in the jejunum. (**B**): Same jejunal lesion marked with activated charcoal.

Enteroscopy allowed to advance along the entire length of the small bowel, even achieving complete visualization of the ileocecal valve from a proximal view (Figure 3).

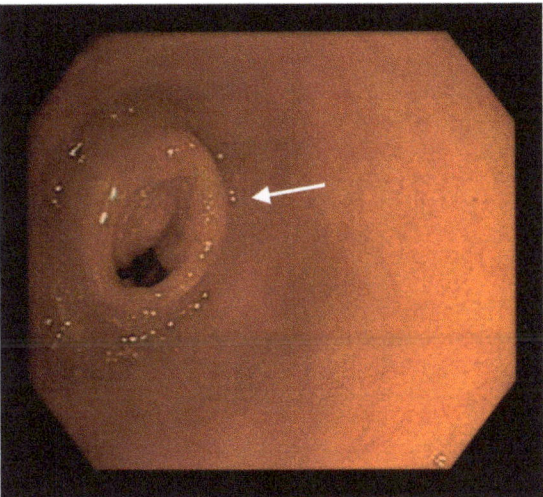

Figure 3. Endoscopic image of the ileocaecal valve (indicated with an arrow) from a proximal (oral) approach reached by enteroscopy.

Pathologist reported the finding of a well-differentiated NET grade 1 with intense and diffuse positivity for chromogranin and synaptophysin with low Ki67 (<3%). Full body Positron Emission Tomography Computerized Tomography (PET-CT) scan, as well as hormone blood tests, were performed for staging. The PET-CT scan was performed using 68Ga-DOTATOC, (a somatostatin receptor-targeted ligand). The study showed lesions along the entire length of the jejunum with several bowel segments involved (Figure 4). After these findings, the case was presented to the Multidisciplinary Committee of Digestive Neoplasms. The surgical management of the lesions was decided together with the General Surgery Department. The patient was referred to them for excision of the affected intestinal segment.

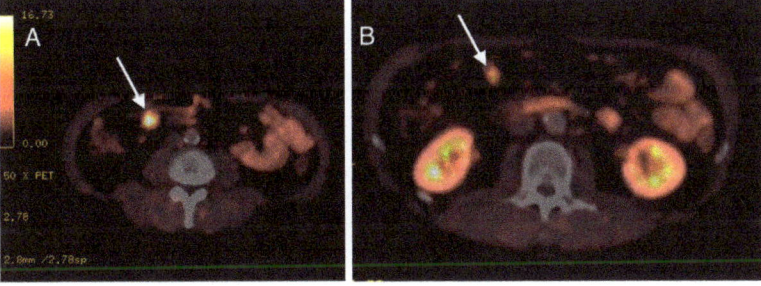

Figure 4. (**A**,**B**): PET-CT scan images showing radiotracer-targeted lesions pointed by arrows.

The surgeons performed a supra-infraumbilical midline laparotomy. Upon entry into the cavity and after exploration of the entire abdomen, multiple lesions in the small intestine (ileum) were evidenced. A segment of small bowel was resected (with distal border about 15 cm from the ileocecal valve) including all the suspicious lesions, and a manual laterolateral anastomosis was performed. The postoperative recovery was satisfactory and the patient was discharged with oral tolerance and digestive transit.

Due to the complete resection of the lesions and the absence of distant disease, the use of adjuvant therapies was not necessary. The patient has not experienced any further episodes of gastrointestinal bleeding with a 5-month follow-up.

3. Discussion

NETs exhibit a wide range of clinical presentations, largely dependent on their location, size, functionality, and hormone production. Functional tumours often lead to hormone-related symptoms, known as syndromes. Carcinoid syndrome, characterized by flushing, diarrhea, and wheezing, is commonly associated with GI tract NETs. Insulinoma syndrome arises from pancreatic NETs (pNETs) and manifests as hypoglycemia due to excessive insulin secretion. Similarly, gastrinoma syndrome results from pNETs secreting gastrin, leading to peptic ulcers and acid hypersecretion. Non-functional tumours, on the other hand, may remain asymptomatic until they reach an advanced stage or cause local symptoms due to mass effect. These can include abdominal pain, obstruction, and bleeding, depending on the tumour's location. The diverse clinical presentations of NETs contribute to the diagnostic challenge they pose [5].

Therefore, the diagnosis of NETs is intricate and necessitates a combination of clinical assessment, imaging studies, and laboratory tests. Imaging techniques play a pivotal role in detecting and localizing NETs. Computed tomography (CT), magnetic resonance imaging (MRI), and somatostatin receptor scintigraphy (SRS) are commonly employed to visualize the tumours and assess their extent [6]. Laboratory tests measure specific biomarkers, such as chromogranin A and 5-hydroxyindoleacetic acid (5-HIAA), which aid in diagnosing and monitoring NETs. Chromogranin A, a protein released by neuroendocrine cells, serves as a valuable marker for disease progression and treatment response. 5-HIAA, a breakdown product of serotonin, is elevated in carcinoid syndrome and assists in diagnosing GI tract NETs. A histopathological analysis of biopsy specimens is essential for confirming the diagnosis and determining the tumour's grade and stage. Immunohistochemical staining can help identify neuroendocrine markers, further characterizing the tumour [7].

OGIB can be a challenge for clinical practice, causing a need for recurrent medical procedures usually associated with chronic anemization, and serial tests without finding a causal factor [8]. Furthermore, the use of advanced diagnostic techniques such as VCE and enteroscopy has become essential for the management of these conditions, providing the ability to diagnose lesions that were previously inaccessible by other techniques [9].

The small intestine constitutes approximately 90% of the entire gastrointestinal tract. Despite this, tumours located in this region account for only 3% of all malignant gastrointestinal neoplasms. The most frequent malignancies are adenocarcinoma, representing almost 60% of the total, and gastrointestinal stromal tumours, representing about 17%. Sarcomas, lymphomas and NETs are less frequent entities [10,11].

Accordingly, and in line with the above, GI NETs are rare compared to other types of gastrointestinal tumours. However, their incidence has increased in recent decades, possibly due to better detection and diagnosis. It is estimated that GI NETs account for approximately 2% of all gastrointestinal tumours. The average age at diagnosis is around 50 years, and no clear gender predilection is observed [12].

NETs exhibit a wide spectrum of behaviors, histological features, and hormone production capabilities, leading to a complex classification system based on histology and degree of cell proliferation. They are often characterized by their site of origin, such as gastrointestinal (GI) tract NETs, pNETs, lung NETs, and others. Each of these subtypes possesses unique features and behaviors, further emphasizing the complexity of NET classification. The most commonly used classification is the World Health Organization (WHO) classification [13], which divides NET-GI into three main categories: low-grade well-differentiated neuroendocrine tumours (G1), intermediate-grade well-differentiated neuroendocrine tumours (G2) and high-grade poorly differentiated neuroendocrine tumours (G3). This classification helps to predict the biological behavior and prognosis of the tumours. Additionally, NETs are categorized based on their functionality into functional and non-functional tumours. Functional tumours produce excessive amounts of hormones, resulting in distinct clinical syndromes, whereas non-functional tumours do not exhibit hormone-related symptoms [14].

The precise etiology of NETs remains enigmatic, although several factors have been implicated in their development. Genetic predisposition, exposure to certain environmental factors, and sporadic mutations may contribute to the initiation of NETs. In some cases, NETs are associated with inherited syndromes, such as multiple endocrine neoplasia type 1 (MEN1), von Hippel-Lindau (VHL) syndrome, and neurofibromatosis type 1 (NF1), highlighting the role of genetic abnormalities in their pathogenesis [15].

The prognosis of NET-GI varies according to histologic grade, tumour stage, location, and other clinical factors. Low-grade (G1) well-differentiated tumours generally have a more indolent clinical course and a better prognosis compared to high-grade (G3) poorly differentiated tumours. Accurate staging is crucial in determining prognosis and guiding treatment [12,16]. Early diagnosis, accurate staging, and appropriate treatment selection play crucial roles in determining prognosis. Regular surveillance and follow-up are essential for monitoring disease progression, treatment response, and the emergence of any new symptoms. Long-term follow-up is especially important given the potential for recurrence and metastasis, even after successful treatment [17].

Nevertheless, the absence of symptoms until advanced stages means that, in many cases, there is a delay in diagnosis. As a result, liver metastases are seen in 61–91% of cases at diagnosis. In patients with hepatic involvement by malignancy, it is frequent to see, in up to 10% of cases the association with carcinoid syndrome, with varied symptoms such as facial flushing, diarrhea, abdominal cramps, heart valve disease, telangiectasia, wheezing and edema [1,18]. In line with this and since no distant disease was found in our case, our patient did not present any of these symptoms.

The management of NETs involves a multidisciplinary approach, with treatment strategies tailored to the tumour's grade, stage, functionality, and patient-specific factors. Surgical resection is the primary treatment for localized NETs, aiming to remove the tumour and prevent its progression. However, for metastatic or inoperable cases, a range of therapeutic options is available [6]. Somatostatin analogs, such as octreotide and lanreotide, are frequently used to control hormonal symptoms and slow tumour growth by binding to somatostatin receptors on the tumour cells. Targeted therapies, including tyrosine kinase inhibitors and mTOR inhibitors, have shown efficacy in certain cases by disrupting pathways that are essential for tumour growth and survival. Peptide receptor radionuclide therapy (PRRT) is an emerging treatment modality that combines a somatostatin analog with a radioactive compound, selectively delivering radiation to neuroendocrine tumour cells. PRRT has demonstrated promising results in managing advanced NETs, particularly those expressing somatostatin receptors. For high-grade, poorly differentiated NETs, chemotherapy and immunotherapy may be considered, although their efficacy is generally limited. Clinical trials exploring novel therapeutic approaches, including immunotherapies and combination therapies, are ongoing and hold potential for improving outcomes [1,19].

VCE is a non-invasive diagnostic procedure that utilizes a small, ingestible capsule equipped with a miniature camera and a light source. As the capsule traverses the gastrointestinal tract, it captures high-resolution images, which are wirelessly transmitted to a data recorder worn by the patient. These images provide a comprehensive view of the small intestine's mucosa, allowing for the detection of abnormalities, such as tumours, lesions, and bleeding sources. VCE has meant a breakthrough in the evaluation of pathology located in the small intestine. However, this technique does not allow for any type of intervention, facilitating visualization but not biopsy of suspicious lesions. In addition, the dependence of VCE on passive propulsion by peristalsis may result in variable transit times and incomplete visualization [9].

On the other hand, enteroscopy involves the insertion of a flexible, thin tube equipped with a camera and instruments through the mouth or rectum to directly visualize and access the small intestine [4]. Enteroscopy plays a key role in the diagnosis of GI NETs due to its ability to visualize and obtain tissue samples in regions of the small bowel that are difficult to reach with other examination methods. Nevertheless, it requires specialized training and equipment and may not be feasible for all patients [20]. A distinctive point in our case was the ability to reach the entire small intestine, even being able to visualize the ileocecal valve from a proximal view, a differential fact with these new therapies that provides a wide variety of possibilities.

NETs can be located anywhere in the digestive system, but approximately 50% are found in the small intestine, making detection and adequate sampling difficult. Enteroscopy has proven to be a valuable technique for evaluating the small bowel and detecting suspicious lesions [21].

Regarding the diagnostic accuracy of the techniques described above, VCE and enteroscopy would have a diagnostic yield of 10% and 83%, respectively. In cases in which the tumour is hidden in the small intestine, capsule endoscopy may be more sensitive than enteroscopy, although it varies depending on the scope of the observer [1,22].

Due to the higher technical complexity compared to conventional endoscopy, enteroscopy may have a higher risk of complications such as intestinal perforations, pancreatitis and bronchoaspiration. In spite of this, these complications only correspond to 0.72% of all interventions [23].

The utility of enteroscopy in the diagnosis of NET-GI has been supported by some studies. For example, a study by Manguso et al. (2018) evaluated 85 patients with a diagnosis of NET in the small bowel who underwent multiple imaging techniques including CT, MRI, SRS, and enteroscopy. Enteroscopy was the technique that achieved the highest sensitivity with 88% [24].

In addition to screening and diagnosis, enteroscopy also plays an important role in the staging of NET-GI. Accurate staging is essential to determine prognosis and guide appropriate treatment. Enteroscopy can help identify the presence of small bowel metastases and assess the extent of the disease, which is crucial in determining the optimal therapeutic approach [25].

Research in the field of NETs continues to expand our understanding of their molecular mechanisms and potential therapeutic targets. Advances in genomic profiling have provided insights into the genetic alterations driving NET development, enabling the exploration of precision medicine approaches. Immunotherapies, which harness the body's immune system to target and destroy tumour cells, are a promising avenue for NET treatment. Clinical trials investigating immune checkpoint inhibitors and other immunotherapeutic strategies are shedding light on their potential role in managing NETs. Furthermore, the development of patient-derived xenograft models and three-dimensional cell culture systems is enhancing our ability to study NET biology and test new treatment regimens [26,27].

4. Conclusions

In conclusion, enteroscopy plays a pivotal role in the diagnosis of gastrointestinal neuroendocrine tumours. It provides a direct and detailed visualization of lesions in the small bowel, which facilitates the detection and sampling of neuroendocrine tumours. In addition, it contributes to accurate staging of the disease, which aids in treatment planning. Enteroscopy, along with other diagnostic and evaluation methods, is essential to ensure the accurate diagnosis and optimal management of NET-GI, as described in our case. Its ability to provide a complete visualization of the mucosa, contribute to accurate diagnosis and facilitate therapeutic interventions offers substantial advantages to patients. As these techniques continue to evolve, their role in improving patient outcomes and our understanding of these complex tumours will expand further.

Author Contributions: Conceptualization, A.O.L., S.F.V. and C.G.M.; methodology, A.O.L.; validation, A.O.L., S.F.V. and C.G.M.; investigation, A.O.L.; resources, S.F.V. and L.B.J.; data curation, A.O.L.; writing—original draft preparation, A.O.L., S.F.V. and C.G.M.; writing—review and editing, A.O.L., S.F.V. and C.G.M.; visualization, A.O.L.; supervision, M.J.M.R., P.S.-F.C., D.C.B., A.V.S. and J.C.P.C. All authors have read and agreed to the published version of the manuscript.

Funding: This research received no external funding.

Institutional Review Board Statement: Not applicable.

Informed Consent Statement: Informed consent was obtained from all subjects involved in the study.

Data Availability Statement: Not applicable.

Conflicts of Interest: The authors declare no conflict of interest.

References

1. Gonzalez, R.S. Diagnosis and Management of Gastrointestinal Neuroendocrine Neoplasms. *Surg. Pathol. Clin.* **2020**, *13*, 377–397. [CrossRef] [PubMed]
2. Soto-Solís, R.; Romano-Munive, A.F.; Santana de Anda, K.; Barreto-Zuñiga, R. Factores relacionados a tumores neuroendocrinos gástricos. *Rev. Gastroenterol. México* **2019**, *84*, 52–56. [CrossRef] [PubMed]
3. Volante, M.; Grillo, F.; Massa, F.; Maletta, F.; Mastracci, L.; Campora, M.; Ferro, J.; Vanoli, A.; Papotti, M. Neuroendocrine neoplasms of the appendix, colon and rectum. *Pathologica* **2021**, *113*, 19–27. [CrossRef] [PubMed]
4. Rondonotti, E.; Spada, C.; Adler, S.; May, A.; Despott, E.J.; Koulaouzidis, A.; Panter, S.; Domagk, D.; Fernandez-Urien, I.; Rahmi, G.; et al. Small-bowel capsule endoscopy and device-assisted enteroscopy for diagnosis and treatment of small-bowel disorders: European Society of Gastrointestinal Endoscopy (ESGE) Technical Review. *Endoscopy* **2018**, *50*, 423–446. [CrossRef]
5. Oronsky, B.; Ma, P.C.; Morgenszstern, D.; Carter, C.A. Nothing But NET: A Review of Neuroendocrine Tumors and Carcinomas. *Neoplasia* **2017**, *19*, 991–1002. [CrossRef]
6. Sanli, Y.; Garg, I.; Kandathil, A.; Kendi, T.; Zanetti, M.J.B.; Kuyumcu, S.; Subramaniam, R.M. Neuroendocrine Tumor Diagnosis and Management: ^{68}Ga-DOTATATE PET/CT. *AJR Am. J. Roentgenol.* **2018**, *211*, 267–277. [CrossRef]
7. Lamberts, S.W.; Hofland, L.J.; Nobels, F.R. Neuroendocrine tumor markers. *Front. Neuroendocrinol.* **2001**, *22*, 309–339. [CrossRef]
8. Patel, A.; Vedantam, D.; Poman, D.S.; Motwani, L.; Asif, N. Obscure Gastrointestinal Bleeding and Capsule Endoscopy: A Win-Win Situation or Not? *Cureus* **2022**, *14*, e27137. [CrossRef]
9. Singeap, A.-M.; Cojocariu, C.; Girleanu, I.; Huiban, L.; Sfarti, C.; Cuciureanu, T.; Chiriac, S.; Stanciu, C.; Trifan, A. Clinical Impact of Small Bowel Capsule Endoscopy in Obscure Gastrointestinal Bleeding. *Medicina* **2020**, *56*, 548. [CrossRef]
10. Bozhkov, V.; Magjov, R.; Chernopolsky, P.; Arnaudov, P.; Plachkov, I.; Ivanov, T. Small Intestinal Tumors. *Khirurgiia* **2015**, *81*, 4–8.
11. Abu-Hamda, E.M.; Hattab, E.M.; Lynch, P.M. Small bowel tumors. *Curr. Gastroenterol. Rep.* **2003**, *5*, 386–393. [CrossRef] [PubMed]
12. Dasari, A.; Shen, C.; Halperin, D.; Zhao, B.; Zhou, S.; Xu, Y.; Shih, T.; Yao, J.C. Trends in the Incidence, Prevalence, and Survival Outcomes in Patients With Neuroendocrine Tumors in the United States. *JAMA Oncol.* **2017**, *3*, 1335–1342. [CrossRef] [PubMed]
13. Assarzadegan, N.; Montgomery, E. What is New in the 2019 World Health Organization (WHO) Classification of Tumors of the Digestive System: Review of Selected Updates on Neuroendocrine Neoplasms, Appendiceal Tumors, and Molecular Testing. *Arch. Pathol. Lab. Med.* **2021**, *145*, 664–677. [CrossRef] [PubMed]
14. Rindi, G.; Mete, O.; Uccella, S.; Basturk, O.; La Rosa, S.; Brosens, L.A.A.; Ezzat, S.; de Herder, W.W.; Klimstra, D.S.; Papotti, M.; et al. Overview of the 2022 WHO Classification of Neuroendocrine Neoplasms. *Endocr. Pathol.* **2022**, *33*, 115–154. [CrossRef]
15. Ito, T.; Masui, T.; Komoto, I.; Doi, R.; Osamura, R.Y.; Sakurai, A.; Ikeda, M.; Takano, K.; Igarashi, H.; Shimatsu, A.; et al. JNETS clinical practice guidelines for gastroenteropancreatic neuroendocrine neoplasms: Diagnosis, treatment, and follow-up: A synopsis. *J. Gastroenterol.* **2021**, *56*, 1033–1044. [CrossRef]
16. Rindi, G.; Klöppel, G.; Alhman, H.; Caplin, M.; Couvelard, A.; de Herder, W.W.; Eriksson, B.; Falchetti, A.; Falconi, M.; Komminoth, P.; et al. TNM staging of foregut (neuro)endocrine tumors: A consensus proposal including a grading system. *Virchows Arch.* **2006**, *449*, 395–401. [CrossRef]
17. Cha, B.; Shin, J.; Ko, W.J.; Kwon, K.S.; Kim, H. Prognosis of incompletely resected small rectal neuroendocrine tumor using endoscope without additional treatment. *BMC Gastroenterol.* **2022**, *22*, 293. [CrossRef] [PubMed]
18. Barsouk, A.; Rawla, P.; Barsouk, A.; Thandra, K.C. Epidemiology of Cancers of the Small Intestine: Trends, Risk Factors, and Prevention. *Med. Sci.* **2019**, *7*, 46. [CrossRef]
19. Pavel, M.; O''Toole, D.; Costa, F.; Capdevila, J.; Gross, D.; Kianmanesh, R.; Krenning, E.; Knigge, U.; Salazar, R.; Pape, U.-F.; et al. ENETS Consensus Guidelines Update for the Management of Distant Metastatic Disease of Intestinal, Pancreatic, Bronchial Neuroendocrine Neoplasms (NEN) and NEN of Unknown Primary Site. *Neuroendocrinology* **2016**, *103*, 172–185. [CrossRef]
20. Kunovský, L.; Dastych, M.; Robek, O.; Svaton, R.; Vlazny, J.; Husty, J.; Eid, M.; Poredska, K.; Kysela, P.; Kala, Z. Multiple neuroendocrine tumor of the small bowel: A case report and a review of literature. *Vnitr. Lek.* **2018**, *64*, 966–969. [CrossRef]
21. Zhang, Z.-H.; Qiu, C.-H.; Li, Y. Different roles of capsule endoscopy and double-balloon enteroscopy in obscure small intestinal diseases. *World J. Gastroenterol. WJG* **2015**, *21*, 7297–7304. [CrossRef]
22. Ethun, C.G.; Postlewait, L.M.; Baptiste, G.G.; McInnis, M.R.; Cardona, K.; Russell, M.C.; Kooby, D.A.; Staley, C.A.; Maithel, S.K. Small bowel neuroendocrine tumors: A critical analysis of diagnostic work-up and operative approach. *J. Surg. Oncol.* **2016**, *114*, 671–676. [CrossRef] [PubMed]
23. Park, S.B. Application of double-balloon enteroscopy for small bowel tumors. *Clin. Endosc.* **2023**, *56*, 53–54. [CrossRef] [PubMed]

24. Manguso, N.; Gangi, A.; Johnson, J.; Harit, A.; Nissen, N.; Jamil, L.; Lo, S.; Wachsman, A.; Hendifar, A.; Amersi, F. The role of pre-operative imaging and double balloon enteroscopy in the surgical management of small bowel neuroendocrine tumors: Is it necessary? *J. Surg. Oncol.* **2018**, *117*, 207–212. [CrossRef] [PubMed]
25. Köseoğlu, H.; Duzenli, T.; Sezikli, M. Gastric neuroendocrine neoplasms: A review. *World J. Clin. Cases* **2021**, *9*, 7973–7985. [CrossRef] [PubMed]
26. Ito, T.; Lee, L.; Jensen, R.T. Treatment of Symptomatic Neuroendocrine Tumor Syndromes: Recent Advances and Controversies. *Expert Opin. Pharmacother.* **2016**, *17*, 2191–2205. [CrossRef] [PubMed]
27. Patient-Derived Xenograft (PDX) Models, Applications and Challenges in Cancer Research—PMC. Available online: https://www.ncbi.nlm.nih.gov/pmc/articles/PMC9088152/ (accessed on 8 August 2023).

Disclaimer/Publisher's Note: The statements, opinions and data contained in all publications are solely those of the individual author(s) and contributor(s) and not of MDPI and/or the editor(s). MDPI and/or the editor(s) disclaim responsibility for any injury to people or property resulting from any ideas, methods, instructions or products referred to in the content.

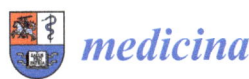

Systematic Review

Efficacy and Safety of Endoscopic Ultrasound-Guided Radiofrequency Ablation for Pancreatic Neuroendocrine Tumors: A Systematic Review and Metanalysis

Elia Armellini [1,*], Antonio Facciorusso [2] and Stefano Francesco Crinò [3]

1. Gastroenterology Unit, Asst-Bergamoest, 24068 Bergamo, Italy
2. Gastroenterology Unit, Department of Medical and Surgical Sciences, University of Foggia, 71122 Foggia, Italy
3. Digestive Endoscopy Unit, University of Verona, 37129 Verona, Italy
* Correspondence: elia.armellini@asst-bergamoest.it

Abstract: *Introduction*: The development of dedicated endoscopes and the technical evolution of endoscopic ultrasound (EUS) have allowed a direct approach to pancreatic neoplastic lesions both for diagnosis and treatment. Among the more promising targets are pancreatic neuroendocrine tumors (Pan-NETs). *Aim*: to describe the evolution of endoscopic ultrasound-guided radiofrequency ablation (EUS-RFA) with particular attention to the treatment of PanNETs, focusing on safety and clinical efficacy of the technique. *Methods*: MEDLINE, Scopus, and Cochrane Library databases were searched for studies reporting about EUS-RFA for the treatment of PanNETs. Studies with outcomes of interest were selected and results were reported to describe clinical success, complications, fol-low-ups, and electrodes used. Clinical success was defined as the disappearance of clinical symp-toms for functional (F-) PanNETs and as complete ablation per nonfunctional (NF-) PanNETs. The pooled data were analyzed by a random-effects model. *Results*: Nineteen studies were selected, including 183 patients (82 males, 44.8%) with 196 lesions (101 F-PanNETs and 95 NF-PanNETs). Pooled estimates for the overall AE rates for the clinical efficacy were 17.8% (95% CI 9.1–26.4%) and 95.1% (95% CI 91.2–98.9%) for F-PanNETs and 24.6% (95% CI 7.4–41.8%) and 93.4% (95% CI 88.4–98.4%) for NF-PanNETs. *Conclusions*: EUS-RFA appears to be a mini-invasive technique with a good safety and efficacy profile for the treatment of F- and NF-PanNETs. EUS-RFA could be of-fered as possible alternative to surgery for the treatment of low-grade NF- or F-PanNETs, especially for those patients that are not eligible or are at high-risk for surgery.

Keywords: endoscopic ultrasound; pancreatic neuroendocrine tumors; insulinoma; radiofrequency ablation; RFA; pancreas; EUS-guided ablation; PanNETs

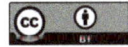

1. Introduction

Radiofrequency ablation (RFA) has been used for years for the treatment of solid malignancies, both with an intraoperative and percutaneous technique [1,2].

Pancreatic lesion ablation using thermal energy or through the injection of substances under EUS guidance is one of the recent applications of EUS [3,4]. EUS-RFA includes among the more promising targets PanNETs (others are pancreatic metastasis from renal cancer and pancreatic adenocarcinoma in the appropriate setting) [5,6].

The use of RFA in medicine is ubiquitous and dates back over 75 years. Energy produced from RFA has been used for the cautery of tissues or vessels and destruction of tumors or hypertrophic tissues, as well to ablate accessory conduction pathways in the heart to improve atrial fibrillation and other conditions. Ultrasound-guided percutaneous RFA has become one of the mainstays in treatment of hepatocellular carcinoma since the 1990s, as stated by Barcelona Clinic Liver Cancer (BCLC) guidelines, and it is used also for tumors of the lung, bone, prostate, and kidney [2]. Principles of RFA are explained in the following Figure 1 reproducing the relation between the main variables during RFA:

change in Time (Seconds) of Current (Ampere, A), red line, and Impedance (Ohm, Ω), green line, at a constant Power (Watt, W), blue line.

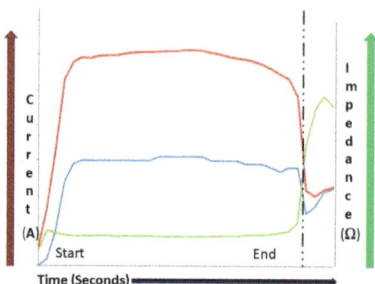

Figure 1. Basic principles of RFA (Courtesy of L. Portella).

Approaches to the treatment of pancreatic neoplastic lesions have been delayed because of the pancreas anatomy and of unsatisfactory results obtained by surgical or percutaneous treatments [7,8].

The evolution of EUS devices with the development of linear-array technology expanded the clinical utility of EUS. EUS guidance allows the precise placement of needles within focal mass lesions, hence therapeutic interventions represent a logical and inevitable advance in the development of EUS. The principal aim of this review is to provide a comprehensive overview on the main outcomes (safety and efficacy) of EUS-RFA for the treatment of pancreatic neuroendocrine tumors (PanNETs), both functional (F-) and non-functional (NF-).

2. Materials and Methods

This systematic review and metanalysis was performed in agreement with PRISMA guidelines [9]. MEDLINE, Scopus, and Cochrane Library databases were searched for studies reporting about EUS-RFA for treatment of PanNETs. The literature search was performed and verified by two independent reviewers (E.A. and A.F.) using the following index terms: "pancreatic neuroendocrine neoplasms" OR "pancreatic neuroendocrine tumors" OR "insulinoma" OR "PanNET" AND "endoscopic ultrasound-guided RFA" OR "EUS-RFA". The inclusion criteria for studies were as follows: (1) Study subjects were adult (≥18 years old); (2) Prospective or retrospective study design, conference proceedings, case reports, and abstracts; (3) Reporting on safety and efficacy of EUS-RFA for the treatment of F- and NF-PanNETs; (4) The manuscript was written in English. The search included reports published until November 2022. A manual search of the reference lists of all review articles and primary studies retrieved was also performed. The flow-chart of the study is shown in Figure 2.

Studies with outcomes of interest were selected and results are reported to describe technical success, procedural details, adverse events (AEs) rate, and clinical efficacy.

Data were extracted independently and entered into standardized Excel spreadsheets (Microsoft Inc., Redmond, WC, USA). The following data were extracted from each study: first author; year of publication; number, gender, and age of patients; number of Pan-NETs; type of PanNETs (F- or NF-); tumor size (mean size in mm) and location; number of RFA sessions; clinical efficacy; occurrence and severity of AEs; and duration of follow-up.

Clinical success was defined as complete ablation (i.e., disappearance on cross-sectional imaging during follow-up) for NF-PanNETs and as disappearance of clinical symptoms for F-PanNETs. Safety was defined as the absence of AEs. AEs were defined and graded in accordance with an international lexicon [10].

Crude rates were extracted as outcome measures. Pooled estimates were obtained using a random-effects model because a high between-study variance in effect size was expected. Heterogeneity was assessed with the Pearson χ^2 test and the I^2 statistic.

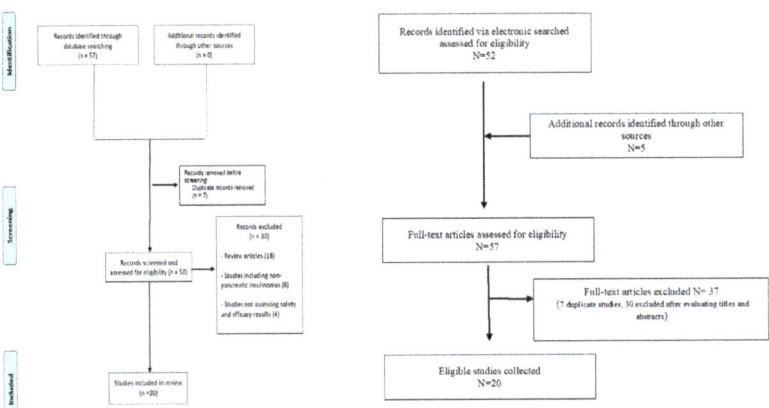

Figure 2. Study flow-chart.

3. Results

Fifty-seven potentially relevant studies were retrieved from the databases. Subsequently, seven duplicates and thirty studies were excluded after reviewing the titles and abstracts, as they were irrelevant articles and were not suitable for the research topic. Finally, we included 20 studies [5,11–29].

Overall, 183 patients (82 males, 44.8%) with 196 lesions (101 F-PanNETs and 95 NF-PanNETs) were included. Most of the cases were treated using a 18/19 G electrode-needle (EUSRA RF-electrode coupled with the VIVA RF generator, by Starmed, Taewoong Medical, South Korea) and a few cases were treated by a through-the-needle 1 Fr, monopolar, electrode-catheter (EndoHPB, Emcision UK, London, UK).

Diameters of the tumors widely varied between 4.5 mm and 30 mm and all but one F-PanNETs were insulinomas. Most of cases were treated by one single session; only a minority required multiple sessions (up to three). Follow-up time ranged between 1 and 41 months. Demographics, lesion features and the technical procedural details of F-PanNETs and NF-Pan NETs are summarized in Tables 1 and 2, respectively.

Table 1. Results from studies reporting the efficacy and safety of EUS-RFA for the treatment of F-PanNETs included in the meta-analysis **.

Study, Year	Study Design	N of Patients/ N of F-PanNET	Male/ Female	Age	Tumor Size (Mean, mm)	Location	Device	N of RFA Sessions /Nodule	Efficacy *	Adverse Events	Follow-Up Months
Lakhtakia [14], 2016	Retrospective	3/3	M	45	19	H	19 G, Starmed	1	100	0	11.5
Waung [15], 2016	Retrospective	1/1	F	70	18	H	Habib EUS RFA	3	100	0	10
Bas-Cutrina [16], 2017	Retrospective	1/1	F	63	10	NR	Habib EUS RFA	1	100	0	10
Choi [17], 2018	Prospective	1/1	M	34	12	H	19 G, Starmed	1	100	0	13
Thosani [18], 2018	Retrospective	3/3	NR	NR	NR	NR	NR	1.6 °	100	1	5
Gueneau de Mussy [19], 2018	Retrospective	1/1	F	69	12	T	19 G, Starmed	1	100	1	2
Klutz [20], 2019	Retrospective	1/1	M	40	9	H	19 G, Starmed	1	100	1	6
Oleinikov [21], 2019	Retrospective	7/7	4M, 3F	60.4	14.9	H:7, T:2	19 G, Starmed	1	100	0	9.7

Table 1. Cont.

Study, Year	Study Design	N of Patients/ N of F-PanNET	Male/ Female	Age	Tumor Size (Mean, mm)	Location	Device	N of RFA Sessions /Nodule	Efficacy *	Adverse Events	Follow-Up Months
De Nucci [22], 2020	Prospective	5/5	2M, 3F	80	12.8	T	19 G, Starmed	1	100	0	12
Brown [23], 2020	Retrospective	1/1	F	66	18	H	19 G, Starmed	1	100	0	8
Marx [24], 2022	Retrospective	7/7	1M, 6F	66	13.3	H:1; T:6	19 G, Starmed	1	85.7	4	21
Rizzatti [25], 2022	Prospective	30/30	10M, 20F	61.9	11.9	H:12, T:18	19 G, Starmed	25:1, 4:2, 1:3	95.8	3	6
Lakhtakia [26]	Retrospective	12/12	NR	NR	NR	NR	19 G, Starmed	NR	100	NR	31.5
Nabi [27], 2022	Retrospective	12/15	7M, 8F	46.7	NR	H:8, T:7	19 G, Starmed	1:10 >1:2	100	1	41
Borrelli deAndreis [28] in press	Retrospective	10/10	7M, 3F	11.9	11.9	H:3, T:7	19 G, Starmed	9:1, 1:2	100	3	3
Rossi [29], 2022	Retrospective	3/3	2M, 1F	82.7	12	H:1, T:2	19 G, Starmed	1:2, 2:1	100	1	24

* Clinical efficacy was defined as disappearance of symptoms. ** table legend. N: number, H: pancreatic head, T: pancreatic tail, NR: not reported. ° in this case, a mean value was indicated.

Table 2. Results from studies reporting the efficacy and safety of EUS-RFA for the treatment of NF-PanNETs included in the meta-analysis **.

Study, Year	Study Design	N of Patients/ N of NF-PanNETs	Male/ Female	Age	Tumor Size (Mean, mm)	Location	Device	N of RFA Sessions per Nodule	Efficacy *	N of Adverse Events	Follow-Up (Months)
Rossi [11], 2014	Retrospective	1/1	M	72	9	T	Habib EUS RFA	1	100	0	34
Armellini [13], 2015	Retrospective	1/1	M	76	20	T	18 G, Starmed	1	100	0	1
Pai [12], 2015	Prospective	2/2	F	69.5	27.5	H	Habib EUS RFA	1:1, 1:2	100	2	6
Choi [17], 2018	Retrospective	7/7	3M, 4F	56.1	20	H:2, T:5	19 G, Starmed	1:3, 2:2, 3:2	75	2	13
Barthet [5], 2018	Prospective	12/14	7M, 5F	59.9	13.1	H:3, T:11	19 G, Starmed	NR	86	2	12
Oleinikov [21], 2019	Retrospective	11/18	6M, 5F	65.8	14.2	H;11, T:7	19 G, Starmed	1	94.5	2	8.7
De Nucci [22], 2020	Prospective	5/6	3M, 2F	77.2	14.2	H:3, T:3	19 G, Starmed	1	100	2	12
Rizzatti [25], 2022	Prospective	32/32	22M, 10F	70.1	14.2	H:11, T:21	19 G, Starmed	1:24, 2:7, 3:1	96.3	0	8
Lakhtakia [26], 2022	Retrospective	14/14	NR	NR	NR	NR	19 G, Starmed	NR	85.7	NR	31.5

* Clinical efficacy was defined as complete disappearance of the lesion upon cross-sectional imaging during follow-up. ** table legend. N: number, H: pancreatic head, T: pancreatic tail, NR: not reported.

In the subgroups of F-PanNETs and NF-PanNETs, the pooled estimates for the overall AE rates were 17.8% (95% CI 9.1–26.4%) and 24.6% (95% CI 7.4–41.8%), respectively (Figure 3a,b).

The most common AEs were mild pancreatitis and abdominal pain. Overall, mild AEs were observed in 21/142 (14.7%) patients; moderate and severe AEs were observed in one patient each (0.007%).

The pooled estimates for the clinical efficacy in the subgroups of F-PanNETs and NF-PanNETs were 95.1% (95% CI 91.2–98.9%) and 93.4% (95% CI 88.4–98.4%), respectively (Figure 4a,b).

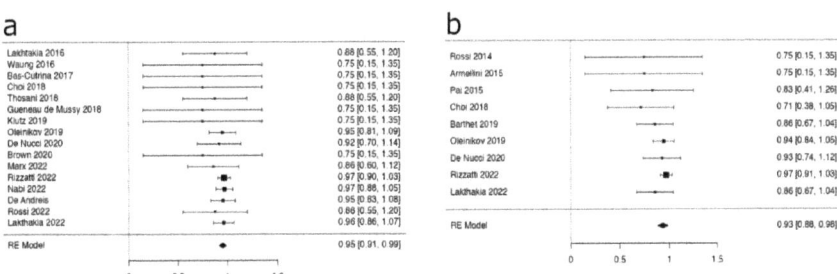

Figure 3. Forest plots reporting estimates for overall adverse event rates in F- (**a**) and NF- PanNETs (**b**). The pooled AE rates were 17.8% (95% CI 9.1–26.4%) and 24.6% (95% CI 7.4–41.8%) in F- and NF-PanNETs, respectively.

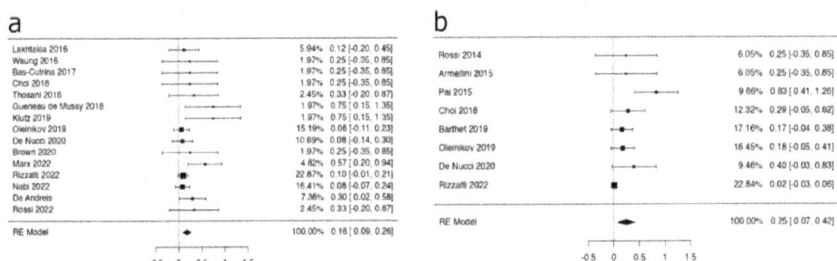

Figure 4. Forest plots reporting estimates for clinical efficacy of F- (**a**) and NF- PanNETs (**b**). The pooled efficacy rates were 95.1% (95% CI 91.2–98.9%) and 93.4% (95% CI 88.4–98.4%) in F- (**a**) and NF-PanNETs (**b**), respectively.

4. Discussion

The term "radiofrequency" originates from the frequency of the electricity used which is like that of radio waves. RFA can be delivered by monopolar or bipolar electrodes. Monopolar electrodes have an insulated electrode needle with an active tip in connection to a grounding pad (passive electrode) placed on the patient's body. It was the first developed model and has the advantage of deep penetration in tissues.

Bipolar electrodes use two active electrodes, adjacent at the tip of the needle; this characteristic implies less penetration and more limited volume of action. In both cases, the radiofrequency current translates into ion agitation within the surrounding tissue, which is converted by friction into heat and induces cellular death by means of coagulation necrosis. Energy transfer is dictated by Ohm's Law: energy (J) = $I^2 \times R \times T$ (where "I" is the current, "R" is the tissue resistance (or properly impedance), and "T" is the time of application). Electrical energy is converted to thermal energy as resistance in the tissue is met [30].

Impendence depends on tissue hydration, electrolyte composition, collagen content, temperature, and other variables and becomes, in the end, the limiting step to the volume of the induced lesion. While energy is applied and radiofrequency acts, the charred tissue becomes an electrical insulator in the end, as shown by the rise in impedance. This phenomenon indicates inefficiency in further ablation (i.e., energy delivery) and marks the end of the procedure [30].

In 1999, Brugge et al. [31] reported the first experimental EUS-RFA in a pig model. They could easily foresee the possible application of ultrasound-guided therapies: "the development of endosonographically placed therapeutic devices may provide a unique alternative for the management of premalignant pancreatic lesions (e.g., islet cell tumors and cystic neoplasms) and potentially may offer palliative therapy for surgically unresectable malignant pancreatic tumors".

These innovative ideas required ten years to come true. After Brugge's first experimental model, years were needed to develop efficient EUS endoscopes and RFA devices, testing devices and accumulating experience on animal models in the meantime [32–34].

Finally, in 2008, a 2.2 mm needle-shaped bipolar hybrid cryotherm probe was used for experimental protocols in animal models [35,36] and humans [37] (Hybrid-therm, ERBE, Tubingen, Germany). These early experiences in patients with advanced pancreatic cancer showed that EUS-RFA could be applied in 16 patients (72.8%); amylase arose in 3 of 16 patients, and none had clinical signs of pancreatitis. Late complications arose in four cases: three were mostly related to tumor progression. A CT scan was performed on all patients, but only in 6 of 16 it was possible to clearly define the tumor margins after ablation.

In 2014, an Italian group reported treatment of a 9 mm NF-PanNET by EUS-guided monopolar RFA [11], preceding the description in 2015 by Pai et al. of the use of a monopolar "trough the needle" electrode for the treatment of cystic and solid lesions [12]. The device was the Habib EUS-guided RFA probe derived from the endovascular application concept: the Habib EUS-guided RFA probe (EndoHPB, Emcision UK, London, UK) was a 220 cm long, 1 Fr (0.33 mm), monopolar catheter that could be inserted through a regular 22-gauge FNA needle (Figure 2) and used in combination with commonly available radiofrequency generators. Its limitations are the limited penetration of energy and the small volume of tissue ablation.

In the same year, a water-cooled monopolar RFA needle with an active tip with different lengths was made commercially available after preliminary experiences on animal models [38].

Early experiences conducted between 2015 and 2016 offered satisfactory results in different fields of application ranging from pancreatic adenocarcinoma [39] to PanNETs [13,14] and extra-pancreatic solid lesions [40–42]. As we are writing this paper, the EUSRA RF Electrode is the only one available on the market. The concept of monopolar RFA that made the success of RFA in percutaneous ultrasound-guided procedure was translated into an EUS device by Taewoong Medical that produced the EUSRA RF-electrode. The volume of ablation corresponds to the length of the active needle, and the cooling system works to avoid fast charring of the tissues.

The EUSRA system is a monopolar radiofrequency needle consisting of a 19-gauge needle (18-gauge was the diameter of the first electrode-needle) with a 140 cm-long electrode lacking insulation over the terminal 5 to 20 mm tip, a dedicated RF current generator (VIVA RF generator) which allows control of power and impedance, and an inner cooling system intended to avoid fast tissue charring and to obtain large volume ablations circulating chilled saline through the needle.

Focusing on EUS-RFA of PanNETs, in 2015, a case of non-functioning PanNET (G2, diameter 20 mm, Ki 67 < 5%) fully ablated by a 10 mm EUSRA RF-electrode in one session with no complications and complete radiological response was reported [13]. In 2016, Lakhtakia et al. [14] treated three patients with symptomatic pancreatic insulinomas, not eligible for surgery. All had rapid symptom relief with biochemical improvement and remained symptom-free at 11–12 months of follow-up. There were no procedure-related adverse events.

Barthet et al. [5] in 2018 published a French prospective multicenter study aiming to assess the technical feasibility and safety of EUS-RFA for treatment of PanNETs and pancreatic cystic lesions. The study population included 12 patients that had 14 PanNETs (mean size 13.1 mm, range 10–20 mm). Among the 14 PanNETs, at 1-year follow-up, 12 had completely disappeared (86% tumor resolution), with three patients having a delayed response. After three complications (two pancreatitis and one small bowel perforation), a change in the original protocol reduced the complications rate: rectal diclofenac was used as recommended before endoscopic retrograde cholangiopancreatography (ERCP) to prevent post-endoscopic pancreatitis.

Antibiotic prophylaxis (2 g of amoxicillin and clavulanic acid intravenously) was used to prevent infection. At six months and one year, the success rates were 71.4 and 85.7, respectively.

J.A. Waung [15] in 2016 described successful treatment of an F-PanNET by the Habib needle; the procedure required multiple sessions to achieve a substantial response. Again, no complications were observed, and in 2017, Bas-Cutrina et al. [16] treated a small F-PanNET similarly.

In 2018, Choi [17] reported a single-center prospective study of seven NF-PanNETs and one insulinoma treated by EUSRA needle. Efficacy was reported in 75% after one year with mild adverse events in 25%. In the same year, Thosani et al. [18] described successful treatment of three F-PanNETs with 100% efficacy achieved at five months and Gueneau de Mussy et al. [19] and Kluz et al. [20] reported, respectively, the successful treatment of a 12 mm and a 9 mm F-PanNET.

In 2019, Oleinikov et al. [21] published a large retrospective series of cases treated in two tertiary centers in Israel to assess the feasibility, safety, and efficacy of EUS-RFA in a cohort of patients with F- and NF-PanNETs. The cohort included eighteen adults (eight women, ten men), aged 60.4 ± 14.4 years (mean $\pm$ SD), seven insulinoma patients, and eleven patients with NF-PanNETs. Twenty-seven lesions with a mean diameter of 14.3 mm (range 4.5 to 30) were treated. Technical success, defined as typical post-ablative changes on surveillance imaging, was achieved in 26 out of 27 lesions. Clinical response with normalization of glucose levels was observed in all (seven of seven) insulinoma cases within 24 h of treatment. Overall, there were no major complications 48 h post-procedure. No clinically significant recurrences were observed during follow-up (range 2 to 21 months).

In 2020, de Nucci et al. [22] published a prospective study of 10 consecutive patients with PanNETs $\leq$ 20 mm treated with EUS-RFA, and they were followed-up for at least 12 months. The mean size of the PanNETs was 14.5 mm (range 9–20 mm). Complete ablation of PanNETs was reached using a single-session RFA with a mean of 2.3 treatment applications per session. At both 6- and 12-month follow-ups, all lesions had disappeared on the CT scan. No major complications were observed. Brown et al. described the successful treatment of an 18 mm insulinoma in 2020 [23].

More recently, M. Marx et al. [24] analyzed the clinical course of patients with pancreatic insulinomas treated by EUS-RFA at two French tertiary referral centers. This study included seven patients, with a mean age of 66 years. EUS-RFA was feasible in all patients with immediate hypoglycemia relief after only one single treatment session; six of seven achieved a complete response by cross-sectional imaging and remained asymptomatic. Three patients had minor adverse events. One elderly patient developed a peripancreatic fluid collections and died consequently. This was a retrospective series collected over three years between 2017 and 2020, so it is difficult to ascertain if the significant complications rate and the serious adverse event were due to changes in operators, in the technique, or to other factors.

Finally, during the United European Gastroenterology Week 2022, the preliminary results of RAPNEN study [25] were shown in poster format. This large multicenter study included 62 patients treated from October 2019 to September 2022 at seven European centers. The results show a high rate of technical success and a good safety profile of the procedure.

In the same meeting, Lakhtakia et al. [26] reported a retrospective study of 26 patients, (mean age 49.3 ± 13.8, 12 males), 29 nodules, affected by F- and NF-PanNETs that were treated between 2014 and 2022 at the Asian Institute of Gastroenterology, Hyderabad, India. They reported significant improvement in mean fasting serum insulin (pre-RFA 39.4 ± 8.9 vs. post-RFA 13.1 ± 5.1; $p < 0.001$) and fasting blood glucose (pre-RFA 30.3 ± 7.3 vs. post-RFA 78.2 ± 7.7; $p < 0.001$) after a median follow-up of 31.5 months, and clinical response was seen in all the cases with insulinomas. In NF-PanNETs, significant responses on imaging were seen in 12 (85.7%) cases. Moreover, the same group [27] described the treatment of 12 patients affected by 15 insulinomas, obtaining a 100% clinical success.

In 2022, two papers by Borrelli de Andreis [28] (in press) and Rossi et al. [29] described the treatment of ten and three insulinomas, achieving complete clinical success with only mild complications in four cases.

In the reported experiences, EUS-RFA was used to treat both F- and NF-PanNETs.

The WHO 2019 classification morphologically distinguishes two groups of pancreatic neuroendocrine neoplasias (PanNENs): well-differentiated tumors or pancreatic neuroendocrine tumors (PanNETs) based on degree of differentiation and Ki67 index, further divided into PanNETs-G1 (Ki67 index $\leq$ 3%), PanNETs-G2 (Ki67 index between 4% and 20%), PanNETs-G3 (Ki67 index above 20%), and poorly differentiated neoplasms, so called neuroendocrine carcinomas (PanNECs) and mixed adenoneuroendocrine carcinomas (MiNen) [43].

The presence or absence of a hormonal hypersecretion syndrome further classifies PanNETs into functional and nonfunctional, which require different therapeutic approaches. However, which PanNETs should be treated by RFA and who should we treat? [44].

Most PanNETs (up to 70%) are nonfunctional, at least a half of which are asymptomatic and discovered on cross-sectional imaging requested for other reasons. International guidelines [45] suggest active surveillance for NF-PanNETs that are <2 cm and well-differentiated. Still, even in small PanNETs, the possibility of disease progression exists [46].

The traditional management of PanNETs has been surgical since excision of a potentially resectable lesion appeared to be a curative option. This is the treatment of choice in accordance with the Vienna Consensus Conference in 2016 [45], but limitations can be found in patient performance status, comorbidities, rate of progression, tumor size and grade, and in the non-negligible complication rate of the surgical option, even in cases of parenchyma sparing procedure [47–51]. However, the same guidelines define "a grey zone of hesitation" which encompasses patients affected by NF-PanNETs < 20 mm, G1-G2, where the choice between surveillance and treatment is affected by doubts and by the patient's preference [52]. In these cases, the presence of disease may negatively affect the emotional well-being and become a substantial reason to favor treatment.

Addressing this topic, a time trends analysis conducted in an Italian high-volume center involving 587 patients from 1990 to 2015 showed that the number of resected PanNETs has increased in recent years, while the size (from 25 to 20 mm) decreased during the study period, but the G1 proportion (from 65% to 49%) still represented half of the resected tumors. After a mean follow-up of 75 months, recurrence analysis revealed that regardless of size, G1 NF-PanNETs with no nodal involvement and vascular invasion had a negligible risk of recurrence at 5 years [53]. Another interesting multicenter analysis showed how a surgical approach seems unnecessary for small G1 sporadic PanNETs [54]. Therefore, a mini-invasive option such as EUS-RFA appears desirable.

For F-PanNETs, the goal of EUS-RFA treatment is to reduce the hormonal hypersecretion syndrome with cessation of symptoms. This can be achieved by inducing necrosis of a sufficient amount of the secerning cells, and the complete ablation of the tumor is not required because of their very low malignant potential, although it would be advisable. On the contrary, for NF-PanNETs, the aim must be complete tumor ablation, with no vital neoplastic tissue left. Therefore, the definition, evaluation, technique, and effectiveness of the radiofrequency procedure vary in accordance with which type of PanNET is targeted.

This is a crucial aspect since the rate AEs may be influenced by the need to pursue complete ablation or, otherwise, if a partial debulking of the lesion is sufficient (i.e., partial ablation of a central area in a functioning tumor). In NF-PanNETs, the goal of complete ablation compels us to treat the margins of the tumor, and proximity to the normal pancreatic parenchyma potentially increases the risk of pancreatitis. In this setting, the availability of an RFA needle with different length active tips (EUSRA 19G needle has active tips ranging from 5 to 20 mm) and a careful selection based on pre-operative imaging and real time visualization is imperative for the success of the procedure and for abating adverse events.

For non-metastatic NF-PanNETs, the definition by which patients can benefit the most from RFA treatment is more complex than for F-PanNETs, as it is difficult to define which patients may benefit from careful follow-up or from surgical treatment, aiming to a balance between overtreatment (RFA/surgery in incidentally discovered PanNETs < 2 cm, that might not progress) and undertreatment (locoregional treatment in patients with undetected metastases).

It is not the aim of this review to discuss staging and prognostic factors of PanNETs, but exclusion of liver, lung, or lymph nodes metastases as well a careful evaluation of tumor grading, the Ki-67 proliferation index, and other prognostic factors, which are of paramount importance to indicate or rule out EUS-RFA [55–64].

A good guide for the selection of patients will probably be, in the future, the inclusion criteria indicated by the RAPNEN study, especially for NF-PanNETs: diameter of the lesion between 15 and 25 mm, ki-67 $\leq$ 5%, absence of distant metastases, symptoms, and inner calcifications. Considering functional lesions, multiple F-PanNETs do not look like a contraindication to EUS-RFA; on the contrary, treatment of multiple lesions in the same session appears feasible and this might become a further indication for EUS-RFA.

Our metanalysis showed pooled estimates for EUS-RFA clinical efficacy in the subgroups of F-PanNETs and NF-PanNETs of 95.1% (95% CI 91.2–98.9%) and 93.4% (95% CI 88.4–98.4%), respectively, which are consistent with a high rate of success in both categories. The subgroups of F-PanNETs and NF-PanNETs showed significant pooled estimate AE rates of 17.8% (95% CI 9.1–26.4%) and 24.6% (95% CI 7.4–41.8%), respectively, but notably, most of the AEs were mild (transient abdominal pain and mild pancreatitis) with a very limited incidence of severe AEs, and some of these were recorded among the earliest procedure of EUS-RFA. This should imply a good chance of improving these results in the future. Moreover, the alternative surgical treatment shows non-negligible rates of complications, even in cases of parenchyma sparing procedures, as reported in literature.

5. Conclusions

PanNETs are rare neoplasms with outcomes varying by stage, grade, and clinical presentation. A growth of PanNET incidence has been observed in the last few decades, with an increase in the low stage rate, as most patients are diagnosed at an initial stage of the disease. Therefore, a rise of the number of patients entering the "grey zone of hesitation" is expected.

About 70% of the PanNETs are nonfunctioning, and up to 50% are discovered in consequence of diagnostic imaging performed for other reasons, as asymptomatic lesions. International guidelines suggest active surveillance for small (1.5 to 2 cm), well-differentiated, asymptomatic, and NF-PanNETs, although they still entail the possibility of disease progression.

The need of an alternative approach to standard surgical treatment is obvious if we consider low-grade < 20 mm PanNETs, patients that are not eligible for surgery or are at high perioperative risk, or when a functional tumor requires debulking of hormone secreting cells. EUS-RFA appears to be a valuable alternative with high efficacy, a low adverse events rate, and major advantages such as low invasiveness and repeatability.

Moreover, the availability of different treatment options requires the involvement of different professional figures and shared decisions when therapeutic interventions are tailored in accordance with disease pathology, overall prognosis, and individual patient wishes.

Ongoing studies are expected to contribute to the final proof of concept and, in the long run, to define the appropriate indications for EUS-RFA.

Author Contributions: E.A., conceptualization, data extraction, drafting of the manuscript, and final revision; A.F., data extraction, methodology, and statistical analysis; S.F.C., conceptualization, data extraction, and final revision. All authors have read and agreed to the published version of the manuscript.

Funding: This research received no external funding.

Institutional Review Board Statement: Not applicable.

Informed Consent Statement: Not applicable.

Data Availability Statement: The data presented in this study are available on request from the corresponding author.

Conflicts of Interest: The authors declare no conflict of interest.

References

1. Goldberg, S.N. Radiofrequency tumor ablation: Principles and techniques. *Eur. J. Ultrasound* **2001**, *13*, 129–147. [CrossRef]
2. Livraghi, T. Radiofrequency ablation of hepatocellular carcinoma. *Surg. Oncol. Clin. N. Am.* **2011**, *20*, 281–299. [CrossRef] [PubMed]
3. Lakhtakia, S. Therapy of Pancreatic Neuroendocrine Tumors: Fine Needle Intervention including Ethanol and Radiofrequency Ablation. *Clin. Endosc.* **2017**, *50*, 546–551. [CrossRef]
4. Signoretti, M.; Valente, R.; Repici, A.; Delle Fave, G.; Capurso, G.; Carrara, S. Endoscopy-guided ablation of pancreatic lesions: Technical possibilities and clinical outlook. *World J. Gastrointest. Endosc.* **2017**, *16*, 41–54. [CrossRef] [PubMed]
5. Barthet, M.; Giovannini, M.; Lesavre, N.; Boustiere, C.; Napoleon, B.; Koch, S.; Gasmi, M.; Vanbiervliet, G.; Gonzalez, J.M. Endoscopic ultrasound-guided radiofrequency ablation for pancreatic neuroendocrine tumors and pancreatic cystic neoplasms: A prospective multicenter study. *Endoscopy* **2019**, *51*, 836–842. [CrossRef] [PubMed]
6. Crinò, S.F.; D'Onofrio, M.; Bernardoni, L.; Frulloni, L.; Iannelli, M.; Malleo, G.; Paiella, S.; Larghi, A.; Gabbrielli, A. EUS-guided Radiofrequency Ablation (EUS-RFA) of Solid Pancreatic Neoplasm Using an 18-gauge Needle Electrode: Feasibility, Safety, and Technical Success. *J. Gastrointest. Liver Dis.* **2018**, *27*, 67–72. [CrossRef]
7. Girelli, R.; Frigerio, I.; Salvia, R.; Barbi, E.; Tinazzi Martini, P.; Bassi, C. Feasibility and safety of radiofrequency ablation for locally advanced pancreatic cancer. *Br. J. Surg.* **2010**, *97*, 220–225. [CrossRef]
8. D'Onofrio, M.; Crosara, S.; De Robertis, R.; Butturini, G.; Salvia, R.; Paiella, S.; Bassi, C.; Mucelli, R.P. Percutaneous Radiofrequency Ablation of Unresectable Locally Advanced Pancreatic Cancer: Preliminary Results. *Technol. Cancer Res. Treat.* **2017**, *16*, 285–294. [CrossRef]
9. Page, M.J.; McKenzie, J.E.; Bossuyt, P.M.; Boutron, I.; Hoffmann, T.C.; Mulrow, C.D.; Shamseer, L.; Tetzlaff, J.M.; Akl, E.A.; Brennan, S.E.; et al. The PRISMA 2020 statement: An updated guideline for reporting systematic reviews. *BMJ* **2021**, *29*, n71. [CrossRef]
10. Cotton, P.B.; Eisen, G.M.; Aabakken, L.; Baron, T.H.; Hutter, M.M.; Jacobson, B.C.; Mergener, K.; Nemcek, A., Jr.; Petersen, B.T.; Petrini, J.L.; et al. A lexicon for endoscopic adverse events: Report of an ASGE workshop. *Gastrointest. Endosc.* **2010**, *71*, 446–454. [CrossRef]
11. Rossi, S.; Viera, F.T.; Ghittoni, G.; Cobianchi, L.; Rosa, L.L.; Siciliani, L.; Bortolotto, C.; Veronese, L.; Vercelli, A.; Gallotti, A.; et al. Radiofrequency ablation of pancreatic neuroendocrine tumors: A pilot study of feasibility; efficacy; and safety. *Pancreas* **2014**, *43*, 938–945. [CrossRef]
12. Pai, M.; Habib, N.; Senturk, H.; Lakhtakia, S.; Reddy, N.; Cicinnati, V.R.; Kaba, I.; Beckebaum, S.; Drymousis, P.; Kahaleh, M.; et al. Endoscopic ultrasound guided radiofrequency ablation; for pancreatic cystic neoplasms and neuroendocrine tumors. *World J. Gastrointest. Surg.* **2015**, *7*, 52–59. [CrossRef]
13. Armellini, E.; Crinò, S.F.; Ballarè, M.; Occhipinti, P. Endoscopic ultrasound-guided radiofrequency ablation of a pancreatic neuroendocrine tumor. *Endoscopy* **2015**, *47* (Suppl. S1), E600–E601. [CrossRef] [PubMed]
14. Lakhtakia, S.; Ramchandani, M.; Galasso, D.; Gupta, R.; Venugopal, S.; Kalpala, R.; Reddy, D.N. EUS-guided radiofrequency ablation for management of pancreatic insulinoma by using a novel needle electrode (with videos). *Gastrointest. Endosc.* **2016**, *83*, 234–239. [CrossRef] [PubMed]
15. Waung, J.A.; Todd, J.F.; Keane, M.G.; Pereira, S.P. Successful management of a sporadic pancreatic insulinoma by endoscopic ultrasound-guided radiofrequency ablation. *Endoscopy* **2016**, *48* (Suppl. S1), E144–E145. [CrossRef]
16. Bas-Cutrina, F.; Bargalló, D.; Gornals, J.B. Small pancreatic insulinoma: Successful endoscopic ultrasound-guided radiofrequency ablation in a single session using a 22-G fine needle. *Dig. Endosc.* **2017**, *29*, 636–638. [CrossRef]
17. Choi, J.H.; Seo, D.W.; Song, T.J.; Park, D.H.; Lee, S.S.; Lee, S.K.; Kim, M.H. Endoscopic ultrasound-guided radiofrequency ablation for management of benign solid pancreatic tumors. *Endoscopy* **2018**, *50*, 1099–1104. [CrossRef]
18. Thosani, N.; Sharma, N.R.; Raiman, I.; Thosani, A.J.; Kannadath, B.S.; Guider, G.C.; Raza, A.; Guha, S. Safety and efficacy of endoscopic ultrasound guided radiofrequency ablation (EUS-RFA) in the treatment of pancreatic lesions: A multi-center experience. *Gastrointest. Endosc.* **2018**, *87*, AB84. [CrossRef]
19. Gueneau de Mussy, P.; Lamine, F. A case of benign insulinoma successfully treated with endoscopic ultrasound guided radiofrequency ablation. *Endocr. Abstr.* **2018**, *56*, 121. [CrossRef]
20. Kluz, M.; Staroń, R.; Krupa, Ł.; Partyka, M.; Polkowski, M.; Gutkowski, K. Successful endoscopic ultrasound-guided radiofrequency ablation of a pancreatic insulinoma. *Pol. Arch. Intern. Med.* **2020**, *130*, 145–146. [CrossRef]
21. Oleinikov, K.; Dancour, A.; Epshtein, J.; Benson, A.; Mazeh, H.; Tal, I.; Matalon, S.; Benbassat, C.A.; Livovsky, D.M.; Goldin, E.; et al. Endoscopic Ultrasound-Guided Radiofrequency Ablation: A New Therapeutic Approach for Pancreatic Neuroendocrine Tumors. *J. Clin. Endocrinol. Metab.* **2019**, *104*, 2637–2647. [CrossRef]

22. de Nucci, G.; Imperatore, N.; Mandelli, E.D.; di Nuovo, F.; d'Urbano, C.; Manes, G. Endoscopic ultrasound-guided radiofrequency ablation of pancreatic neuroendocrine tumors: A case series. *Endosc. Int. Open.* **2020**, *8*, E1754–E1758. [CrossRef]
23. Brown, N.G.; Patel, A.A.; Gonda, T.A. Immediate and durable therapeutic response after EUS-guided radiofrequency ablation of a pancreatic insulinoma. *VideoGIE* **2020**, *5*, 676–678. [CrossRef]
24. Marx, M.; Trosic-Ivanisevic, T.; Caillol, F.; Demartines, N.; Schoepfer, A.; Pesenti, C.; Ratone, J.P.; Robert, M.; Giovannini, M.; Godat, S. EUS-guided radiofrequency ablation for pancreatic insulinoma: Experience in 2 tertiary centers. *Gastrointest. Endosc.* **2022**, *95*, 1256–1263. [CrossRef]
25. Rizzatti, G.; de Nucci, G.; Crino', S.F.; Caillol, F.; Palazzo, L.; Pham, K.D.C.; Larghi, A.; Napolenon, B. Safety and efficacy of endoscopic ultrasound-guided radiofrequency ablation for the treatment of functional and non-functional pancreatic neuroendocrine neoplasms: Preliminary results of a multicentre prospective study. UEG Week 2022 Moderated Posters. *United Eur. Gastroenterol. J.* **2022**, *10* (Suppl. S8), 321–322.
26. Lakhtakia, S.; Nabi, Z.; Fathima, S.; Basha, J.; Gupta, R.; Reddy, N. Long term outcomes of EUS-guided RFA in pancreatic neuroendocrine tumors: A tertiary care centre experience. UEG Week 2022 Moderated Posters. *United Eur. Gastroenterol. J.* **2022**, *10* (Suppl. S8), 322–323.
27. Nabi, Z.; Lakhtakia, S.; Fathima, S.; Basha, J.; Gupta, R.; Negashwar Reddy, D. Long-term outcomes of EUS-guided RFA in pancreatic cancer neuroendocrine tumors: A tertiary care centre experience UEG Week 2022 E-Posters. *United Eur. Gastroenterol. J.* **2022**, *10* (Suppl. S8).
28. Borrelli de Andreis, F.; Boskoski, I.; Mascagni, P.; Bianchi, A.; Schinzari, G.; Annichiarico, E.B.; Quero, G.; Tortora, G.; Alfieri, S.; Gasbarrini, A.; et al. Safety and efficacy of EUS-guided radiofrequency ablation for unresectable pancreatic insulinoma: A single-center experience. *Eur. PMC* **2022**, in press.
29. Rossi, G.; Petrone, M.C.; Capurso, G.; Partelli, S.; Falconi, M.; Arcidiacono, P.G. Endoscopic ultrasound radiofrequency ablation of pancreatic insulinoma in elderly patients: Three case reports. *World J. Clin. Cases* **2022**, *10*, 6514–6519. [CrossRef]
30. Yoon, W.J.; Brugge, W.R. Endoscopic ultrasonography-guided tumor ablation. *Gastrointest. Endosc. Clin. N. Am.* **2012**, *22*, 359–369. [CrossRef]
31. Goldberg, S.N.; Mallery, S.; Gazelle, G.S.; Brugge, W.R. EUS-guided radiofrequency ablation in the pancreas: Results in a porcine model. *Gastrointest. Endosc.* **1999**, *50*, 392–401. [CrossRef] [PubMed]
32. Varadarajulu, S.; Jhala, N.C.; Drelichman, E.R. EUS-guided radiofrequency ablation with a prototype electrode array system in an animal model (with video). *Gastrointest. Endosc.* **2009**, *70*, 372–376. [CrossRef] [PubMed]
33. Gaidhane, M.; Smith, I.; Ellen, K.; Gatesman, J.; Habib, N.; Foley, P.; Moskaluk, C.; Kahaleh, M. Endoscopic Ultrasound-Guided Radiofrequency Ablation (EUS-RFA) of the Pancreas in a Porcine Model. *Gastroenterol. Res. Pract.* **2012**, *2012*, 431451. [CrossRef] [PubMed]
34. Sethi, A.; Ellrichmann, M.; Dhar, S.; Hadeler, K.G.; Kahle, E.; Seehusen, F.; Klapper, W.; Habib, N.; Fritscher-Ravens, A. Endoscopic ultrasound-guided lymph node ablation with a novel radiofrequency ablation probe: Feasibility study in an acute porcine model. *Endoscopy* **2014**, *46*, 411–415. [CrossRef]
35. Carrara, S.; Arcidiacono, P.G.; Albarello, L.; Addis, A.; Enderle, M.D.; Boemo, C.; Neugebauer, A.; Campagnol, M.; Doglioni, C.; Testoni, P.A. Endoscopic ultrasound-guided application of a new internally gas-cooled radiofrequency ablation probe in the liver and spleen of an animal model: A preliminary study. *Endoscopy* **2008**, *40*, 759–763. [CrossRef] [PubMed]
36. Carrara, S.; Arcidiacono, P.G.; Albarello, L.; Addis, A.; Enderle, M.D.; Boemo, C.; Campagnol, M.; Ambrosi, A.; Doglioni, C.; Testoni, P.A. Endoscopic ultrasound-guided application of a new hybrid cryotherm probe in porcine pancreas: A preliminary study. *Endoscopy* **2008**, *40*, 321–326. [CrossRef]
37. Arcidiacono, P.G.; Carrara, S.; Reni, M.; Petrone, M.C.; Cappio, S.; Balzano, G.; Boemo, C.; Cereda, S.; Nicoletti, R.; Enderle, M.D.; et al. Feasibility and safety of EUS-guided cryothermal ablation in patients with locally advanced pancreatic cancer. *Gastrointest Endosc.* **2012**, *76*, 1142–1151. [CrossRef]
38. Kım, H.J.; Seo, D.W.; Hassanuddin, A.; Kim, S.H.; Chae, H.J.; Jang, J.W.; Park, D.H.; Lee, S.S.; Lee, S.K.; Kim, M.H. EUS-guided radiofrequency ablation of the porcine pancreas. *Gastrointest. Endosc.* **2012**, *76*, 1039–1043. [CrossRef] [PubMed]
39. Song, T.J.; Seo, D.W.; Lakhtakia, S.; Reddy, N.; Oh, D.W.; Park, D.H.; Lee, S.S.; Lee, S.K.; Kim, M.H. Initial experience of EUS-guided radiofrequency ablation of unresectable pancreatic cancer. *Gastrointest. Endosc.* **2016**, *83*, 440–443. [CrossRef]
40. Armellini, E.; Leutner, M.; Stradella, D.; Ballarè, M.; Occhipinti, P. EUS-guided radiofrequency ablation: An option for the extrapancreatic region. *Endosc. Ultrasound* **2018**, *7*, 282–283. [CrossRef]
41. Jiang, T.A.; Deng, Z.; Tian, G.; Zhao, Q.Y.; Wang, W.L. Efficacy and safety of endoscopic ultrasonography-guided interventional treatment for refractory malignant left-sided liver tumors: A case series of 26 patients. *Sci. Rep.* **2016**, *6*, 36098. [CrossRef]
42. Lee, S.H.; Seo, D.W.; Oh, D.; Song, T.J.; Park, D.H.; Lee, S.S.; Kim, M.H. Cushing's syndrome managed by endoscopic ultrasound-guided radiofrequency ablation of adrenal gland adenoma. *Endoscopy* **2017**, *49*, E1–E2. [CrossRef]
43. Nagtegaal, I.D.; Odze, R.D.; Klimstra, D.; Paradis, V.; Rugge, M.; Schirmacher, P.; Washington, K.M.; Carneiro, F.; Cree, I.A.; WHO Classification of Tumours Editorial Board. The 2019 WHO classification of tumours of the digestive system. *Histopathology* **2020**, *76*, 182–188. [CrossRef]
44. Larghi, A.; Rizzatti, G.; Rimbaş, M.; Crino, S.F.; Gasbarrini, A.; Costamagna, G. EUS-guided radiofrequency ablation as an alternative to surgery for pancreatic neuroendocrine neoplasms: Who should we treat? *Endosc. Ultrasound* **2019**, *8*, 220–226. [CrossRef]

45. Falconi, M.; Eriksson, B.; Kaltsas, G.; Bartsch, D.K.; Capdevila, J.; Caplin, M.; Kos-Kudla, B.; Kwekkeboom, D.; Rindi, G.; Klöppel, G.; et al. Vienna Consensus Conference participants. ENETS Consensus Guidelines Update for the Management of Patients with Functional Pancreatic Neuroendocrine Tumors and Non-Functional Pancreatic Neuroendocrine Tumors. *Neuroendocrinology* **2016**, *103*, 153–171. [CrossRef]
46. Rosenberg, A.M.; Friedmann, P.; Del Rivero, J.; Libutti, S.K.; Laird, A.M. Resection versus expectant management of small incidentally discovered nonfunctional pancreatic neuroendocrine tumors. *Surgery* **2016**, *159*, 302–309. [CrossRef]
47. Falconi, M.; Zerbi, A.; Crippa, S.; Balzano, G.; Boninsegna, L.; Capitanio, V.; Bassi, C.; Di Carlo, V.; Pederzoli, P. Parenchyma-preserving resections for small nonfunctioning pancreatic endocrine tumors. *Ann. Surg. Oncol.* **2010**, *17*, 1621–1627. [CrossRef]
48. Falconi, M.; Mantovani, W.; Crippa, S.; Mascetta, G.; Salvia, R.; Pederzoli, P. Pancreatic insufficiency after different resections for benign tumours. *Br. J. Surg.* **2008**, *95*, 85–91. [CrossRef]
49. Aranha, G.V.; Shoup, M. Nonstandard pancreatic resections for unusual lesions. *Am. J. Surg.* **2005**, *189*, 223–228. [CrossRef] [PubMed]
50. Jilesen, A.P.; van Eijck, C.H.; in't Hof, K.H.; van Dieren, S.; Gouma, D.J.; van Dijkum, E.J. Postoperative Complications; In-Hospital Mortality and 5-Year Survival after Surgical Resection for Patients with a Pancreatic Neuroendocrine Tumor: A Systematic Review. *World J. Surg.* **2016**, *40*, 729–748. [CrossRef]
51. Partelli, S.; Maurizi, A.; Tamburrino, D.; Baldoni, A.; Polenta, V.; Crippa, S.; Falconi, M. GEP-NETS update: A review on surgery of gastro-entero-pancreatic neuroendocrine tumors. *Eur. J. Endocrinol.* **2014**, *171*, R153–R162. [CrossRef]
52. Leyden, S.; Kolarova, T.; Bouvier, C.; Caplin, M.; Conroy, S.; Davies, P.; Dureja, S.; Falconi, M.; Ferolla, P.; Fisher, G.; et al. Unmet needs in the international neuroendocrine tumor (NET) community: Assessment of major gaps from the perspective of patients; patient advocates and NET health care professionals. *Int. J. Cancer* **2020**, *146*, 1316–1323. [CrossRef]
53. Landoni, L.; Marchegiani, G.; Pollini, T.; Cingarlini, S.; D'Onofrio, M.; Capelli, P.; De Robertis, R.; Davì, M.V.; Amodio, A.; Impellizzeri, H.; et al. The Evolution of Surgical Strategies for Pancreatic Neuroendocrine Tumors (Pan-NENs): Time-trend and Outcome Analysis from 587 Consecutive Resections at a High-volume Institution. *Ann. Surg.* **2019**, *269*, 725–732. [CrossRef]
54. Ricci, C.; Partelli, S.; Landoni, L.; Rinzivillo, M.; Ingaldi, C.; Andreasi, V.; Nessi, C.; Muffatti, F.; Fontana, M.; Tamburrino, D.; et al. Sporadic non-functioning pancreatic neuroendocrine tumours: Multicentre analysis. *Br. J. Surg.* **2021**, *108*, 811–816. [CrossRef]
55. Papaefthymiou, A.; Laskaratos, F.M.; Koffas, A.; Manolakis, A.; Gkolfakis, P.; Coda, S.; Sodergren, M.; Suzuki, N.; Toumpanakis, C. State of the Art in Endoscopic Therapy for the Management of Gastroenteropancreatic Neuroendocrine Tumors. *Curr. Treat. Options Oncol.* **2022**, *23*, 1014–1034. [CrossRef]
56. Khanna, L.; Prasad, S.R.; Sunnapwar, A.; Kondapaneni, S.; Dasyam, A.; Tammisetti, V.S.; Salman, U.; Nazarullah, A.; Katabathina, V.S. Pancreatic Neuroendocrine Neoplasms: 2020 Update on Pathologic and Imaging Findings and Classification. *Radiographics* **2020**, *40*, 1240–1262. [CrossRef]
57. Paiella, S.; Landoni, L.; Tebaldi, S.; Zuffante, M.; Salgarello, M.; Cingarlini, S.; D'Onofrio, M.; Parisi, A.; Deiro, G.; Manfrin, E.; et al. Dual-Tracer (68Ga-DOTATOC and 18F-FDG-)-PET/CT Scan and G1-G2 Nonfunctioning Pancreatic Neuroendocrine Tumors: A Single-Center Retrospective Evaluation of 124 Nonmetastatic Resected Cases. *Neuroendocrinology* **2022**, *112*, 143–152. [CrossRef]
58. Crinó, S.F.; Brandolese, A.; Vieceli, F.; Paiella, S.; Conti Bellocchi, M.C.; Manfrin, E.; Bernardoni, L.; Sina, S.; D'Onofrio, M.; Marchegiani, G.; et al. Endoscopic Ultrasound Features Associated with Malignancy and Aggressiveness of Nonhypovascular Solid Pancreatic Lesions: Results from a Prospective Observational Study. *Ultraschall Med.* **2021**, *42*, 167–177. [CrossRef]
59. Paiella, S.; De Pastena, M.; D'Onofrio, M.; Crinò, S.F.; Pan, T.L.; De Robertis, R.; Elio, G.; Martone, E.; Bassi, C.; Salvia, R. Palliative therapy in pancreatic cancer-interventional treatment with radiofrequency ablation/irreversible electroporation. *Transl. Gastroenterol. Hepatol.* **2018**, *3*, 80. [CrossRef]
60. Paiella, S.; Landoni, L.; Rota, R.; Valenti, M.; Elio, G.; Crinò, S.F.; Manfrin, E.; Parisi, A.; Cingarlini, S.; D'Onofrio, M.; et al. Endoscopic ultrasound-guided fine-needle aspiration for the diagnosis and grading of pancreatic neuroendocrine tumors: A retrospective analysis of 110 cases. *Endoscopy* **2020**, *52*, 988–994. [CrossRef]
61. Tacelli, M.; Bina, N.; Crinò, S.F.; Facciorusso, A.; Celsa, C.; Vanni, A.S.; Fantin, A.; Antonini, F.; Falconi, M.; Monica, F.; et al. Reliability of grading preoperative pancreatic neuroendocrine tumors on EUS specimens: A systematic review with meta-analysis of aggregate and individual data. *Gastrointest. Endosc.* **2022**, *96*, 898–908.e23. [CrossRef]
62. Hallet, J.; Law, C.H.; Cukier, M.; Saskin, R.; Liu, N.; Singh, S. Exploring the rising incidence of neuroendocrine tumors: A population-based analysis of epidemiology; metastatic presentation; and outcomes. *Cancer* **2015**, *121*, 589–597. [CrossRef]
63. Melita, G.; Pallio, S.; Tortora, A.; Crinò, S.F.; Macrì, A.; Dionigi, G. Diagnostic and Interventional Role of Endoscopic Ultrasonography for the Management of Pancreatic Neuroendocrine Neoplasms. *J. Clin. Med.* **2021**, *10*, 2638. [CrossRef]
64. Rimbaş, M.; Horumbă, M.; Rizzatti, G.; Crinò, S.F.; Gasbarrini, A.; Costamagna, G.; Larghi, A. Interventional endoscopic ultrasound for pancreatic neuroendocrine neoplasms. *Dig. Endosc.* **2020**, *32*, 1031–1041. [CrossRef]

Disclaimer/Publisher's Note: The statements, opinions and data contained in all publications are solely those of the individual author(s) and contributor(s) and not of MDPI and/or the editor(s). MDPI and/or the editor(s) disclaim responsibility for any injury to people or property resulting from any ideas, methods, instructions or products referred to in the content.

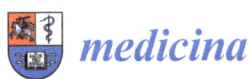

Article

Efficacy and Safety of Electrohydraulic Lithotripsy Using Peroral Cholangioscopy under Endoscopic Retrograde Cholangiopancreatography Guidance in Older Adults: A Single-Center Retrospective Study

Koji Takahashi [1,2,*], Hiroshi Ohyama [1], Yuichi Takiguchi [2], Yu Sekine [1], Shodai Toyama [1], Nana Yamada [1], Chihei Sugihara [1], Motoyasu Kan [1], Mayu Ouchi [1], Hiroki Nagashima [1], Yotaro Iino [1], Yuko Kusakabe [1], Kohichiroh Okitsu [1], Izumi Ohno [1,2] and Naoya Kato [1]

[1] Department of Gastroenterology, Graduate School of Medicine, Chiba University, Chiba 260-8670, Japan
[2] Department of Medical Oncology, Graduate School of Medicine, Chiba University, Chiba 260-8670, Japan
* Correspondence: takahashi.koji@chiba-u.jp; Tel.: +81-43-226-2083

Abstract: *Background and objectives:* The safety of electrohydraulic lithotripsy (EHL) in older adults remains unclear. We aimed to investigate the efficacy and safety of EHL using peroral cholangioscopy (POCS) under endoscopic retrograde cholangiopancreatography (ERCP) guidance in older adults aged ≥80 years. *Materials and Methods:* This retrospective clinical study was conducted at a single center. Fifty patients with common bile duct stones who underwent EHL using POCS under ERCP guidance at our institution, between April 2017 and September 2022, were enrolled in this study. The eligible patients were divided into an elderly group ($n = 21$, age ≥80 years) and a non-elderly group ($n = 29$, age ≤79 years), and were analyzed. *Results:* A total of 33 and 40 EHL procedures were performed in the elderly and non-elderly groups, respectively. After excluding cases in which stone removal was performed at other institutions, complete removal of common bile duct stones was confirmed in 93.8% and 100% of the elderly and non-elderly groups, respectively ($p = 0.20$). The mean number of ERCPs required for complete removal of bile duct stones was 2.9 and 4.3 in the elderly and non-elderly groups, respectively ($p = 0.17$). In the EHL session, the overall occurrence of adverse events was eight and seven in the elderly (24.2%) and non-elderly (17.5%) groups, respectively; however, the difference was insignificant ($p = 0.48$). *Conclusions:* EHL using POCS under ERCP guidance is effective in patients aged ≥80 years and there was no significant increase in adverse event rates compared to those aged ≤79 years.

Keywords: common bile duct stone; elderly; electrohydraulic lithotripsy; endoscopic retrograde cholangiopancreatography; safety

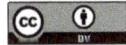

1. Introduction

Choledocholithiasis is often encountered in daily clinical practice and is a potential risk factor for acute cholangitis, pancreatitis, or obstructive jaundice. The European Society of Gastrointestinal Endoscopy recommends stone removal for patients with common bile duct (CBD) stones, symptomatic or not, who are fit enough to tolerate the intervention [1]. Endoscopic retrograde cholangiopancreatography (ERCP) is the standard procedure used for CBD stone removal. Various techniques have been developed for CBD stone dissolution, including balloon extraction, basket extraction, papillary balloon dilatation, mechanical lithotripsy, and stent insertion [2]. However, CBD stone removal remains challenging in some cases. Difficult CBD stones often require multiple ERCP sessions, which increases the risk of adverse events. Electrohydraulic lithotripsy (EHL) using peroral cholangioscopy (POCS) under ERCP guidance is considered an option for the treatment of difficult CBD stones. EHL is particularly effective in patients with large stones that are difficult to grasp due to breakup using a mechanical lithotripter or in those with bile duct strictures [3]. To date, there have been several reports on the safety of ERCP in the elderly; however, there are few comprehensive reports on the efficacy and safety of EHL using POCS under ERCP guidance in the elderly. To investigate this issue, we retrospectively evaluated the clinical outcomes and procedure-related adverse event rates of EHL using POCS under ERCP guidance in an elderly group (age $\geq$80 years) and non-elderly group (age $\leq$79 years) at our institution.

2. Patients and Methods

2.1. Study Design

This retrospective clinical study was conducted at a single center. Fifty consecutive patients with CBD stones who underwent EHL using POCS under ERCP guidance at our institution, between April 2017 and September 2022, were enrolled in this study. The exclusion criteria were as follows: (1) patients aged <20 years; (2) patients with surgical altered gastrointestinal anatomy, other than the distal gastrectomy Billroth I reconstruction; (3) patients with unclear background and treatment information; and (4) patients judged as inappropriate by the investigators.

The baseline characteristics of eligible patients included age, sex, Eastern Cooperative Oncology Group performance status (ECOG-PS), Charlson comorbidity index, previously attempted methods of stone removal, maximum CBD stone diameter, and presence of multiple stones. Clinical outcomes included the total number of EHL per patient, confirmation of complete removal of the CBD stone, procedure time, and adverse events. Patients were retrospectively examined using their medical records and data from an endoscopic database at our institution. The data were analyzed by patient and EHL session. Eligible patients were then divided into an elderly group (aged $\geq$80 years) and a non-elderly group (aged $\leq$79 years) and compared.

2.2. Definitions

The size and number of CBD stones were evaluated by cholangiography. The procedure time from duodenoscope insertion to removal was measured. The complete removal of CBD stones was defined as the confirmation of the absence of stones in the bile duct by cholangiography. The definitions and severity of each adverse event were defined according to the lexicon of the American Society for Gastrointestinal Endoscopy [4]. To explain the details, an adverse event was defined as an event that caused a prolongation of the hospital stay, medical consultation, or another procedure. Severity was defined as follows: an event requiring unplanned transfusion, ventilation support, additional endoscopic or radiological intervention, intensive care unit admission, or prolonged hospitalization for 4–10 days, which was defined as moderate. An adverse event which required surgical intervention, an intensive care unit stay of >1 day, or prolonged hospitalization for >10 nights was defined as severe. If an adverse event did not correspond to any of these, it was defined as mild. The ECOG-PS is a score that expresses the patient's daily living abilities, and the key elements of the ECOG-PS scale first appeared in the medical literature in 1960 [5]. The Charlson comorbidity index, which was proposed in 1987, is an index that evaluates comorbidities that contribute to death and is reported to be correlated with short-term mortality risk [6]. The ECOG-PS and Charlson comorbidity index were calculated from the patient's status records immediately prior to their first EHL.

2.3. Techniques

For patients with acute cholangitis, EHL was not performed in the state of cholangitis, but was performed after it subsided by stent placement or nasobiliary drainage. All patients fasted from the morning of the day of the treatment. EHL using POCS under ERCP guidance was performed as follows: prophylactic intravenous antibiotics were administered prior to the ERCP. Carbon dioxide insufflation was used during the procedure unless contraindicated. All patients underwent conscious sedation with the administration of a combination of midazolam and pethidine hydrochloride, or fentanyl and propofol. An oblique-viewing duodenoscope (TJF-260V, TJF-Q290V, Olympus Corporation, Tokyo, Japan) was inserted orally to reach the duodenal papilla, and an ERCP catheter (PR-104Q-1, Olympus, Tokyo, Japan; MTW ERCP catheter, ABIS, Hyogo, Japan) was inserted into the bile duct followed by cholangiography. After imaging the bile duct with a contrast medium, a 0.025-inch guidewire (VisiGlide2, Olympus Corporation, Tokyo, Japan; M-Through, ASAHI INTECC, Aichi, Japan; EndoSelector; Boston Scientific, Marlborough, MA, USA) was placed in the bile duct. Then, a cholangioscope (CHF-B260, CHF-B290, Olympus Corporation, Tokyo, Japan; SpyScope DS, SpyScope DS II; Boston Scientific, Marlborough, MA, USA) was inserted into the bile duct. An electrohydraulic shock wave generator was used to generate shock waves. EHL was performed under POCS guidance using a 1.9 French gauge EHL probe. After fragmentation, CBD stone removal was performed using ERCP techniques, such as a basket or balloon extraction (Figure 1). After treatment, the patient rested in bed for 2 h, and a blood test was performed the following day. Imaging tests, such as ultrasonography and computed tomography, were promptly performed if procedure-related adverse events were suspected.

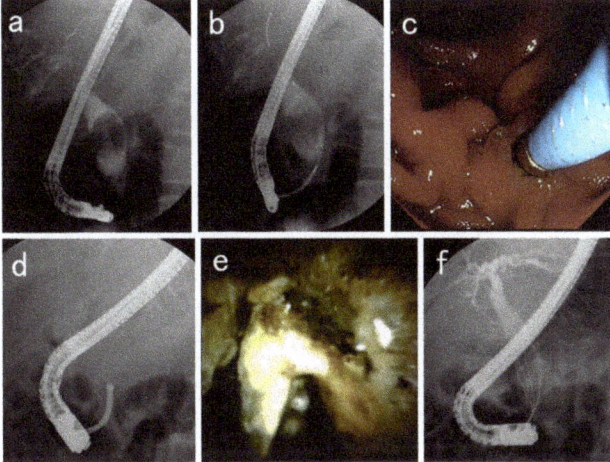

Figure 1. Electrohydraulic lithotripsy techniques using peroral cholangioscopy under endoscopic retrograde cholangiopancreatography guidance. (**a**) Cholangiography image showing a large common bile duct stone. (**b**) Stone removal is impossible using standard techniques. (**c**,**d**) A cholangioscope is inserted into the bile duct. (**e**) Electrohydraulic lithotripsy was performed under cholangioscopic guidance using an electrohydraulic lithotripsy probe. (**f**) Stone removal was performed using the standard technique after fragmentation of the common bile duct stone.

2.4. Statistical Analysis

The data are presented as means with standard deviations or numbers with percentages. Pearson's chi-squared test was used to assess the categorical data, whereas the Mann–Whitney U test was used to assess the quantitative data. Statistical significance was set at $p < 0.05$. All statistical analyses were performed using the bell curve for Excel (Social Survey Research Information Co., Ltd., Tokyo, Japan).

3. Results

Fifty eligible patients (28 men and 22 women) were included in this study. The age range of the patients was 36–94 years, with a mean age of 75.1 years. All eligible patients had previously attempted non-EHL stone removal, but it was unsuccessful. Endoscopic sphincterotomy (EST) had been performed previously on all eligible patients. Table 1 shows the baseline characteristics of all the eligible patients. The mean ECOG-PS was

1.0. The mean Charlson comorbidity index was 1.3. As previously attempted methods of stone removal, removal by a basket catheter, balloon catheter, or both was performed in all cases. Endoscopic papillary balloon dilatation was performed in 16.0% of patients, and an endoscopic mechanical lithotripsy was attempted in 56.0% of patients. The mean maximum diameter of the bile duct stones was 15.0 mm. The proportion of patients with multiple stones was 70.0%. The mean number of EHL was 1.4 times. In 42 patients, excluding 8 who underwent stone removal at another hospital after EHL, 41 patients (97.6%) had complete CBD stone removal. The mean number of ERCP procedures performed prior to complete stone removal was 3.5 times.

Table 1. Baseline characteristics of all eligible patients.

Variable	$n = 50$
Age, year, mean (SD)	75.1 (11.5)
Sex, male, n (%)	28 (56)
ECOG-PS, mean (SD)	1.0 (1.1)
Charlson comorbidity index, mean (SD)	1.3 (1.1)
Previously attempted methods for stone removal, n (%)	
Endoscopic papillary balloon dilatation	8 (16.0)
Endoscopic mechanical lithotripsy	28 (56.0)
Maximum diameter of bile duct stones, mm, mean (SD)	15.0 (4.8)
Multiple stones, n (%)	35 (70.0)
Total number of EHL per patient, mean (SD)	1.4 (1.0)
Number of cases in which complete stone removal was finally confirmed, n (%)	41/42 (97.6)
Number of ERCPs before complete stone removal, mean (SD)	3.5 (2.4)

SD: standard deviation; ECOG-PS: Eastern Cooperative Oncology Group performance status; EHL: electrohydraulic lithotripsy; ERCP: endoscopic retrograde cholangiopancreatography.

The procedure times and adverse events per EHL session are shown in Table 2. In total, 73 EHL sessions were conducted. The mean procedure time was 57.7 min. Adverse events occurred in 20.5% of all EHL procedures. Cholangitis occurred in 12 patients (16.4%), and its severity was mild in all patients. Pancreatitis occurred in two patients (2.7%) with mild severity. Peritonitis occurred in one patient (1.4%) with moderate severity. Pneumonia occurred in one patient (1.4%) with mild severity. No procedure-related deaths or sedation-related problems were reported.

Table 2. The procedure time and adverse events per electrohydraulic lithotripsy session.

Variable	$n = 73$
Procedure time, minutes, mean (SD)	57.7 (17.0)
Adverse events, n (%)	15 (20.5)
Cholangitis	12 (16.4)
mild	12 (16.4)
Pancreatitis	2 (2.7)
mild	2 (2.7)
Peritonitis	1 (1.4)
moderate	1 (1.4)
Pneumonia	1 (1.4)
mild	1 (1.4)

SD: standard deviation.

All eligible patients were divided into an elderly group (age ≥ 80 years) and a non-elderly group (age ≤ 79 years). Table 3 shows the results of the comparison of baseline characteristics and final treatment results of the elderly and non-elderly groups. There were 21 and 29 patients in the elderly and non-elderly groups, respectively. The mean age was 84.6 and 68.2 years in the elderly and the non-elderly groups, respectively ($p < 0.001$). The proportion of males was 57.1% and 55.2% in the elderly and non-elderly groups, respectively ($p = 0.89$). The mean ECOG-PS was 1.7 and 1.0 in the elderly and non-elderly groups, respectively ($p < 0.001$). The mean Charlson comorbidity index was 1.5 and 1.3 in the elderly and non-elderly groups, respectively ($p = 0.17$). Regarding previously attempted methods of stone removal, other than basket catheters and balloon catheters, the proportion of attempted endoscopic papillary balloon dilatation was 23.8% and 10.3% in the elderly and non-elderly groups, respectively ($p = 0.20$). The proportion of attempted endoscopic mechanical lithotripsy was 47.6% and 62.1% in the elderly and non-elderly groups, respectively ($p = 0.31$). The mean maximum diameter of the CBD stones was 16.1 mm and 14.1 mm in the elderly and non-elderly groups, respectively ($p = 0.085$). The percentage of patients with multiple CBD stones was 61.9% and 75.9% in the elderly and non-elderly groups, respectively ($p = 0.29$). A total of 33 and 40 EHL procedures were performed in the elderly and non-elderly groups, respectively. The proportion of patients who underwent stone removal at another hospital after EHL was 23.8% and 10.3% in the elderly and non-elderly groups, respectively ($p = 0.35$). Complete removal of CBD stones was confirmed in 15 of 16 cases (93.8%) and in all 26 cases (100%) in the elderly and non-elderly groups, respectively ($p = 0.20$). The mean number of ERCPs required for complete removal of bile duct stones was 2.9 and 4.3 in the elderly and non-elderly groups, respectively ($p = 0.17$).

Table 3. Comparison of baseline characteristics and final treatment results between the elderly and non-elderly groups.

Variable	Elderly $n = 21$	Non-Elderly $n = 29$	p-Value
Age, year, mean (SD)	84.6 (4.2)	68.2 (10.1)	<0.001
Sex, male, n (%)	12 (57.1)	16 (55.2)	0.89
ECOG-PS, mean (SD)	1.7 (1.0)	1.0 (1.0)	<0.001
Charlson comorbidity index, mean (SD)	1.5 (1.0)	1.3 (1.0)	0.17
Previously attempted methods for stone removal, n (%)			
Endoscopic papillary balloon dilatation	5 (23.8)	3 (10.3)	0.20
Endoscopic mechanical lithotripsy	10 (47.6)	18 (62.1)	0.31
Maximum diameter of bile duct stones, mm, mean (SD)	16.1 (4.3)	14.1 (5.0)	0.085
Multiple stones, n (%)	13 (61.9)	22 (75.9)	0.29
Total number of performing EHL	33	40	
Total number of performing EHL per patients, mean (SD)	1.3 (0.6)	1.5 (1.2)	0.86
Number of patients who underwent stone removal at another hospital after EHL, n (%)	5 (23.8)	3 (10.3)	0.35
Number of cases in which complete stone removal was finally confirmed, n (%)	15/16 (93.8)	26/26 (100)	0.20
Number of ERCPs before complete stone removal, mean (SD)	2.9 (1.4)	4.3 (2.9)	0.17

SD: standard deviation; ECOG-PS: Eastern Cooperative Oncology Group performance status; EHL: electrohydraulic lithotripsy; ERCP: endoscopic retrograde cholangiopancreatography.

The clinical outcomes for each EHL session are shown in Table 4. The mean procedure time was 54.4 and 60.4 min in the elderly and non-elderly groups, respectively ($p = 0.15$). The overall occurrence of adverse events was eight and seven in the elderly (24.2%) and non-elderly (17.5%) groups, respectively, with no significant difference ($p = 0.48$). Cholangitis occurred in both the elderly and non-elderly groups. Pancreatitis occurred only in the non-elderly group, whereas peritonitis and pneumonia occurred only in the elderly group. However, these differences were not statistically significant between the two groups.

Table 4. Clinical outcomes per electrohydraulic lithotripsy session.

Variable	Elderly n = 33	Non-Elderly n = 40	p-Value
Procedure time, minutes, mean (SD)	54.4 (15.7)	60.4 (17.6)	0.15
Adverse events, n (%)	8 (24.2)	7 (17.5)	0.48
Cholangitis	6 (18.2)	6 (15.0)	0.72
mild	6 (18.2)	6 (15.0)	0.72
Pancreatitis	0	2 (5.0)	0.19
mild	0	2 (5.0)	0.19
Peritonitis	1 (3.0)	0	0.27
moderate	1 (3.0)	0	0.27
Pneumonia	1 (3.0)	0	0.27
mild	1 (3.0)	0	0.27

SD: standard deviation.

4. Discussion

The present study investigated the efficacy and safety of EHL using POCS under ERCP guidance in patients aged ≥80 years. Even in patients in whom CBD stone removal was impossible using ERCP without EHL, 97.6% of the CBD stones were completely removed, finally. The adverse event rates were relatively high (20.5%), with mild cholangitis being the most common adverse event. There were no significant differences in the adverse event rates between patients aged >80 years and those aged ≤79 years. Furthermore, no procedure-related deaths occurred.

In EHL, a cholangioscope is inserted into the bile duct using ERCP and then, a probe for EHL is inserted into the bile duct to generate shock waves to crush the CBD stones. Because EHL is relatively labor intensive and costly, it is typically performed only when stone removal is difficult using other techniques. If the distal bile duct diameter is larger than that of the CBD stone, it can be removed with endoscopic papillary balloon dilatation, and if the CBD stone can be grasped with a mechanical lithotripter, it can be crushed and removed. EHL is indicated for CBD stones that are difficult to remove using endoscopic papillary balloon dilatation or endoscopic mechanical lithotripsy. In this study, EST was performed in all eligible patients, and endoscopic papillary balloon dilatation was performed in a small proportion of patients (16.0%); however, endoscopic mechanical lithotripsy was attempted in more than half of the patients. The contents of the endoscopic treatment prior to EHL depended on the environment of each facility where ERCP was performed. Some facilities do not have the devices for endoscopic papillary balloon dilatation or endoscopic mechanical lithotripsy. At our institution, EHL may be performed without endoscopic papillary balloon dilatation or endoscopic mechanical lithotripsy in cases where the stone is larger than the diameter of the distal bile duct or it is expected to be difficult to grasp with a mechanical lithotripter.

In this study, the overall EHL-related adverse event rate was 20.5%, which was higher than that of the conventional ERCP-related procedure. Among the adverse events, cholangitis was the most common at 16.4%. Cholangitis is presumed to be caused by increasing intraductal pressure of the bile duct due to washing the bile duct by injecting saline during the EHL. In this study, all cases of EHL-related cholangitis were mild in severity and improved rapidly without additional intervention. The pancreatitis was presumed to be caused by temporary edema of the duodenal papilla, due to the stimulation by the insertion of the cholangioscope and improved rapidly after the procedure without additional treatment. Peritonitis occurred in one case. Although the cause was not clear, EHL was performed within a short period after cholecystectomy in this case, and it was speculated that this occurred because the severed part of the cystic duct was partially released due to the increasing intraductal pressure of the bile duct. Pneumonia occurred in one case and was considered to be caused by saliva or gastric juice entering the airway during EHL.

Several reports have shown the efficacy of EHL using POCS under ERCP guidance for the removal of CBD stones. Conventionally, reusable cholangioscopes were used for EHL. Single-use cholangioscopes have recently been developed. A reusable cholangioscope can be used repeatedly; therefore, it is cost-effective if it is not broken down. However, even in facilities that have a reusable cholangioscope, most facilities have only one, and it is necessary to interrupt or stop treatment if it breaks down. The disadvantage of single-use cholangioscopes is their high cost. However, the risk of infection through the scope is very low. In 2018, Kamiyama reported that the complete CBD stone removal rate was 98%, with an adverse event rate of 12% for cholangitis and 2.4% for pancreatitis in EHL using single-use cholangioscopes. [3]. In 2020, Murabayashi compared the clinical outcomes of reusable cholangioscopy and single-use cholangioscopes in EHL and found no significant difference in the rate of final stone removal and adverse events between both groups; however, the procedure time was significantly shorter in the single-use cholangioscopy group, and the mean number of endoscopic sessions was significantly lower in the single-use cholangioscopy group [7].

Although there are few reports on the safety of EHL using POCS under ERCP guidance in older adults, there are several reports on the safety of ERCP in older adults. In 2015, a retrospective study showed that ERCP could be safely performed even in those aged ≥80 years, however the sedation-related adverse events increased in a retrospective analysis of 758 patients who underwent ERCP [8]. In 2018, a retrospective study comparing patients aged ≥80 years to those aged ≤65 years who underwent therapeutic ERCP, showed that the rate of difficult cannulation was higher in the ≥80 years group, the mean procedure time was longer in the aged ≥80 years group, and second ERCPs were performed more frequently in the aged ≥80 years group. The overall success and adverse event rates were not significantly different between the two groups [9]. In 2018, a retrospective study comparing patients aged ≥85 years to those aged <85 years who underwent therapeutic ERCP for CBD stones showed no difference in the recurrence rate of stones, adverse event and mortality rates, and the length and cost of hospitalization between the two groups [10]. In older adults, attention should be paid to post-procedural pneumonia. In 2023, a retrospective study showed that patients aged ≥90 years who underwent ERCP for CBD stone removal had a higher incidence of post-ERCP pneumonia than those aged 65–89 years [11]. In addition, there is a report that patients aged ≥90 years require particular attention among the elderly. In 2018, a retrospective study of 137 patients aged ≥85 years who underwent therapeutic ERCP showed that the incidence of adverse events significantly increased in those aged ≥90 years [12].

It is also characteristic of the elderly that the ECOG-PS is often lower than that of the non-elderly. There are several reports on the effect of ECOG-PS on ERCP. In 2019, a retrospective study showed that comparing 287 patients who underwent therapeutic ERCP divided into ECOG-PS 3–4 group and ECOG-PS 0–2 group, the overall adverse events did not significantly differ; however, aspiration pneumonia and heart failure were more likely to occur among patients with ECOG-PS 3–4 [13]. In a retrospective study reported in 2021, 1845 patients who underwent ERCP were divided into two groups: ECOG-PS 0–3 patients and ECOG-PS 4 patients. The pulmonary adverse event rate and severe adverse event rate were significantly higher in the ECOG-PS 4 group [14]. In a retrospective study reported in 2022, 1343 native papillae who underwent therapeutic ERCP for CBDS were divided into two groups: ECOG-PS 0–2 and those with ECOG-PS 3–4. No significant difference was observed between the therapeutic success rates and the overall ERCP-related adverse event rates; however, adverse events were significantly more severe in the ECOG-PS 3–4 group than in the ECOG-PS 0–2 group [15].

In our study, although there was no significant difference in the Charlson comorbidity index between the two groups, the ECOG-PS was significantly lower in the elderly group. In addition, although there was no significant difference, the elderly group tended to have multiple stones. However, there was no significant difference in clinical outcomes, including the occurrence rate of adverse events, between the two groups, and there were no treatment-related deaths. No duodenal perforation or bleeding occurred in this study. EHL does not require a large sphincterotomy because the CBD stones are crushed in the bile duct before stone removal. In addition, EHL does not require excessive dilation of the duodenal papilla, so it is a procedure with relatively little irritation to the duodenal papilla. Therefore, even if mild cholangitis occurs relatively frequently, serious adverse events, such as hemorrhage, perforation, and pancreatitis, may occur less frequently. Currently, EHL is not the first choice for difficult stones because it is costlier and more complicated to prepare than EML or EPBD. If it is resolved, depending on the case, EHL can be the first choice for CBD stones that are difficult to remove with basket or balloon extraction.

In this study, CBD stones, which were difficult to remove using other methods, were completely removed using EHL at a very high rate. The mean procedure time for EHL was 57.7 min, and the occurrence rates of post-procedure cholangitis were 16.4%. Compared to other ERCP procedures, EHL has a relatively long procedure time and a relatively high adverse event rate. However, EHL enables complete removal of difficult stones at a high rate and can be said to be a very useful procedure. There was no significant difference in the clinical outcomes and occurrence rates of adverse events in EHL between patients aged ≥ 80 years and those aged ≤ 79 years. EHL can be safely performed in individuals aged >80 years. However, attention should be given to the onset of post-procedural pneumonia.

This study has several limitations. First, it is a retrospective study. Second, the sample size of this study is small. Third, there are case-to-case differences in the endoscopic treatment before EHL. Fourth, there is a difference in the background characteristics between the elderly group and the non-elderly group because propensity score matching was not performed. Finally, the long-term outcomes, such as the recurrence rate of CBD stones after EHL treatment, are unclear.

5. Conclusions

In our study, we found that EHL using POCS under ERCP guidance enabled the efficient removal of CBD stones in the elderly group aged ≥ 80 years, and there was no significant increase in adverse event rates compared with those aged ≤ 79 years. Our analysis suggests that EHL using POCS under ERCP guidance can be performed equally effectively and safely in the elderly and non-elderly.

Author Contributions: Conceptualization, K.T. and H.O.; methodology, K.T. and H.O.; formal analysis, K.T.; investigation, Y.S., S.T., N.Y., C.S., M.K., M.O., H.N., Y.I., Y.K., K.O. and I.O.; data curation, Y.S., S.T., N.Y., C.S., M.K., M.O., H.N., Y.I., Y.K., K.O. and I.O.; writing—original draft preparation, K.T. and H.O.; writing—review and editing, all authors; supervision, Y.T. and N.K.; project administration, K.T., H.O., Y.T. and N.K. All authors have read and agreed to the published version of the manuscript.

Funding: This research received no external funding.

Institutional Review Board Statement: The study was conducted in accordance with the Declaration of Helsinki and approved by the Ethics Committee of Chiba University Hospital (protocol code: M10575 and date of approval: 7 February 2023).

Informed Consent Statement: Written informed consent for the procedure was obtained from all the patients. Consent for study participation was obtained using the opt-out methodology.

Data Availability Statement: The datasets generated during and/or analyzed during the current study are not publicly available but are available from the corresponding author upon reasonable request.

Conflicts of Interest: The authors declare no conflict of interest.

References

1. Manes, G.; Paspatis, G.; Aabakken, L.; Anderloni, A.; Arvanitakis, M.; Ah-Soune, P.; Barthet, M.; Domagk, D.; Dumonceau, J.M.; Gigot, J.F.; et al. Endoscopic management of common bile duct stones: European Society of Gastrointestinal Endoscopy (ESGE) guideline. *Endoscopy* **2019**, *51*, 472–491. [CrossRef] [PubMed]
2. Kedia, P.; Tarnasky, P.R. Endoscopic Management of Complex Biliary Stone Disease. *Gastrointest. Endosc. Clin.* **2019**, *29*, 257–275. [CrossRef] [PubMed]
3. Kamiyama, R.; Ogura, T.; Okuda, A.; Miyano, A.; Nishioka, N.; Imanishi, M.; Takagi, W.; Higuchi, K. Electrohydraulic Lithotripsy for Difficult Bile Duct Stones under Endoscopic Retrograde Cholangiopancreatography and Peroral Transluminal Cholangioscopy Guidance. *Gut Liver* **2018**, *12*, 457–462. [CrossRef] [PubMed]
4. Cotton, P.B.; Eisen, G.M.; Aabakken, L.; Baron, T.H.; Hutter, M.M.; Jacobson, B.C.; Mergener, K.; Nemcek, A., Jr.; Petersen, B.T.; Petrini, J.L.; et al. A lexicon for endoscopic adverse events: Report of an ASGE workshop. *Gastrointest. Endosc.* **2010**, *71*, 446–454. [CrossRef] [PubMed]
5. Oken, M.M.; Creech, R.H.; Tormey, D.C.; Horton, J.; Davis, T.E.; McFadden, E.T.; Carbone, P.P. Toxicity and response criteria of the Eastern Cooperative Oncology Group. *Am. J. Clin. Oncol.* **1982**, *5*, 649–655. [CrossRef] [PubMed]
6. Charlson, M.E.; Pompei, P.; Ales, K.L.; MacKenzie, C.R. A new method of classifying prognostic comorbidity in longitudinal studies: Development and validation. *J. Chronic. Dis.* **1987**, *40*, 373–383. [CrossRef] [PubMed]
7. Murabayashi, T.; Ogawa, T.; Koshita, S.; Kanno, Y.; Kusunose, H.; Sakai, T.; Masu, K.; Yonamine, K.; Miyamoto, K.; Kozakai, F.; et al. Peroral Cholangioscopy-guided Electrohydraulic Lithotripsy with a SpyGlass DS Versus a Conventional Digital Cholangioscope for Difficult Bile Duct Stones. *Intern. Med.* **2020**, *59*, 1925–1930. [CrossRef] [PubMed]
8. Finkelmeier, F.; Tal, A.; Ajouaou, M.; Filmann, N.; Zeuzem, S.; Waidmann, O.; Albert, J. ERCP in elderly patients: Increased risk of sedation adverse events but low frequency of post-ERCP pancreatitis. *Gastrointest. Endosc.* **2015**, *82*, 1051–1059. [CrossRef] [PubMed]
9. Yang, J.H.; Li, W.; Si, X.K.; Zhang, J.X.; Cao, Y.J. Efficacy and Safety of Therapeutic ERCP in the Elderly: A Single Center Experience. *Surg. Laparosc. Endosc. Percutan. Tech.* **2018**, *28*, e44–e48. [CrossRef] [PubMed]
10. Iida, T.; Kaneto, H.; Wagatsuma, K.; Sasaki, H.; Naganawa, Y.; Nakagaki, S.; Satoh, S.; Shimizu, H.; Nakase, H. Efficacy and safety of endoscopic procedures for common bile duct stones in patients aged 85 years or older: A retrospective study. *PLoS ONE* **2018**, *13*, e0190665. [CrossRef] [PubMed]
11. Jalal, M.; Khan, A.; Ijaz, S.; Gariballa, M.; El-Sherif, Y.; Al-Joudeh, A. Endoscopic removal of common bile duct stones in nonagenarians: A tertiary centre experience. *Clin. Endosc.* **2023**, *56*, 92–99. [CrossRef] [PubMed]
12. Takahashi, K.; Tsuyuguchi, T.; Sugiyama, H.; Kumagai, J.; Nakamura, M.; Iino, Y.; Shingyoji, A.; Yamato, M.; Ohyama, H.; Kusakabe, Y.; et al. Risk factors of adverse events in endoscopic retrograde cholangiopancreatography for patients aged ≥85 years. *Geriatr. Gerontol. Int.* **2018**, *18*, 1038–1045. [CrossRef] [PubMed]
13. Takahashi, K.; Nihei, T.; Aoki, Y.; Nakagawa, M.; Konno, N.; Munakata, A.; Okawara, K.; Kashimura, H. Efficacy and safety of therapeutic endoscopic retrograde cholangiopancreatography in patients with native papillae with a performance status score of 3 or 4: A single-center retrospective study. *J. Rural Med.* **2019**, *14*, 226–230. [CrossRef] [PubMed]
14. Kitano, R.; Inoue, T.; Ibusuki, M.; Kobayashi, Y.; Ohashi, T.; Sumida, Y.; Nakade, Y.; Ito, K.; Yoneda, M. Safety and Efficacy of Endoscopic Retrograde Cholangiopancreatography in Patients with Performance Status 4. *Dig. Dis. Sci.* **2021**, *66*, 1291–1296. [CrossRef] [PubMed]
15. Saito, H.; Kadono, Y.; Shono, T.; Kamikawa, K.; Urata, A.; Nasu, J.; Imamura, H.; Matsushita, I.; Kakuma, T.; Tada, S. Endoscopic retrograde cholangiopancreatography for bile duct stones in patients with a performance status score of 3 or 4. *World J. Gastrointest. Endosc.* **2022**, *14*, 215–225. [CrossRef] [PubMed]

Disclaimer/Publisher's Note: The statements, opinions and data contained in all publications are solely those of the individual author(s) and contributor(s) and not of MDPI and/or the editor(s). MDPI and/or the editor(s) disclaim responsibility for any injury to people or property resulting from any ideas, methods, instructions or products referred to in the content.

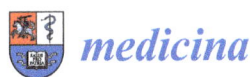

Article

Endosonography-Guided Versus Percutaneous Gallbladder Drainage Versus Cholecystectomy in Fragile Patients with Acute Cholecystitis—A High-Volume Center Study

Hayato Kurihara [1,†], Francesca M. Bunino [2,3,†], Alessandro Fugazza [4], Enrico Marrano [5], Giulia Mauri [2,3], Martina Ceolin [2], Ezio Lanza [6], Matteo Colombo [4], Antonio Facciorusso [7], Alessandro Repici [3,4] and Andrea Anderloni [8,*]

1. Emergency Surgery Unit, Fondazione IRCCS Ca' Granda Ospedale Maggiore Policlinico, 20122 Milan, Italy
2. Emergency Surgery and Trauma Section, Department of Surgery, IRCCS—Humanitas Research Hospital, 20089 Rozzano, Italy
3. Department of Biomedical Sciences, Humanitas University, 20090 Pieve Emanuele, Italy
4. Division of Gastroenterology and Digestive Endoscopy, Department of Gastroenterology, IRCCS—Humanitas Research Hospital, 20089 Rozzano, Italy
5. General Surgery, Hospital Universitari Parc Taulí, 08208 Sabadell, Spain
6. Department of Diagnostic and Interventional Radiology, IRCCS—Humanitas Research Hospital, 20089 Rozzano, Italy
7. Department of Medical and Surgical Sciences, Gastroenterology Unit, University of Foggia, 71122 Foggia, Italy
8. Gastroenterology and Digestive Endoscopy Unit, Fondazione IRCCS Policlinico San Matteo, 27100 Pavia, Italy
* Correspondence: andrea_anderloni@hotmail.com
† Shared first authorship.

Abstract: *Background and Objectives:* Acute cholecystitis is a frequent cause of admission to the emergency department, especially in old and frail patients. Percutaneous drainage (PT-GBD) and endosonographic guided drainage (EUS-GBD) could be an alternative option for relieving symptoms or act as a definitive treatment instead of a laparoscopic or open cholecystectomy (LC, OC). The aim of the present study was to compare different treatment groups. *Materials and Methods:* This is a five-year monocentric retrospective study including patients ≥65 years old who underwent an urgent operative procedure. A descriptive analysis was conducted comparing all treatment groups. A propensity score was estimated based on the ACS score, incorporated into a predictive model, and tested by recursive partitioning analysis. *Results:* 163 patients were included: 106 underwent a cholecystectomy (81 laparoscopic (LC) and 25 Open (OC)), 33 a PT-GBD and 21 EUS-GBD. The sample was categorized into three prognostic groups according to the adverse event occurrence rate. All patients treated with EUS-GBD or LC resulted in the low risk group, and the adverse event rate (AE) was 10/96 (10.4%). The AE was 4/28 (14.2%) and 21/36 (58.3%) in the middle- and high-risk groups respectively ($p < 0.001$). These groups included all the patients who underwent an OC or a PT-GBD. The PT-GBD group had a lower clinical success rate (55.5%) and higher RR (16,6%) when compared with other groups. *Conclusions:* Surgery still represents the gold standard for AC treatment. Nevertheless, EUS-GBD is a good alternative to PT-GBD in terms of clinical success, RR and AEs in all kinds of patients.

Keywords: cholecystitis; percutaneous gallbladder drainage; endosonography-guided gallbladder drainage; cholecystectomy; frailty; ACS score

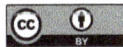

1. Introduction

Acute cholecystitis (AC) is one of the common differential diagnoses for patients presenting with abdominal pain in the emergency department. The risk of developing symptomatic episodes of biliary colic and cholecystitis is higher in the older population. Early cholecystectomy is the gold standard of treatment for AC [1,2]. However, in elderly, polymorbid and high-risk patients, alternative therapies should be considered such as percutaneous gallbladder drainage (PT-GBD) or endoscopic ultrasound-guided gallbladder drainage (EUS-GBD) [3]. Several studies reported comparisons between surgery and alternatives techniques such as the CHOCOLATE trial [4] and more recently Teoh et al. [5,6]. Current guidelines do not provide definitive recommendations on how to manage high-risk patients with AC who would not be considered for surgery [2,7]. Due to the lack of evidence, we decided to investigate our series by comparing all treatment populations for AC.

2. Materials and Methods

Data were collected from a prospectively maintained database at the Humanitas Research Hospital, IRCCS, Rozzano, Italy (with approval of the Ethical Committee of the IRCSS Humanitas Research Hospital of Rozzano – Milan; NCT02855151 (20 January 2016)). All patients ≥ 65 years old accepted at the emergency department with AC who underwent an urgent operative procedure (PT-GBD, EUS-GBD, LC or OC) between January 2015 and December 2020 were included. Data included: sociodemographic and preoperative data and medical history (previous episodes of AC, nonoperative management (NOM) failure, previous ERCP, anticoagulant medications, laboratory tests). The severity of the disease was calculated according to the latest Tokyo guidelines (TG18) that state AC into three severity grades. Each AC case was evaluated and its severity scored according to TG18 [2]. The American College of Surgeons National Surgical Quality Improvement Program Surgical Risk Calculator (ACS NSQIP score SRC) was used to estimate the serious complication risk and the death risk compared with the average risk of the procedure [8]. We defined it as ACS score. The Clinical Frailty Scale Score (CFSS) was used to define the fragility level [9]. The failure of nonoperative management (NOM) was reported even if patients were included independent of the fact that a conservative treatment had been previously attempted.

The therapeutic strategy was decided by a multidisciplinary group composed of surgeons, endoscopists, and radiologists choosing for each patient the best procedure according to the above-mentioned score and the best practice habits. If surgery was the choice, the laparoscopic or open approach was chosen by the attending surgeon considering the patient physiology, the TG18 score, the AAST score, and lastly the laparoscopy expertise (although at our center, all the senior surgeons have good laparoscopy expertise, and if a difficult LC was performed by a surgery resident, a further laparoscopic procedure was attempted by the senior surgeon before converting to open surgery).

Ongoing anticoagulant therapy was considered a risk factor for complications.

Postoperative variables were classified as: adverse events (AE), technical success (TS), clinical success (CS), need for rescue procedure, kind of rescue procedure, recurrence rate (RR), length of hospital stay, 90-day mortality.

2.1. Outcomes Definitions

The first outcome was technical success (TS), and it was defined differently for each technique: the ability to drain the gallbladder with the placement of a lumen-apposing metal stent (LAMS) in the EUS-GBD group; performing a complete cholecystectomy, laparoscopic or open; or placing a percutaneous catheter in the PT-GBD group.

The second outcome was the clinical success, considered the improvement of clinical symptoms and laboratory tests within the first week after the procedure [5,10].

The third outcome was the recurrence rate (RR), considered a further AC episode within one year from the first procedure or the immediate need of a rescue procedure due to a lack of clinical improvement.

As a last but major outcome, we considered the adverse event (AE) rate and the serious adverse event (SAE) rate. We registered AEs according to the Clavien Dindo scale (CD) considering them severe if CD ≥ 3 [11]. We considered infective complications all cases that required antibiotics, both oral and intravenous; we defined septic shock according to the last 2016 Sepsis-3 consensus [12].

Patients were followed up through both clinical visits and phone calls.

2.2. Procedures

LC or OC: In case of a laparoscopic approach, the procedure was performed using a four-trocar technique [2], while the open technique was performed through subcostal incision [13]. The critical view of safety [7] was always required before the cystic duct and cystic artery were transected after clipping them. The gallbladder was subsequently removed from its bed by electrocautery. Preoperative antibiotic prophylaxis was administered (2 gr. cefazolin e.v. or piperacilline-tazobactam in more severe grades of AC) [2].

PT-GBD: A percutaneous catheter was placed under image guidance (US or CT scan). The puncture was performed transhepatic or transperitoneal, and the pigtail catheter (8–10 Fr) was placed either with one-step using a trocar or with the Seldinger technique. The drain would stay in place for almost three weeks and required an antegrade cholangiography before its removal [4–6,14].

EUS-GBD: This procedure provides a connection between the gastrointestinal lumen and the gallbladder by placing a LAMS. Under EUS guidance, the gallbladder was studied and drained from either the stomach or duodenum. It consisted in accessing the gallbladder directly by puncturing it with the device on the pure-cut setting, followed by deployment of a 8–8 mm or a 10–10 mm stent without any exchange of devices [10,15].

2.3. Statistical Analysis

Patient characteristics were summarized using median and interquartile range (IQR) for continuous variables and absolute frequencies and percentages for categorical ones. Variables were compared with chi square test in the case of categorical variables and ANOVA in the case of continuous ones. To assess the prognostic role of the baseline variables on AE rate and to rank the relevance of each predictor variable, we estimated random-forest variable importance measures through the permutation of variable values. To control for pretreatment imbalances on observed variables and better estimate the causal effects of interventions, a propensity score was estimated with a generalized boosted model on the following variables: age, sex, ACS, previous episode of AC, antithrombotic therapy, WBC, and CRP. The propensity score was then incorporated into the predictive model through inverse probability weighting [16–18]. The predictor variables were then tested by recursive partitioning analysis (RPA) [19]. Once risk groups were identified in the model, they were compared to determine whether sufficient divergences in terms of adverse event rate and severe adverse event rate were present across identified risk classes, by means of chi square test. The model was then internally validated using bootstrap resampling and the performance validation was expressed through the area under the receiver-operating characteristic curve (AUC, or c-statistic) [20]. Calibration was assessed by means of a plot showing the correlation between the mean predicted AE probability versus the mean observed AE rate in deciles of patients with increasing values of the predicted probability. Differences between predicted probability and observed AE rate were assessed by the Hosmer–Lemeshow test [21]. All statistical tests were 2-tailed, and differences were considered significant at a p value < 0.05. The statistical analysis was run using the rpart and performance packages in R Statistical Software 3.0.2 (Foundation for Statistical Computing, Vienna, Austria).

3. Results

In this study, 163 patients were included. Surgery was performed in 106 patients (81 LC, 25 OC), PT-GBD on 33 cases and EUS-GBD on 21 cases. Among the group, 90 patients (56%) were males, with significant difference in sex distribution amongst groups. Median age was 77 (IQR 71–82) ($p < 0.001$). Patients who underwent surgery were younger. The same was for the ACS score distribution: it was higher in the PT-GBD group and in the OC group ($p < 0.001$). The width range was 1.00–8.00, and the median CFSS was 3, but it was higher in the PT-GBD groups, and its difference was statistically significant ($p < 0.001$).

Considering the pretreatment laboratory values, a significant difference was found amongst groups for WBC count ($p = 0.002$) and CRP ($p = 0.004$). Differences in INR values were not significant, but our study outlined relevant differences in distribution among groups. A statistically significant distribution was observed for the anticoagulant therapy: over half (57%) of the patients who underwent EUS-GBD were on active antithrombotic therapy ($p = 0.02$) and the therapy wasn't suspended before the procedure.

The failure of eventual nonoperative management was reported with a statistically significant difference among groups: patients from PT-GBD group resulted in a higher rate of NOM failure (51.5%).

The preoperative baseline characteristics of patients are outlined in Table 1.

Table 1. Baseline patients' characteristics.

Variable	Total ($n = 163$)	PT-GBD ($n = 33$)	EUS-GBD ($n = 21$)	LC ($n = 81$)	OC ($n = 25$)	p Value
Age Median (IQR)	77 (71–82)	83 (75–87)	84 (81–89)	74 (70–79)	74 (69–80)	**<0.001**
Male No (%)	90 (56%)	12 (36%)	10 (48%)	51 (63%)	17 (68%)	**0.03**
BMI Median (IQR)	26.2 (24.2–29.1)	26.7 (23.6–29.6)	25.8 (21.6–28)	25.8 (24.3–25.8)	27.3 (25.2–31.2)	0.24
Clinical Fraility Scale Score (median [range])	3.00 [1.00, 8.00]	6.00 [2.00, 8.00]	4.00 [2.00, 8.00]	3.00 [1.00, 8.00]	3.00 [2.00, 7.00]	**<0.001**
ACS score Median (IQR)	6.45 (3.88–17.02)	17.6 (16.4,23)	6.1 (5.3–7.3)	4 (2.8–6)	17.5 (12.9–20.6)	**<0.001**
Non operative management (NOM) failure	36 (22.5)	17 (51.5)	4 (19.0)	11 (13.6)	4 (16.0)	**<0.001**
Previous AC No (%)	41 (26%)	12 (38%)	8 (38%)	17 (21%)	4 (16%)	0.10
Previous ERCP No (%)	17 (11%)	3 (9%)	6 (29%)	7 (9%)	1 (4%)	0.12
Anticoagulant therapy No (%)	47 (29%)	10 (30%)	12 (57%)	18 (22%)	7 (28%)	**0.02**
WBC No ($\times 1000$)	12 (8.5–16.5)	6.9 (0.7–16.1)	14.7 (7.5–17.1)	12.6 (10.4–17)	11.7 (10.7–14.4)	**0.02**
Hb [g/dl] Median (IQR)	12.9 (10.3–13.4)	NR	NR	13.1 (10.3–14.2)	12.4 (11–14.3)	0.11
CRP [mg/dl] Median (IQR)	11.5 (4–22.7)	15 (11.2–24)	6.15 (1.87–25)	8.32 (2.4–19.1)	13.5 (7.16–24.8)	**0.04**
Total Bilirubin [mg/dl] Median (IQR)	1.2 (0.73–2)	1.2 (0.7–2.4)	1.1 (0.62–1.53)	1.32 (0.88–2.08)	0.9 (0.68–1.87)	0.43
INR Median (IQR)	1.21 (1.1–1.37)	1.32 (1.21–1.69)	1.23 (1.1–1.36)	1.15 (1.07–1.31)	1.2 (1.13–1.29)	**0.008**

Continuous variables were reported as median values and interquartile range. Comparisons were performed with ANOVA for continuous variables and chi square test for categorical ones. Significances were reported in bold. Previous AC: previous episode of acute cholecystitis; ERCP: Endoscopic retrograde cholangiopancreatography; WBC: white blood cells; Hb: Hemoglobin; CPR: c-reactive protein; INR: International Normalized Ratio. Bold values are statistically significant.

A detailed list of patient outcomes is reported in Table 2.

Table 2. Postoperative Outcomes.

	Total (163 pts)	PT-GBD (n = 33)	EUS-GBD (n = 21)	LC (n = 81)	OC (n = 25)	
Technical Success (TS) No (%)	162 (99)	33 (100)	20 (95)	81 (100)	25 (100)	0.084
Clinical success (CS) No (%)	124 (78)	21 (64)	18 (85)	69 (85)	16 (64)	**0.02**
Recurrence Rate (RR) No (%)	11 (9)	7 (24)	3 (14)	0	1 (4)	**<0.001**
Adverse event rate No (%)	41 (26)	13 (9)	2 (10)	13 (16)	13 (52)	**<0.001**
Severe Adverse Event rate No (%)	17 (11)	9 (27)	0	2 (2)	4 (16)	**0.001**
Type of adverse event						
Drainage Displacement No (%)	6 (12)	5 (18)	0	-	-	NC
Sepsis/Septic Shock No (%)	8 (19)	4 (12)	1 (5)	2 (2)	2 (8)	NC
Cystic duct obstruction No (%)	1 (2)	1 (3)	-			NC
.cBiliary leak No (%)	6 (15)	1 * (3)	-	-	5 * (20)	NC
Cholangitis No (%)	1 (2)	-	-	-	1 (4)	NC
Medical complications (cardiological, respiratory, renal failure) No (%)	17 (41)	1 (3)	1 (5)	6 (7)	4 (16)	NC
Lenght of stay (day) (median [range])	6.00 [1.00, 167.69]	15.26 [5.00, 57.53]	5.00 [1.00, 167.69]	4.61 [1.12, 70.90]	8.12 [3.00, 53.82]	**<0.001**
90-Day mortality No (%)	5 (4)	3 (27)	-	2 (2)	0 (0)	**0.004**

* 1 secondary biliary duct. Bold values are statistically significant.

TS was reached in 100% of cases except in the EUS-GBD group, where in one case, the device positioning was not feasible due to the migration of the device between the gallbladder lumen and the stomach. A rescue surgery was performed with the repair of a microscopic antral wall defect.

In the surgical group, four patients were converted from LC to OC, but all the surgeries were completed successfully without cases of incomplete cholecystectomy. All the AC that required a change of surgical plan had an AAST score of more than 3 and a TG18 score of 2 or 3. Furthermore, during surgery they badly tolerated pneumoperitoneum, and the surgical team finally decide to convert. One of them was a severely ill patient with a frailty score of 8 who failed NOM and was surgically treated. He finally died during intensive care hospitalization due to his extremely poor physiological status.

Overall CS rate was 124/163 (78%), and RR was 15/163 (9%). The overall AE rate was 41/163 (26%). Of all AEs (41), only 17 were graded as severe and required invasive treatment. We registered five cases of PT-GBD displacement managed by the repositioning of the drain.

Six patients experienced a biliary leak (five in the OC group and one PT-GBD). Of these, the one from the PT-GBD group was due to a Luschka duct and was surgically treated, while the others resolved by leaving the drains in place. In five cases (all from the PT-GBD group), patients experienced severe septic shock. In one of them, a rescue EUS-GBD was performed, and the others patients were surgically treated.

No bleeding complications occurred, and the EUS-GBD series patients on active anticoagulant therapy were not burdened by a higher number of AEs. Infective complications occurred in 10 patients; 3 cholangitis and 7 severe septic shocks: 4 from the PT-GBD group, 1 from the EUS-GBD group, 2 from OC group and 1 from the LC. The 4 patients from the PT-GBD group, underwent a rescue procedure: 2 surgeries, 1 repositioning of percutaneous drainage and 1 EUS-GBD. The endoscopically treated patient and one of the two surgically treated patients died due to medical complications (pneumonia and cardiac failure).

In the results, 90-day mortality was 5/163 (3%): 3 patients from the PT-GBD group and 2 from the surgical group. Of the PT-GBD group, two patients died after a rescue cholecystectomy due to a serious septic status. The others died because of medical complications. One case of cholangitis was reported after surgery, and it was treated with antibiotics.

Additional data about adverse events are presented in Supplementary Table S1.

Looking at the RR, 11 patients returned to the emergency department for a new AC episode. Of these, 7 were from the PT-GBD group, 3 from the EUS-GBD group. Patients from PT-GBD group were managed with EUS-GBD in 2 cases and LC in 2 cases, and the others were treated non-operatively with antibiotics. Furthermore, a case of cholangitis was described in the LC group causing readmission of the patient. It was managed with antibiotics with no complications.

Patients from the EUS-GBD groups who developed a recurrent AC episode were all treated non-operatively with good response.

The median LOS for PT-GBD patients was 15,26 days while it was 5 days for patients who underwent EUS-GBD, 4.61 for LC and 8.12 for OC. All the hospitalization was considered and not only the time after the procedure. Most patients who underwent PT-GBD were severely comorbid and frail, and they developed AC during the hospitalization for other issues.

3.1. Recursive Partitioning Analysis

As reported in Figure 1, random forest analysis found that greater importance in predicting AE occurrence was related to treatment used and ACS score. In fact, the greater permutation accuracy importance was observed in the treatment (EUS-GBD, PC-GBD, open surgery or VLS) and ACS score, followed by clinical frailty score and age. RPA of prognostic factors demonstrated that the risk of AE was stratified according to treatment used and ACS score, as in Figure 2. These factors split the series into three classes: low, intermediate, and high risk. Patients treated with EUS-GBD and patients with ACS score <17.4 treated with LC fall in the low-risk group (AE 10.4%, SAE 3.1%). Patients with ACS score <17.4 treated with open surgery or PT-GBD are classified at intermediate risk (AE 14.2%, SAE 7.1%), whereas patients with ACS score >17.4 treated with surgical (either LC or open) or percutaneous approach were at high risk of AE (AE 58.3%, SAE 25%). Of note, patients in the high-risk group experienced also poorer efficacy outcomes, with a success rate of 55.5% (versus 87.5% and 89.2% of low and intermediate risk groups; $p < 0.001$) and RR of 16.6%, again significantly superiors (7.3% and 0%, respectively; $p < 0.001$). Higher values of mean decrease in accuracy importance indicate variables that are more important to the classification.

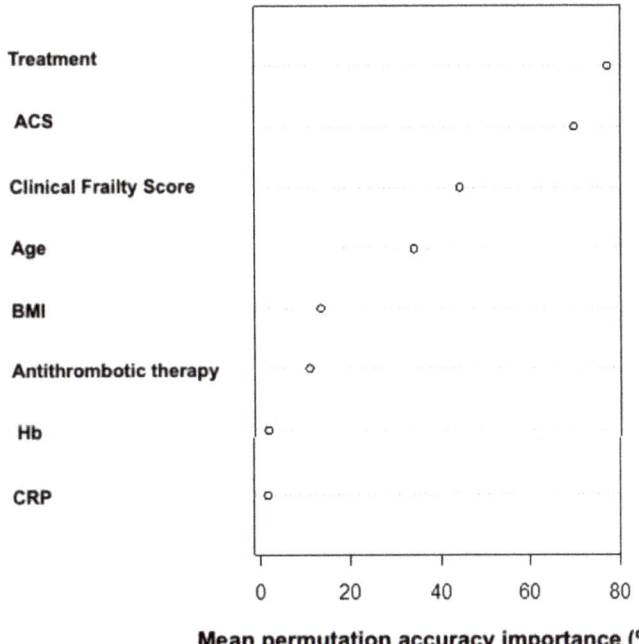

Figure 1. Variable importance estimated by permutation-based mean decreased accuracy importance considering adverse event rate as outcome.

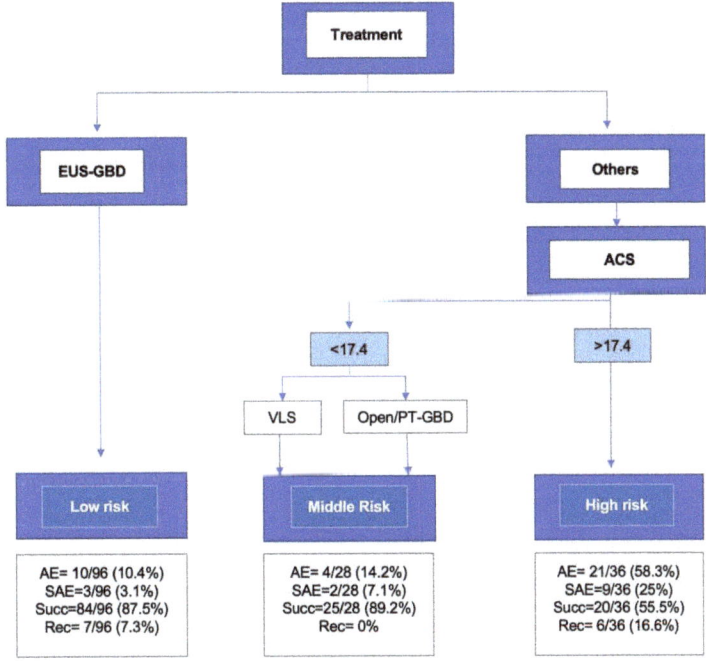

Figure 2. Recursive partitioning classification tree for adverse event occurrence. The terminal nodes

categorized the study sample into three prognostic groups according to the adverse event occurrence rate. Adverse event rate was 10/96 (10.4%) in the low-risk group, 4/28 (14.2%) and 21/36 (58.3%) in the middle and high-risk groups, respectively ($p < 0.001$). Abbreviations: VLS: Videolaparoscopy, PT-GBD: Percutaneous Gallbladder drainage; EUS-GBD: Endoscopic ultrasound guided gallbladder drainage; ACS: American College of Surgeons risk score; AE: Adverse Event; SAE: Severe adverse event; Succ: Clinical success (CS); Rec: Recurrence (RR).

3.2. Performance of the Model and Validation

The model showed a c-index of 74.3% (95% CI: 71.1%-78.2%; Figure 3) and a proper calibration (Hosmer–Lemeshow p value = 0.58 and mean error rate 3.3%) as shown by the calibration plot (Wald test for calibration slope p = 0.55; Figure 4). The internal validation of the model based on a bootstrap method (250 repetitions), showed a c-index of 72.5% (95% CI 70.3%–75.4%) (Figure 3) thus excluding the risk of overfitting.

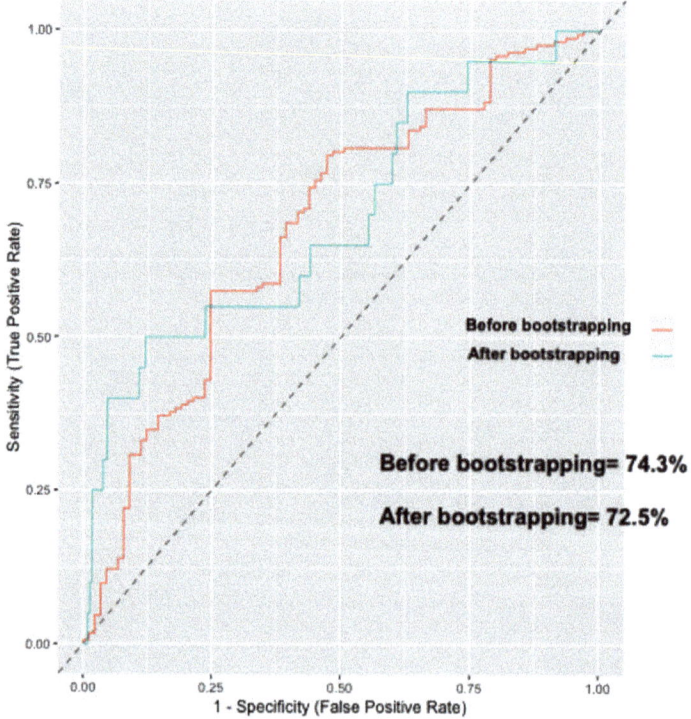

Figure 3. Receiver operating characteristic (ROC) curve and the corresponding area of the predictive model. Red line corresponded to the analysis before internal validation and green line corresponded to the analysis after bootstrapping-based internal validation.

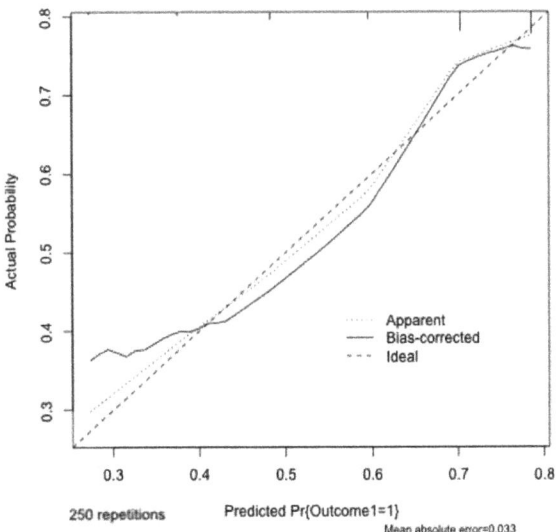

Figure 4. Calibration plot. Smoothed (loess) calibration plots reporting increasing predicted probability of adverse events by the assessed model. The diagonal line indicates the ideal line of perfect correspondence of predicted to observed adverse event rate. Mean absolute error rate was 3.3%.

4. Discussion

The aim of the current study was to compare outcomes of EUS-GBD, PT-GBD and surgery (both Laparoscopic and Open approach) considering and comparing technical and clinical success, complications rate and recurrence [13,14,22–25]. In the last few years, an increasing interest for alternative treatments of AC in frail patients was registered and many studies focused on this topic [10,14,22,26–29].

From the baseline characteristics analysis, a different distribution amongst frailty and age was outlined; patients treated with PT-GBD were older than patients submitted to surgery and had a higher ACS score. CFS score was calculated for all patients and it outlined, at first, an extremely heterogenous distribution of fragility among the population, second, that patients undergoing PT-GBD resulted being frailer than others. Such a difference highlight, in our opinion, a good evaluation and treatment choice. In fact, these PT-GBD patients would have been expected to have a poor surgery response due to their frailty level. It must be noticed that patients undergoing EUS-GBD had a 2-point-lower CFSS. This is probably due to the retrospective nature of the current study and the short-time experience in EUS-GBD field. Patients with AC, candidate to an invasive procedure, were evaluated by surgeon, endoscopist and radiologist and frail patients should have been avoided from surgery and addressed to PT vs EUS guided drainage. However, the short-time expertise could have compelled the multi-disciplinary team to avoid EUS-GBD if not completely safe. In the end, the different distribution of treatments reflects the clinical practice where surgical treatment continues to be considered the gold standard also thanks to increased quality of anesthesiologic assistance [3,7]. The AE rate for the surgical branch did not result in a higher severe complication rate when compared to PT-GBD. The interim analysis of the CHOCOLATE trial recently demonstrated that patients who undergo surgery have a lower rate of major complications (12%) when compared with PT-GBD (44% of AE) [4]. In our series, 16% of the LC group had AEs vs 39% of the PT-GBD group [4]. A higher number of AEs was observed in the OC group (52%). Revising the OC series many cases of AC with high ASST and TG18 score were observed. Moreover, the ACS score was usually higher in patients undergoing an open approach, either due to the inner risk of the procedure and to the physio pathological state of the patient. The AE rate was quite high suggesting that these patients could have been good candidates to EUS-GBD instead of a surgical approach.

We choose the ACS as score considering its widespread use in the surgical community [8]. Patients with an ACS >17.4 had higher AE rate; all the patients treated with PT-GBD were part of this group (high risk of AE). On the other hand, patients who underwent LC had an ACS <17.4 and a lower AE rate. Considering this finding we may assume that the therapeutic strategy was correct and based on a valid risk estimation. Recently, Teoh et al., promoted EUS-GBD use, demonstrating that it may reduce the risk of gallstone-related adverse events. They demonstrated, using a propensity score matching, an AE rate of 13.3%, a RR of 10% with a clinical success of 93.3%. When compared to PT-GBD, they found that EUS-GBD significantly reduced 1-year AEs (10 (25.6%) vs. 31 (77.5%), $p < 0.001$) and 30-day AEs (5 (12.8%) vs. 19 (47.5%), $p = 0.001$). Based on our results we can support their findings (AE 10.4% vs. 14.2% in patients with ACS <17.4 and 58.3 in patients with ACS > 17.4) [5,6]. Similar were RR and CS (in our population respectively 7.3% and 87.5%). The main difference was the population selection, in Teoh's series only patients excluded from surgery with an AC grade 2 and 3 were considered for EUS-GBD. In our study we considered all patients admitted with AC independently from the grade. This way EUS-GBD represents a real alternative to surgery in frail patients and not a second line procedure. In our center TS ranged almost 100% in all groups. However, multicentric study may be desirable to compare these procedures, also pondering the lack of experience, especially in EUS-GBD positioning [25–29].

CS was achieved in 64% of PT-GBDs, against 85% of both the EUS-GBD and LC groups. It may be assumed that EUS-GBD and LC are the best strategies, when looking at the first postoperative period. If we exclude the LC patients (RR = 0), the lower RR was observed in the EUS-GBD group (RR = 14% vs. 24% in PT-GBD). This could be due to the ease of displacement of the gallbladder drain or the higher risk of obstruction in a small drain lumen. 5 cases of dislodgment were registered in PT-GBD series (vs only one case in EUS-GBD group). This finding is in line with the current literature [22–25]. In a recent retrospective study the cholecystostomy tube dislodgment was registered 17,8% [30]. In Teoh's series PT-GBD resulted in a higher rate of dislodgement (35%) while no EUS-GBD drain displaced. Another interesting finding is related to anticoagulant therapy did not influence the AE rate: the safety of this strategy has already been described in our center within a case series and it is confirmed in this setting [30]. Moreover, the device could theoretically stay in place until stones and sludge are completely drained and then removed or left in place lifelong if well tolerated by the patient. In our center no devices have been removed and until now any issue or complication or affection to the QoL have been reported. We are aware that a longer follow up could be desirable to better evaluate the efficiency of the device, recurrence rate and lastly the possible technical difficulty in performing future surgery. Our experience up to now provide results on the safety of the EUS-GBD procedure, on the clinical improvement and in shortening hospitalization. Future studies and the extension of the follow up on our patients will provide evidence on long-term efficacy.

5. Conclusions

Surgery for AC remains the gold standard treatment with good outcomes in recurrence rate, complications rate, safety and mortality. This paper evidence the emerging role of EUS-GBD, particularly in patients not fit for surgery. EUS-GBD could be considered a good alternative for treatment, long term results are promising even though still under study. This EUS procedure could represent an innovation, especially facing old and frail patients. Moreover, our results highlight the need for calculating scores and approaching patients in a multidisciplinary way even in an emergency setting.

Supplementary Materials: The following supporting information can be downloaded at: https://www.mdpi.com/article/10.3390/medicina58111647/s1, Table S1: Adverse events (Complications) and Severe Adverse Events (CD > 3).

Author Contributions: H.K. and F.M.B. shared authorship as first authors and they equally contributed to the original draft of the article. H.K. conceptualization, data curation, methodology, validation, writing—original draft, review and editing; F.M.B. conceptualization, data curation, methodology, validation, writing—original draft, review and editing; A.F. (Alessandro Fugazza) conceptualization, methodology, supervision, validation, review and editing; M.C. (Martina Ceolin) methodology, supervision, validation, review and editing; G.M. data curation, writing, review and editing; E.L. data curation, review and editing; M.C. (Matteo Colombo) data curation, methodology; A.F. (Antonio Facciorusso) methodology, supervision, validation, statistical analysis, writing, review and editing; E.M. methodology, supervision, validation, statistical analysis, review and editing; A.R. conceptualization, methodology, supervision, validation, review and editing; A.A. conceptualization, methodology, supervision, validation, review and editing, article correspondence. All authors have read and agreed to the published version of the manuscript.

Funding: This research received no external funding.

Institutional Review Board Statement: The study was conducted in accordance with the Declaration of Helsinki, and the protocol was approved by the Ethics Committee of the IRCSS Humanitas Research Hospital (NCT02855151 (20 January 2016)).

Informed Consent Statement: All subjects gave their informed consent for inclusion before they participated in the study.

Conflicts of Interest: Alessandro Fugazza, Andrea Anderloni, are consultants for Olympus and Boston Scientific. Alessandro Repici is a consultant for Fujifilm, Boston Scientific, ERBE. Hayato Kurihara, Francesca M. Bunino, Martina Ceolin, Giulia Mauri, Ezio Lanza, Matteo Colombo, Antonio Facciorusso, Enrico Marrano have no conflicts of interest or financial ties to disclose.

References

1. Miura, F.; Okamoto, K.; Takada, T.; Strasberg, S.M.; Asbun, H.J.; Pitt, H.A.; Gomi, H.; Solomkin, J.; Schlossberg, D.; Han, H.-S.; et al. Tokyo Guidelines 2018: Initial management of acute biliary infection and flowchart for acute cholangitis. *J. Hepato-Biliary-Pancreat. Sci.* **2017**, *25*, 31–40. [CrossRef]
2. Yokoe, M.; Hata, J.; Takada, T.; Strasberg, S.M.; Bun, T.A.Y.; Wakabayashi, G.; Kozaka, K.; Endo, I.; DeZiel, D.J.; Miura, F.; et al. Tokyo Guidelines 2018: Diagnostic criteria and severity grading of acute cholecystitis (with videos). *J. Hepato-Biliary-Pancreat. Sci.* **2017**, *25*, 41–54. [CrossRef] [PubMed]
3. Pisano, M.; Ceresoli, M.; Cimbanassi, S.; Gurusamy, K.; Coccolini, F.; Borzellino, G.; Costa, G.; Allievi, N.; Amato, B.; Boerma, D.; et al. 2017 WSES and SICG guidelines on acute calcolous cholecystitis in elderly population. *World J. Emerg. Surg.* **2019**, *14*, 10. [CrossRef] [PubMed]
4. Loozen, C.S.; van Santvoort, H.C.; van Duijvendijk, P.; Besselink, M.G.; Gouma, D.J.; Nieuwenhuijzen, G.A.; Kelder, C.J.; Donkervoort, S.C.; van Geloven, A.A.W.; Kruyt, P.M.; et al. Laparoscopic cholecystectomy versus percutaneous catheter drainage for acute cholecystitis in high risk patients (CHOCOLATE): Multicentre randomised clinical trial. *BMJ* **2018**, *2018*, 3965. [CrossRef] [PubMed]
5. Teoh, A.Y.B.; Kitano, M.; Itoi, T.; Pérez-Miranda, M.; Ogura, T.; Chan, S.M.; Serna-Higuera, C.; Omoto, S.; Torres-Yuste, R.; Tsuichiya, T.; et al. Endosonography-guided gallbladder drainage versus percutaneous cholecystostomy in very high-risk surgical patients with acute cholecystitis: An international randomised multicentre controlled superiority trial (DRAC 1). *Gut* **2020**, *69*, 1085–1091. [CrossRef]
6. Teoh, A.Y.B.; Leung, C.H.; Tam, P.T.H.; Yeung, K.K.Y.A.; Mok, R.C.Y.; Chan, D.L.; Chan, S.M.; Yip, H.C.; Chiu, P.W.Y.; Ng, E.K.W. EUS-guided gallbladder drainage versus laparoscopic cholecystectomy for acute cholecystitis: A propensity score analysis with 1-year follow-up data. *Gastrointest. Endosc.* **2020**, *93*, 577–583. [CrossRef]
7. Pisano, M.; Allievi, N.; Gurusamy, K.; Borzellino, G.; Cimbanassi, S.; Boerna, D.; Coccolini, F.; Tufo, A.; Di Martino, M.; Leung, J.; et al. 2020 World Society of Emergency Surgery updated guidelines for the diagnosis and treatment of acute calculus cholecystitis. *World J. Emerg. Surg.* **2020**, *15*, 61. [CrossRef]
8. Bilimoria, K.Y.; Liu, Y.; Paruch, J.L.; Zhou, L.; Kmiecik, T.E.; Ko, C.Y.; Cohen, M.E. Development and Evaluation of the Universal ACS NSQIP Surgical Risk Calculator: A Decision Aid and Informed Consent Tool for Patients and Surgeons. *J. Am. Coll. Surg.* **2013**, *217*, 833–842.e3. [CrossRef]
9. Church, S.; Rogers, E.; Rockwood, K.; Theou, O. A scoping review of the Clinical Frailty Scale. *BMC Geriatr.* **2020**, *20*, 393. [CrossRef]

10. Fugazza, A.; Colombo, M.; Repici, A.; Anderloni, A. Endoscopic Ultrasound-Guided Gallbladder Drainage: Current Perspectives. *Clin. Exp. Gastroenterol.* **2020**, *13*, 193–201. [CrossRef]
11. Dindo, D.; Demartines, N.; Clavien, P.A. Classification of Surgical Complications: A New Proposal With Evaluation in a Cohort of 6336 Patients and Results of a Survey. *Ann. Surg.* **2004**, *240*, 205–213. [CrossRef]
12. Singer, M.; Deutschman, C.S.; Seymour, C.W.; Shankar-Hari, M.; Annane, D.; Bauer, M.; Bellomo, R.; Bernard, G.R.; Chiche, J.-D.; Coopersmith, C.M.; et al. The Third International Consensus Definitions for Sepsis and Septic Shock (Sepsis-3). *JAMA* **2016**, *315*, 801–810. [CrossRef] [PubMed]
13. Coccolini, F.; Catena, F.; Pisano, M.; Gheza, F.; Fagiuoli, S.; Di Saverio, S.; Leandro, G.; Montori, G.; Ceresoli, M.; Corbella, D.; et al. Open versus laparoscopic cholecystectomy in acute cholecystitis. Systematic review and meta-analysis. *Int. J. Surg.* **2015**, *18*, 196–204. [CrossRef] [PubMed]
14. Rerknimitr, R.; Pham, K.C. Practical Approaches for High-Risk Surgical Patients with Acute Cholecystitis: The Percutaneous Approach versus Endoscopic Alternatives. *Clin. Endosc.* **2020**, *53*, 678–685. [CrossRef]
15. Fugazza, A.; Sethi, A.; Trindade, A.J.; Troncone, E.; Devlin, J.; Khashab, M.A.; Vleggaar, F.P.; Bogte, A.; Tarantino, I.; Deprez, P.H.; et al. International multicenter comprehensive analysis of adverse events associated with lumen-apposing metal stent placement for pancreatic fluid collection drainage. *Gastrointest. Endosc.* **2019**, *91*, 574–583. [CrossRef]
16. Facciorusso, A.; Di Maso, M.; Antonino, M.; Del Prete, V.; Panella, C.; Barone, M.; Muscatiello, N. Polidocanol injection decreases the bleeding rate after colon polypectomy: A propensity score analysis. *Gastrointest. Endosc.* **2015**, *82*, 350–358.e2. [CrossRef] [PubMed]
17. McCaffrey, D.F.; Griffin, B.A.; Almirall, D.; Slaughter, M.E.; Ramchand, R.; Burgette, L.F. A tutorial on propensity score estimation for multiple treatments using generalized boosted models. *Stat. Med.* **2013**, *32*, 3388–3414. [CrossRef]
18. Austin, P.C. The performance of different propensity score methods for estimating marginal hazard ratios. *Stat. Med.* **2012**, *32*, 2837–2849. [CrossRef]
19. Strobl, C.; Malley, J.; Tutz, G. An introduction to recursive partitioning: Rationale, application, and characteristics of classification and regression trees, bagging, and random forests. *Psychol. Methods* **2009**, *14*, 323–348. [CrossRef]
20. Steyerberg, E.W.; Harrell, F.E.; Borsboom, G.J.; Eijkemans, M.; Vergouwe, Y.; Habbema, J.F. Internal validation of predictive models: Efficiency of some procedures for logistic regression analysis. *J. Clin. Epidemiol.* **2001**, *54*, 774–781. [CrossRef]
21. Hosmer, D.W.; Hosmer, T.; Le Cessie, S.; Lemeshow, S. A comparison of goodness-of-fit tests for the logistic regression model. *Stat. Med.* **1997**, *15*, 965–980. [CrossRef]
22. McKay, A.; Abulfaraj, M.; Lipschitz, J. Short- and long-term outcomes following percutaneous cholecystostomy for acute cholecystitis in high-risk patients. *Surg. Endosc.* **2011**, *26*, 1343–1351. [CrossRef] [PubMed]
23. Markopoulos, G.; Mulita, F.; Kehagias, D.; Tsochatzis, S.; Lampropoulos, C.; Kehagias, I. Outcomes of percutaneous cholecystostomy in elderly patients: A systematic review and meta-analysis. *Gastroenterol. Rev.* **2020**, *15*, 188–195. [CrossRef]
24. Dimou, F.M.; Adhikari, D.; Mehta, H.B.; Riall, T.S. Outcomes in Older Patients with Grade III Cholecystitis and Cholecystostomy Tube Placement: A Propensity Score Analysis. *J. Am. Coll. Surg.* **2017**, *224*, 502–511e1. [CrossRef]
25. Anderloni, A.; Buda, A.; Vieceli, F.; Khashab, M.A.; Hassan, C.; Repici, A. Endoscopic ultrasound-guided transmural stenting for gallbladder drainage in high-risk patients with acute cholecystitis: A systematic review and pooled analysis. *Surg. Endosc.* **2016**, *30*, 5200–5208. [CrossRef] [PubMed]
26. Mussetto, A.; Anderloni, A. Through the LAMS towards the future: Current uses and outcomes of lumen-apposing metal stents. *Ann. Gastroenterol.* **2018**, *31*, 535–540. [CrossRef] [PubMed]
27. Luk, S.W.-Y.; Irani, S.; Krishnamoorthi, R.; Lau, J.Y.W.; Ng, E.K.W.; Teoh, A.Y.-B. Endoscopic ultrasound-guided gallbladder drainage versus percutaneous cholecystostomy for high risk surgical patients with acute cholecystitis: A systematic review and meta-analysis. *Endoscopy* **2019**, *51*, 722–732. [CrossRef]
28. Choi, J.H.; Lee, S.; Choi, J.; Park, D.; Seo, D.W.; Lee, S.; Kim, M.H. Long-term outcomes after endoscopic ultrasonography-guided gallbladder drainage for acute cholecystitis. *Endoscopy* **2014**, *30*, 656–661. [CrossRef] [PubMed]
29. Fleming, C.A.; Ismail, M.; Kavanagh, R.G.; Heneghan, H.M.; Prichard, R.S.; Geoghegan, J.; Brophy, D.P.; McDermott, E.W. Clinical and Survival Outcomes Using Percutaneous Cholecystostomy Tube Alone or Subsequent Interval Cholecystectomy to Treat Acute Cholecystitis. *J. Gastrointest. Surg.* **2019**, *24*, 627–632. [CrossRef]
30. Anderloni, A.; Attili, F.; Sferrazza, A.; Rimbaș, M.; Costamagna, G.; Repici, A.; Larghi, A. EUS-guided gallbladder drainage using a lumen-apposing self-expandable metal stent in patients with coagulopathy or anticoagulation therapy: A case series. *Endosc. Int. Open* **2017**, *5*, E1100–E1103. [CrossRef]

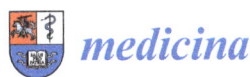 medicina

Article

The Use of PuraStat® in the Management of Walled-Off Pancreatic Necrosis Drained Using Lumen-Apposing Metal Stents: A Case Series

Cecilia Binda [1], Alessandro Fugazza [2], Stefano Fabbri [1], Chiara Coluccio [1], Alessandro Repici [2,3], Ilaria Tarantino [4], Andrea Anderloni [5] and Carlo Fabbri [1,*]

1. AUSL Romagna, Gastroenterology and Digestive Endoscopy Unit, Forlì-Cesena Hospitals, 47121 Forlì-Cesena, Italy
2. Humanitas Research Hospital, Digestive Endoscopy Unit, Division of Gastroenterology, Rozzano, 20089 Milan, Italy
3. Humanitas University, Department of Biomedical Sciences, 20090 Pieve Emanuele, Italy
4. Digestive Endoscopy and Gastroenterology Unit, Department of Gastroenterology, Istituto Mediterraneo per i Trapianti e Terapie ad Alta Specializzazione (IsMeTT/UPMC), 90127 Palermo, Italy
5. Fondazione I.R.C.C.S. Policlinico San Matteo, Gastroenterology and Digestive Endoscopy Unit, 27100 Pavia, Italy
* Correspondence: carlo.fabbri@auslromagna.it

Abstract: *Background and Objectives*: Bleeding is one of the most feared and frequent adverse events in the case of EUS-guided drainage of WOPN using lumen-apposing metal stents (LAMSs) and of direct endoscopic necrosectomy (DEN). When it occurs, its management is still controversial. In the last few years, PuraStat, a novel hemostatic peptide gel has been introduced, expanding the toolbox of the endoscopic hemostatic agents. The aim of this case series was to evaluate the safety and efficacy of PuraStat in preventing and controlling bleeding of WOPN drainage using LAMSs. *Materials and Methods*: This is a multicenter, retrospective pilot study from three high-volume centers in Italy, including all consecutive patients treated with the novel hemostatic peptide gel after LAMSs placement for the drainage of symptomatic WOPN between 2019 and 2022. *Results*: A total of 10 patients were included. All patients underwent at least one session of DEN. Technical success of PuraStat was achieved in 100% of patients. In seven cases PuraStat was placed for post-DEN bleeding prevention, with one patient experiencing bleeding after DEN. In three cases, on the other hand, PuraStat was placed to manage active bleeding: two cases of oozing were successfully controlled with gel application, and a massive spurting from a retroperitoneal vessel required subsequent angiography. No re-bleeding occurred. No PuraStat-related adverse events were reported. *Conclusions*: This novel peptide gel could represent a promising hemostatic device, both in preventing and managing active bleeding after EUS-guided drainage of WON. Further prospective studies are needed to confirm its efficacy.

Keywords: PuraStat; walled-off pancreatic necrosis; pancreatic fluid collection; LAMS; EUS-guided drainage; bleeding; endoscopic hemostasis; endoscopic hemostatic agents

Citation: Binda, C.; Fugazza, A.; Fabbri, S.; Coluccio, C.; Repici, A.; Tarantino, I.; Anderloni, A.; Fabbri, C. The Use of PuraStat® in the Management of Walled-Off Pancreatic Necrosis Drained Using Lumen-Apposing Metal Stents: A Case Series. *Medicina* 2023, 59, 750. https://doi.org/10.3390/medicina59040750

Academic Editor: Áron Vincze

Received: 24 February 2023
Revised: 10 April 2023
Accepted: 11 April 2023
Published: 12 April 2023

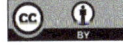

Copyright: © 2023 by the authors. Licensee MDPI, Basel, Switzerland. This article is an open access article distributed under the terms and conditions of the Creative Commons Attribution (CC BY) license (https://creativecommons.org/licenses/by/4.0/).

1. Introduction

Walled-off necrosis (WON) is one of the possible local complications of acute necrotizing pancreatitis (ANP) that could be life-threatening when it becomes symptomatic (e.g., signs of systemic infections, gastric or intestinal outflow obstruction, abdominal pain, compression on major vessels, jaundice) [1]. The management of these collections has been largely studied in the last years, and the paradigm of treatment has changed over the years. The current international guidelines suggest adopting the so called "step-up approach", indicating a gradual increase from a less invasive procedure to a more invasive one [2,3]. The endoscopic ultrasound (EUS)-guided drainage followed by direct endoscopic necrosectomy (DEN) nowadays represents the treatment of choice in the case of symptomatic WON, especially after the introduction on the market of dedicated devices, such as lumen-apposing metal stents (LAMSs) [2]. These stents have been demonstrated to be very effective for the drainage of WON but are burdened by non-negligible rates of adverse events (AEs), up to 20% [4].

Bleeding is one of the most common and feared AEs in the case of EUS-guided drainage of WON using LAMSs and of DEN, and when it occurs, it usually requires urgent interventions, such as endoscopy or radiological embolization or coiling. A large international multicenter series published by Fugazza et al. [5] reported bleeding in 27.8% of all LAMS-related AEs in the setting of pancreatic fluid collections (PFCs), with an overall risk of 7.2% (22/304). In a retrospective analysis involving 30 Italian centers over a 5-year period, including 269 WON, bleeding was reported as the most frequent AEs, occurred in 6% of the patients [6]. When it occurs, the management of bleeding is still a dilemma, mainly because of the difficulties in obtaining effective hemostasis and because of the "extraluminal"/peritoneal location.

In the last few years, a novel hemostatic peptide gel has been introduced, expanding the toolbox of the endoscopic hemostatic agents. PuraStat® (3-D Matrix Europe SAS, Caluire et Cuire, France) is a synthetic hemostatic agent licensed as CE and marketed as a surgical hemostatic agent. PuraStat is a liquid that when applied to a bleeding area acts rapidly to form a gel coat, which induces hemostasis. It is a slightly viscous solution of synthetic peptides. Contact between PuraStat and blood causes the acidic peptide solution to be neutralized and exposed to ions, resulting in the formation of ß-sheets that then form a three-dimensional scaffold structure. For this reason, it has both a role for the treatment of active bleeding and the potential of enhancing endoscopic mucosal wound healing, preventing delayed bleeding.

PuraStat is applied through a small catheter placed through the biopsy channel of the endoscope and can be used in various small spaces. It is supplied in a pre-filled syringe and is currently available in 1 mL, 3 mL, and 5 mL unit doses indicated for hemostasis in several surgical circumstances. On application to tissues, PuraStat forms a fully transparent, slightly viscous aqueous peptide (2.5%) solution over the bleeding or potentially bleeding area. PuraStat has several unique features that distinguish it from existing products. As advantages, it is an inert material with no risk of contamination from a biological source, it is available in single prefilled and ready-to-use syringes, requiring no preparation, and can be used repetitively. The transparent adherent barrier permits further endoscopic therapy to be performed, and it can be applied in the general area of bleeding and does not require precise application on the exact point of bleeding. Moreover, it can be removed easily if desired, and it is applicable to narrow spaces.

For all these reasons, PuraStat could represent a promising hemostatic device for many endoscopic procedures, including EUS-PFCs drainage. Therefore, the aim of this study was to evaluate the safety and efficacy of this new hemostatic agent in preventing and controlling bleeding after LAMSs drainage in the setting of WON.

2. Materials and Methods

The present case series is a multicenter, retrospective pilot study of a prospectively maintained database from three tertiary Italian institutions, including all consecutive patients treated with PuraStat after LAMSs placement for the drainage of symptomatic WON between June 2019 and February 2022.

Mature pancreatic WON was defined as encapsulated collection containing necrotic debris, as defined by the Atlanta classification [1]. Indications for drainage of WON included infections and symptoms of obstruction and abdominal pain attributable to WON.

Baseline characteristics, including age, sex, etiology of pancreatitis, location, and size of WON, percentage of estimated necrosis, and indication to WON intervention, were collected. Preprocedural bleeding risk factors, such as antithrombotic or anticoagulant therapy or presence of a vessel within the WON on cross-sectional imaging, were identified.

2.1. Procedure

All patients signed adequate informed consent prior to any interventional procedure [7]. All the initial drainage procedures were performed by experienced endoscopists with a linear array echoendoscope under general anesthesia. Under EUS and fluoroscopic guidance, the WON was drained from either the stomach or duodenum with the deployment of an electrocautery LAMS (Hot-AXIOS; Boston Scientific Corp, Marlborough, MA, USA) (Figure 1). The optimal puncture site, avoiding vasculature, was confirmed under EUS and Doppler flow guidance. All LAMSs were released using the free-hand technique, with direct access into the collection by puncture with the electrocautery system and without a guidewire. The second flange of the stent was released with the intra-channel stent release technique [8]. The 15 × 10 or 20 × 10 mm LAMSs were chosen according to the size of the collection with the amount of necrosis at the discretion of the endoscopist. Pneumatic dilation of the LAMSs, hydrogen peroxide irrigation of the cavity, placement of double-pigtail stent through the LAMSs, and/or immediate extraction of necrotic debris at the time of WON drainage were left at the discretion of the endoscopist. All patients were under broad-spectrum antibiotic therapy at the moment of LAMS placement.

Then, DEN was performed through LAMS with a forward-viewing endoscope at regular intervals. Endoscopic necrosectomy was performed with a combination of sucking debris through the working channel, removing necrotic material with a removal device, and applying irrigation. Endoscopists could use various accessories for fragmentation and removal of necrotic debris, including conventional cold snares, baskets, roth nets, or novel dedicated devices, such as the EndoRotor Powered Endoscopic Debridement (PED) System® (Interscope Medical, Inc., Worcester, MA, USA) or Necrolit® (Meditalia s.a.s., Palermo, Italy). Finally, debris after copious lavage were aspirated, while hydrogen peroxide irrigation of the cavity was left at the discretion of the endoscopists. DEN sessions were performed until complete debridement of necrotic material was achieved and granulation of pink tissue in almost all walls of the cavity was seen.

PuraStat was then applied both for the treatment of active intraprocedural bleeding and for the prevention of delayed bleeding at the end of the DEN sessions (Figure 1). PuraStat was placed at the bleeding source, alone or in combination with other conventional hemostatic techniques, for the control of intraprocedural active bleeding. Instead, after the DEN sessions, the hemostatic gel was placed inside the WON cavity on the newly exposed granulation tissue after removal of necrotic debris. Thus, PuraStat was applied on the most vascularized areas of granulation tissue to prevent delayed bleeding from microscopic vessels and to promote cystic wall healing.

2.2. Data Collections and Analysis

Intraprocedural bleeding was defined as visible bleeding within the WON cavity or on the gastric wall, identified during the initial drainage procedure or subsequent DENs. Delayed bleeding was defined as the occurrence of clinical signs of bleeding (hematemesis, melena, or a drop in hemoglobin >2 g/dL) and the presence of fresh blood or stigmata of recent bleeding on endoscopic investigation after the procedure when PuraStat was placed to prevent a primary bleeding event. Rebleeding was defined as secondary bleeding event when PuraStat was used alone or in combination with other hemostatic techniques in the management of the primary active bleeding. Technical success of PuraStat application was defined by the ability of gel deployment in the target area. Posology, time for application, and PuraStat-related AEs were recorded. Additional endoscopic or radiological hemostatic techniques were decided by the endoscopist according to severity of the hemorrhage.

The primary endpoints were to assess the clinical success of PuraStat, meaning its ability to achieve immediate hemostasis in the treatment of active bleeding and to prevent delayed bleeding and the rate of PuraStat-related AEs. The secondary outcomes assessed were the severity of bleeding and type and number of additional interventions needed for the management of bleeding in the setting of WON.

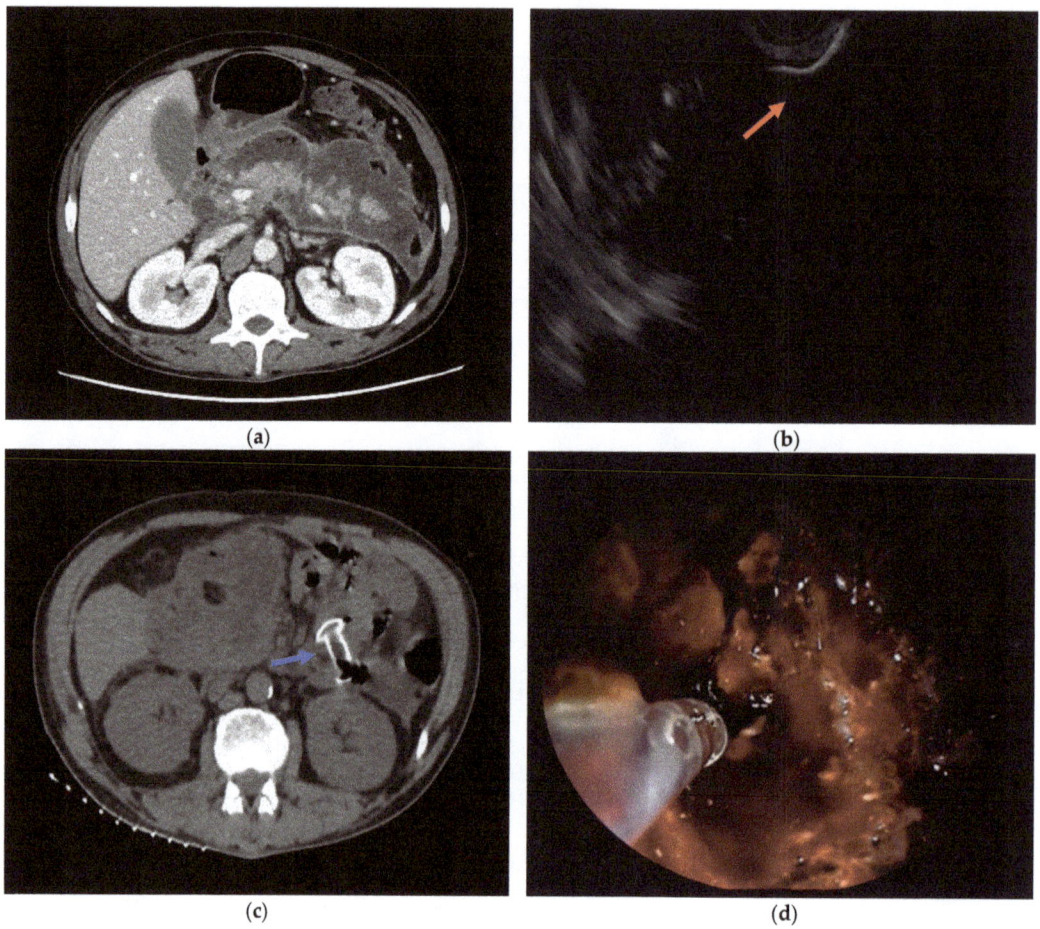

Figure 1. (**a**) CT scan showing a large WON, involving the entire pancreatic gland; (**b**) EUS-WON drainage using LAMS (red arrow); (**c**) CT scan showing LAMS placed between the gastric cavity and the WON (blue arrow); (**d**) PuraStat application on WON walls to treat oozing bleeding from a small intracavitary vessel during DEN.

Technical success of EUS-drainage was defined as placement of the LAMSs for PFC-drainage. Necrotic tissue was debrided during one or more DEN session until complete resolution. Clinical success of DEN was established as WON < 2 cm on cross-sectional imaging and symptoms resolution without need for further interventional radiologic or surgical procedures. All LAMSs were removed within 4 weeks after placement, and the patients were followed up for at least 30 days after LAMS removal.

All AEs related to LAMS placement and DEN procedure, including bleeding, were classified according to the ASGE Lexicon severity grading system [9], and time of occurrence and their management were reported.

3. Results

3.1. Baseline Characteristics

During the study period, a total of ten patients (nine men, one woman) were enrolled (Table 1), with a mean age of 65.7 years (range 24–89 years). The etiologies of acute pancreatitis were 70% gallstones, 20% idiopathic, and 10% alcohol. Indications for EUS-

WON were abdominal pain in six patients (60%), infected WON in six (60%), and gastric outlet obstruction in five (50%), and early satiety in two (20%). At the onset of pancreatitis, two patients were on anticoagulant therapy with Rivaroxaban, which was shifted to low molecular weight heparin (LMWH) during their hospital stays; according to the recent guidelines [10], LMWH was omitted the day of the procedure. Before drainage, all the patients underwent contrast-enhanced abdominal CT-scan to assess WON characteristics. WON was located in the head of the pancreas in two patients (20%), in the body-tail in five (50%), while it affected the entire pancreatic gland in three cases (30%). The medium WON diameter was 126.8 mm (range 82–180 mm). Pancreatic necrosis was estimated to be greater than 50% in four patients (40%). Three patients had vessels within the WON seen on cross-sectional imaging before LAMS placement; after a multidisciplinary discussion with interventional radiologists and surgeons, prophylactic coil embolization of the splenic artery was pursued in one case, while in another patient the DEN procedure was performed in an angiographic room without the need of arterial embolization. The third patient did not require any radiological treatment; thus, conventional EUS-guided drainage and subsequent DEN were performed in the endoscopic room. None of these patients experienced bleeding events during the study period.

Table 1. Baseline Characteristics.

Patients' Characteristics	10 Patients
Gender	
M	9
F	1
Mean Age	65.7 years (24–89)
Etiology of acute pancreatitis	
Gallstones	7
Idiopathic	2
Alcohol	1
Indication for drainage	
Abdominal pain	6
Infected WON	6
Gastric outlet obstruction	5
Early satiety	2
WON Characteristics	**10 WON**
WON location	
Body and Tail	5
Entire Pancreas	3
Head	2
Max WON diameter	126.8 mm (82–180)
% of estimated necrosis	
<50% of necrosis	6
>50% of necrosis	4
Evidence of vessel inside WON	3
Prophylactic Embolization	1
DEN performed in angiographic room	1
No need for radiological treatment	1

3.2. Procedure Details

Details of EUS-drainage, DEN and PuraStat application are shown in Table 2. Technical success of WON drainage using LAMSs was 100%. The 20 × 10 mm LAMSs were used in nine cases, while 15 × 10 mm LAMSs were deployed during three initial drainage procedures. Two patients (20%) were treated with two LAMSs with a multiple gateway drainage strategy, as previously reported [11]. In all cases, LAMSs were deployed through the gastric wall. Pneumatic dilation of the LAMSs were performed in nine patients (90%), while the WON cavity was irrigated with hydrogen peroxide in seven patients (70%).

Table 2. Procedure Details.

EUS-Guided WON Drainage	10 Patients
Technical success	100%
LAMS size	
20 × 10 mm	9
15 × 10 mm	3
Multiple Gateway Drainage	2
Trans-Gastric Drainage	10
LAMS dilation	9
Hydrogen peroxide irrigation	7
Direct Endoscopic Necrosectomy	**10 Patients**
Devices used for DEN	
Snares	10
Dormia baskets	3
EndoRotor®	1
Necrolit®	1
Mean DEN sessions	1.6 (1–3)
Clinical success of DEN	10/10
PuraStat Application	
Technical success	100%
Mean application time	4 min (2–6)
Mean volume	3 mL

DEN was subsequently performed using conventional accessories, including snares and Dormia baskets, respectively, in ten and three cases. In addition, two patients were treated with novel dedicated necrosectomy devices, such as EndoRotor® and Necrolit®. Clinical success of DEN was obtained in 100% of the patients. The mean number of DEN sessions needed to achieve the complete debridement of the WON was 1.6 (range 1–3), with four patients that required more than one DEN session. Double pig-tail plastic stents were placed through the LAMSs at the end of the DEN procedures in five cases (50%). Technical success of PuraStat application was achieved in 100% of patients in the mean time of 4 min (range 2–6 min). The mean posology of PuraStat applied after each DEN session was 3 mL. In two cases, the novel hemostatic gel was used during two sessions.

3.3. Bleeding Management and Prevention with PuraStat

Outcomes of PuraStat application in the management and prevention of WON-related bleeding are reported in Table 3. In three patients out of ten, PuraStat was used in the management of WON-related active bleeding. None of these patients were previously treated with PuraStat for prophylactic purpose. In one patient, blood oozing from the gastric wall was seen during the drainage procedure immediately after LAMS deployment and was successfully treated with PuraStat application after multiple unsuccessful attempts with Trough-The-Scope Clips (TTSC). The second patient experienced blood oozing 12 h after a DEN session from a minor WON vessel, which was effectively treated with PuraStat without the need for additional conventional hemostatic techniques. The third patient had massive spurting bleeding from a large retroperitoneal vessel during a DEN session. Endoscopic hemostasis with clips was initially attempted, but the source of bleeding could not be for certain identified because of the large amount of blood clots within the collection. As hemodynamic instability succeeded, PuraStat was applied inside the cavity as a bridge hemostatic treatment to the subsequent radiological embolization. Indeed, after fluid resuscitation and blood transfusions, the patient was referred to the angiographic room, but as no active bleeding was identified, embolization was not needed. The patient was admitted to the intensive care unit, and no further hemorrhages occurred. No case of re-bleeding occurred.

Table 3. Bleeding Management and Prevention with PuraStat.

Outcomes	Patients
PuraStat in management of active WON-related bleeding	3
Oozing bleedings successfully treated	2
Bridge to embolization in spurting bleeding	1
PuraStat in post-DEN bleeding prevention	7
Delayed Bleeding	1
PuraStat-related adverse events	0/10

In the other seven cases, PuraStat was placed on the WON walls to prevent post-DEN bleeding. Of these seven patients, only one experienced delayed bleeding 36 h after DEN. After blood transfusion, the patients underwent endoscopy examinations, which did not show any active bleeding, without the need for additional hemostatic techniques. No PuraStat-related AEs occurred.

However, two different procedure-related complications were also reported: a severe periprocedural respiratory failure requiring ICU admission and a mild pneumonia conservatively treated.

4. Discussion

The endoscopic management of intracystic bleeding is still a dilemma for the endoscopist because of the difficulties of obtaining adequate hemostasis with the available devices and the lack of dedicated ones. Several endoscopic hemostatic techniques for the management of PFC-related hemorrhage has been reported: epinephrine injection, hemoclip placement, coagulation [12], balloon tamponade [13], fibrin glue injection [14], hemostatic powder application [15], and covered SEMS placement [16,17]. However, there is no consensus on the optimal endoscopic hemostasis.

The use of PuraStat in gastrointestinal endoscopy is approved for the management of bleeding from small vessels and oozing from capillaries of the GI tract and the surrounding tissues. Moreover, PuraStat application showed a reduction of delayed bleeding following gastrointestinal endoscopic submucosal dissection (ESD) procedures in the colon [18,19].

In a recently published prospective multicenter study, Branchi et al. [20] investigated the role of PuraStat in providing hemostasis in 111 patients with acute non-variceal gastrointestinal bleeding. When PuraStat was used as the primary therapy, initial hemostatic success was reached in 94% of patients (74/79, 95% CI 88–99%). PuraStat induced hemostasis in 75% of patients (24/32, 95% CI 59–91%) if used as a secondary treatment option after failure of standard techniques. The volume of gel required to achieve hemostasis was 3 mL in 59% of cases. Overall, the rebleeding rate at the 30-day follow-ups was 16% (18/111). No adverse events due to application of PuraStat or technical failures were reported.

Soriani et al. [21] reported a successfully PuraStat-managed bleeding from intrahepatic biliary ducts that occurred during cholangioscopy-guided lithotripsy. This case report confirmed the opportunity of PuraStat placement also in bleeding sites that are inaccessible using conventional endoscopic hemostatic devices as it could happen inside the necrotic cavities during DEN.

First, in our case series, PuraStat was used in the management of three cases of WON-related active bleeding. The two blood-oozing events, one from the gastric wall and one from inside the cavity, were successfully controlled with PuraStat application. In one case of massive blood spurting causing hemorrhagic shock, PuraStat was used as a bridge hemostatic agent to temporarily control the blood loss, allowing the patient to be referred to the angiographic room after hemodynamic resuscitation. These data are in line with the results of previous studies, which demonstrated that PuraStat is much more effective in achieving initial hemostasis in cases of oozing than for spurting bleeding. In fact, Subramaniam et al. [19] reported that PuraStat could provide hemostasis in 72.6% of oozing bleeding cases but only in 50.0% of spurting bleeding cases in gastrointestinal tract. Moreover, PuraStat can be used as a rescue hemostatic agent to achieve temporary hemostasis of massive arterial bleeding. Likewise to what was reported in our cohort, Branchi et al. [20] described five cases in which PuraStat was used a bridge to surgery in the case of refractory severe bleeding.

The use of PuraStat in the treatment of acute bleeding inside a pseudocyst after EUS-guided drainage using LAMS was anecdotally described for the first time by De Nucci et al. [22]. In their cohort, PuraStat was applied into the pseudocyst cavity as the primary hemostatic agent, and hemorrhage was controlled after the application of 6 mL of gel. After 3 days, a second-look endoscopy revealed granulation tissue on the cyst cavity. No rebleeding occurred, and the LAMS was removed 2 weeks later.

Secondarily, this is the first pilot study to investigate the role of PuraStat in the prevention of WON-related delayed bleeding. In light of the reduction of delayed bleeding following endoscopic resections in the gastrointestinal tract [18], we applied PuraStat on the WON walls as a prophylactic hemostatic agent in seven cases, and only one patient experienced moderate delayed bleeding with no need for subsequent additional endoscopic hemostasis. Heretofore, a technique described for the prevention of bleeding after transmural drainage of PFC was the co-axial DPPSs placement within the LAMS lumen. It has been hypothesized that the placement of the co-axial DPPS through the LAMS could have a protective effect in preventing the impaction and the friction of the distal flange against the adjacent wall of the cavity, which would reduce the risk of bleeding [8]. The role of DPPS in preventing bleeding after LAMS drainage is still matter of debate. The first single center study by Puga et al. [23] demonstrated that adjunctive placement of DPPS resulted in decreased adverse events, particularly bleeding, while a subsequent large multicenter study reported that deployment of pigtail stents across the LAMSs did not significantly reduce overall adverse events (26% with DPPS (Group 1) versus 27% without DPPS (Group 2); $p = 0.88$.) [24].

The rationale for the use of a hemostatic gel, both in prophylaxis and as treatment of active bleeding, comes from the idea that WON bleeding has several mechanisms. Intraprocedural bleeding, indeed, can originate at the puncture site from small missed venous collaterals of the gastric or duodenal wall, from minor vessels within the cavity, or from the large retroperitoneal vessel that may bleed after rapid collapse of the collection or due to iatrogenic damage during necrosectomy [25]. In this setting, the hemostatic gel can therefore be useful both to prevent bleeding, especially when originating from minor vessels within the cavity, or to treat active bleeding of the gastric or duodenal wall or from the vessel of the cystic wall.

Instead, delayed bleeding is usually caused by prolonged contact between the distal flange of the indwelling LAMS and the walls that can lead to the erosion of intracavitary vessels and promote the formation of a pseudoaneurysm [25]. Thus, LAMS removal within 4 weeks of deployment is recommended, especially if imaging shows resolution of the cavity [26,27]. In the case of pseudoaneurysm, the role of Purastat may be marginal, although it may be useful as a bridge to other definitive treatments, namely radiological ones.

Jiang et al. [28] proposed an algorithm for the management of WON-related bleeding based on the stratification of bleeding severity (adapted in Figure 2). Mild bleeding occurring either during initial drainage or during necrosectomy or caused by stent erosion after the procedure could be treated endoscopically with interventional radiology (IR) or surgery as a backup option. Intra- or post-procedural bleeding believed to come from a pseudoaneurysm should be directly managed by IR embolization [28].

Moreover, in the presence of pseudoaneurysms [29] or arterial vessels [30,31] inside the WON, prophylactic coil embolization could be performed to prevent massive arterial bleeding during drainage or subsequent necrosectomy. Indeed, perigastric varices (OR 2.90, 1.31–6.42, $p = 0.008$) or pseudoaneurysm (OR 2.99, 1.75–11.93, $p = 0.002$) have been identified as independent predictors of overall adverse event occurrences in a large multicenter series [32], while the endoscopic identification of a vessel within the cavity has emerged as a strong predictor of bleeding on multivariate analysis (OR 23.3, 4.0–135.1, $p < 0.01$)

in a recent retrospective study by Holmes et al. [33]. In our cohort, prophylactic coil embolization was performed in one of three patients who had evidence of major arterial vessels inside the WON.

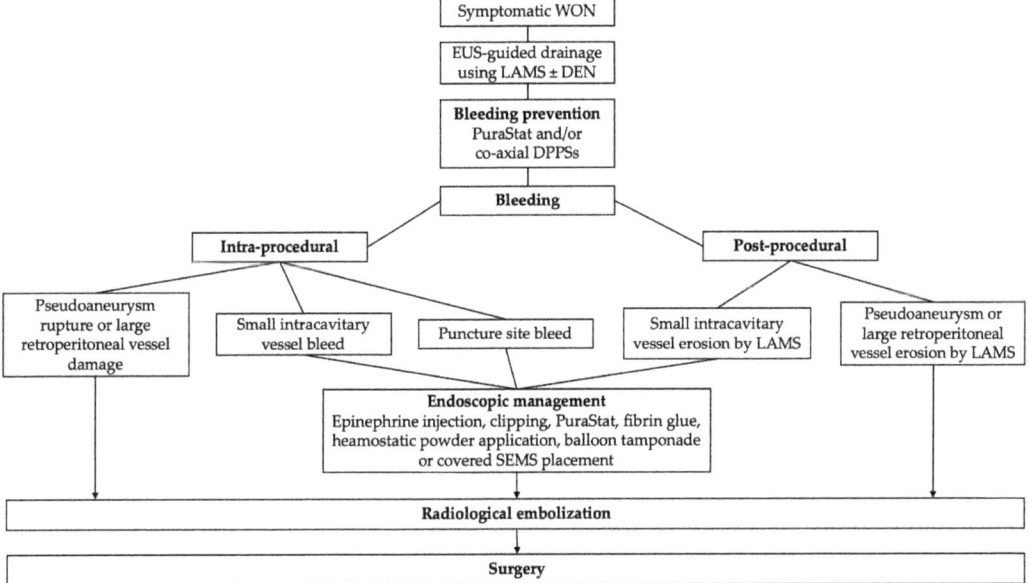

Figure 2. Algorithm for management of WON-related bleeding adapted from Jiang et al. [28] and Rana et al. [25].

In addition to the known hemostatic effect, it has been hypothesized that the Purastat 3-D structure favors the tissue proliferative process during healing, thanks to its similarity with the natural extracellular matrix. Indeed, PuraStat action in promoting mucosal regeneration has been reported in some recent studies [34,35]. Based on this hypothetical re-epithelizing property, PuraStat application on the walls of the cavity could promote resurfacing, enhancing WON resolution.

Our case series does have limitations, mainly owing to the small cohort of patients enrolled, its retrospective design, and the lack of a control group; thus, firm conclusions cannot be drawn. Therefore, the potential role of PuraStat in managing and preventing WON-related bleeding and in improving clinical success during necrosectomy must be validated in larger prospective and comparative studies.

5. Conclusions

The promising results of our case series confirm that PuraStat expanded the toolbox of the endoscopic hemostatic agents, even in the still debated management of WON-related bleeding. This novel peptide gel is particularly effective in achieving hemostasis for oozing-type bleeding but also plays a role in the management of spurting-type bleeding to temporarily control the blood loss as a bridge hemostatic agent to subsequent radiological or surgical treatments. Moreover, PuraStat can be easily and safely applied for the prevention of delayed post-DEN bleeding and might promote cavity resurfacing, enhancing WON resolution, although these hypotheses require confirmation with ad hoc designed trials.

Author Contributions: Conceptualization, C.B., A.F., I.T., A.A. and C.F.; data curation, S.F., C.B. and A.F.; writing—original draft preparation, S.F., C.B. and C.C.; writing—review and editing, C.B., A.F., S.F., C.C., A.R., I.T., A.A. and C.F. All authors have read and agreed to the published version of the manuscript.

Funding: Article Processing Charge was funded by 3-D Matrix Europe SAS, France.

Institutional Review Board Statement: Not applicable.

Informed Consent Statement: Informed consent was obtained from all subjects involved in the study.

Data Availability Statement: All articles cited in this article are listed in PubMed.

Conflicts of Interest: C.B. is a lecturer for Steris, Fujifilm, and Boston Scientific. A.F. is a consultant for Boston Scientific. C.C. is a lecturer for Steris. A.R. has received research grants and speaker's fees from Boston Scientific, Fujifilm, and Norgine; he is also on an advisory board for Fujifilm. A.A is a consultant for Boston Scientific. C.F. is a lecturer for Steris, Fujifilm, and Q3 Medical; he is also a consultant for Boston Scientific. S.F. and I.T. declare no conflicts of interest.

Abbreviations

AEs	adverse events
ASGE	American Society for Gastrointestinal Endoscopy
DEN	direct endoscopic necrosectomy
DPPS	double pigtail plastic stent
EUS	endoscopic ultrasound
IR	interventional radiology
LAMS	lumen apposing metal stent
PFC	pancreatic fluid collection
SEMS	self-expandable metal stent
WON	walled-off necrosis
WOPN	walled-off pancreatic necrosis
SEMS	self-expandable metal stent

References

1. Banks, P.A.; Bollen, T.L.; Dervenis, C.; Gooszen, H.G.; Johnson, C.D.; Sarr, M.G.; Tsiotos, G.G.; Vege, S.S. Classification of Acute Pancreatitis—2012: Revision of the Atlanta Classification and Definitions by International Consensus. *Gut* **2013**, *62*, 102–111. [CrossRef] [PubMed]
2. Arvanitakis, M.; Dumonceau, J.-M.; Albert, J.; Badaoui, A.; Bali, M.; Barthet, M.; Besselink, M.; Deviere, J.; Oliveira Ferreira, A.; Gyökeres, T.; et al. Endoscopic Management of Acute Necrotizing Pancreatitis: European Society of Gastrointestinal Endoscopy (ESGE) Evidence-Based Multidisciplinary Guidelines. *Endoscopy* **2018**, *50*, 524–546. [CrossRef] [PubMed]
3. Baron, T.H.; DiMaio, C.J.; Wang, A.Y.; Morgan, K.A. American Gastroenterological Association Clinical Practice Update: Management of Pancreatic Necrosis. *Gastroenterology* **2020**, *158*, 67–75.e1. [CrossRef] [PubMed]
4. Siddiqui, A.A.; Kowalski, T.E.; Loren, D.E.; Khalid, A.; Soomro, A.; Mazhar, S.M.; Isby, L.; Kahaleh, M.; Karia, K.; Yoo, J.; et al. Fully Covered Self-Expanding Metal Stents versus Lumen-Apposing Fully Covered Self-Expanding Metal Stent versus Plastic Stents for Endoscopic Drainage of Pancreatic Walled-off Necrosis: Clinical Outcomes and Success. *Gastrointest. Endosc.* **2017**, *85*, 758–765. [CrossRef] [PubMed]
5. Fugazza, A.; Sethi, A.; Trindade, A.J.; Troncone, E.; Devlin, J.; Khashab, M.A.; Vleggaar, F.P.; Bogte, A.; Tarantino, I.; Deprez, P.H.; et al. International Multicenter Comprehensive Analysis of Adverse Events Associated with Lumen-Apposing Metal Stent Placement for Pancreatic Fluid Collection Drainage. *Gastrointest. Endosc.* **2020**, *91*, 574–583. [CrossRef]
6. Amato, A.; Tarantino, I.; Facciorusso, A.; Binda, C.; Crinò, S.F.; Fugazza, A.; Forti, E.; Petrone, M.C.; Di Mitri, R.; Macchiarelli, R.; et al. Real-Life Multicentre Study of Lumen-Apposing Metal Stent for EUS-Guided Drainage of Pancreatic Fluid Collections. *Gut* **2022**, *71*, 1050–1052. [CrossRef]
7. Spadaccini, M.; Binda, C.; Fugazza, A.; Repici, A.; Tarantino, I.; Fabbri, C.; Cugia, L.; Anderloni, A.; On Behalf of the Interventional Endoscopy Amp Ultra Sound I-Eus Group. Informed Consent for Endoscopic Biliary Drainage: Time for a New Paradigm. *Medicina* **2022**, *58*, 331. [CrossRef]
8. Anderloni, A.; Attili, F.; Carrara, S.; Galasso, D.; Di Leo, M.; Costamagna, G.; Repici, A.; Kunda, R.; Larghi, A. Intra-Channel Stent Release Technique for Fluoroless Endoscopic Ultrasound-Guided Lumen-Apposing Metal Stent Placement: Changing the Paradigm. *Endosc. Int. Open* **2017**, *5*, E25–E29. [CrossRef]

9. Cotton, P.B.; Eisen, G.M.; Aabakken, L.; Baron, T.H.; Hutter, M.M.; Jacobson, B.C.; Mergener, K.; Nemcek, A.; Petersen, B.T.; Petrini, J.L.; et al. A Lexicon for Endoscopic Adverse Events: Report of an ASGE Workshop. *Gastrointest. Endosc.* 2010, *71*, 446–454. [CrossRef]
10. Veitch, A.M.; Radaelli, F.; Alikhan, R.; Dumonceau, J.-M.; Eaton, D.; Jerrome, J.; Lester, W.; Nylander, D.; Thoufeeq, M.; Vanbiervliet, G.; et al. Endoscopy in Patients on Antiplatelet or Anticoagulant Therapy: British Society of Gastroenterology (BSG) and European Society of Gastrointestinal Endoscopy (ESGE) Guideline Update. *Endoscopy* 2021, *53*, 947–969. [CrossRef]
11. Binda, C.; Dabizzi, E.; Anderloni, A.; Cennamo, V.; Fiscaletti, M.; Fugazza, A.; Jovine, E.; Ercolani, G.; Gasbarrini, A.; Fabbri, C. Single-Step Endoscopic Ultrasound-Guided Multiple Gateway Drainage of Complex Walled-off Necrosis with Lumen Apposing Metal Stents. *Eur. J. Gastroenterol. Hepatol.* 2020, *32*, 1401–1404. [CrossRef] [PubMed]
12. van Brunschot, S.; Fockens, P.; Bakker, O.J.; Besselink, M.G.; Voermans, R.P.; Poley, J.-W.; Gooszen, H.G.; Bruno, M.; van Santvoort, H.C. Endoscopic Transluminal Necrosectomy in Necrotising Pancreatitis: A Systematic Review. *Surg. Endosc.* 2014, *28*, 1425–1438. [CrossRef] [PubMed]
13. Wang, B.-H.; Xie, L.-T.; Zhao, Q.-Y.; Ying, H.-J.; Jiang, T.-A. Balloon Dilator Controls Massive Bleeding during Endoscopic Ultrasound-Guided Drainage for Pancreatic Pseudocyst: A Case Report and Review of Literature. *World J. Clin. Cases* 2018, *6*, 459–465. [CrossRef]
14. Auriemma, F.; Anderloni, A.; Carrara, S.; Fugazza, A.; Maselli, R.; Troncone, E.; Repici, A. Cyanoacrylate Hemostasis for Massive Bleeding After Drainage of Pancreatic Fluid Collection by Lumen-Apposing Metal Stent. *Am. J. Gastroenterol.* 2018, *113*, 1582. [CrossRef]
15. Tarantino, I.; Barresi, L.; Granata, A.; Curcio, G.; Traina, M. Hemospray for Arterial Hemorrhage Following Endoscopic Ultrasound-Guided Pseudocyst Drainage. *Endoscopy* 2014, *46*, E71. [CrossRef] [PubMed]
16. Săftoiu, A.; Ciobanu, L.; Seicean, A.; Tanţău, M. Arterial Bleeding during EUS-Guided Pseudocyst Drainage Stopped by Placement of a Covered Self-Expandable Metal Stent. *BMC Gastroenterol.* 2013, *13*, 93. [CrossRef]
17. Chavan, R.; Basha, J.; Lakhtakia, S.; Nabi, Z.; Reddy, D.N. Large-Caliber Metal Stent Controls Significant Entry Site Bleeding during EUS-Guided Drainage of Walled-off Necrosis. *VideoGIE* 2019, *4*, 27–28. [CrossRef]
18. Pioche, M.; Camus, M.; Rivory, J.; Leblanc, S.; Lienhart, I.; Barret, M.; Chaussade, S.; Saurin, J.-C.; Prat, F.; Ponchon, T. A Self-Assembling Matrix-Forming Gel Can Be Easily and Safely Applied to Prevent Delayed Bleeding after Endoscopic Resections. *Endosc. Int. Open* 2016, *4*, E415–E419. [CrossRef]
19. Subramaniam, S.; Kandiah, K.; Chedgy, F.; Fogg, C.; Thayalasekaran, S.; Alkandari, A.; Baker-Moffatt, M.; Dash, J.; Lyons-Amos, M.; Longcroft-Wheaton, G.; et al. A Novel Self-Assembling Peptide for Hemostasis during Endoscopic Submucosal Dissection: A Randomized Controlled Trial. *Endoscopy* 2021, *53*, 27–35. [CrossRef]
20. Branchi, F.; Klingenberg-Noftz, R.; Friedrich, K.; Bürgel, N.; Daum, S.; Buchkremer, J.; Sonnenberg, E.; Schumann, M.; Treese, C.; Tröger, H.; et al. PuraStat in Gastrointestinal Bleeding: Results of a Prospective Multicentre Observational Pilot Study. *Surg. Endosc.* 2022, *36*, 2954–2961. [CrossRef]
21. Soriani, P.; Biancheri, P.; Deiana, S.; Ottaviani, L.; Manno, M. Off-Label PuraStat Use for the Treatment of Acute Intrahepatic Biliary Duct Bleeding. *Endosc. Int. Open* 2021, *9*, E1926–E1927. [CrossRef] [PubMed]
22. de Nucci, G.; Reati, R.; Arena, I.; Bezzio, C.; Devani, M.; della Corte, C.; Morganti, D.; Mandelli, E.D.; Omazzi, B.; Redaelli, D.; et al. Efficacy of a Novel Self-Assembling Peptide Hemostatic Gel as Rescue Therapy for Refractory Acute Gastrointestinal Bleeding. *Endoscopy* 2020, *52*, 773–779. [CrossRef] [PubMed]
23. Puga, M.; Consiglieri, C.F.; Busquets, J.; Pallarès, N.; Secanella, L.; Peláez, N.; Fabregat, J.; Castellote, J.; Gornals, J.B. Safety of Lumen-Apposing Stent with or without Coaxial Plastic Stent for Endoscopic Ultrasound-Guided Drainage of Pancreatic Fluid Collections: A Retrospective Study. *Endoscopy* 2018, *50*, 1022–1026. [CrossRef] [PubMed]
24. Shamah, S.; Sahakian, A.; Chapman, C.; Buxbaum, J.; Muniraj, T.; Aslanian, H.; Villa, E.; Cho, J.; Haider, H.; Waxman, I.; et al. Double Pigtail Stent Placement as an Adjunct to Lumen-Apposing Metal Stents for Drainage of Pancreatic Fluid Collections May Not Affect Outcomes: A Multicenter Experience. *Endosc. Ultrasound.* 2022, *11*, 53–58. [CrossRef]
25. Rana, S. Complications of Endoscopic Ultrasound-Guided Transmural Drainage of Pancreatic Fluid Collections and Their Management. *Ann. Gastroenterol.* 2019, *32*, 441. [CrossRef]
26. Bang, J.Y.; Navaneethan, U.; Hasan, M.K.; Sutton, B.; Hawes, R.; Varadarajulu, S. Non-Superiority of Lumen-Apposing Metal Stents over Plastic Stents for Drainage of Walled-off Necrosis in a Randomised Trial. *Gut* 2019, *68*, 1200–1209. [CrossRef]
27. Brimhall, B.; Han, S.; Tatman, P.D.; Clark, T.J.; Wani, S.; Brauer, B.; Edmundowicz, S.; Wagh, M.S.; Attwell, A.; Hammad, H.; et al. Increased Incidence of Pseudoaneurysm Bleeding With Lumen-Apposing Metal Stents Compared to Double-Pigtail Plastic Stents in Patients With Peripancreatic Fluid Collections. *Clin. Gastroenterol. Hepatol.* 2018, *16*, 1521–1528. [CrossRef]
28. Jiang, T.-A.; Xie, L.-T. Algorithm for the Multidisciplinary Management of Hemorrhage in EUS-Guided Drainage for Pancreatic Fluid Collections. *WJCC* 2018, *6*, 308–321. [CrossRef]
29. Rana, S.S.; Kumar, A.; Lal, A.; Sharma, R.; Kang, M.; Gorsi, U.; Gupta, R. Safety and Efficacy of Angioembolisation Followed by Endoscopic Ultrasound Guided Transmural Drainage for Pancreatic Fluid Collections Associated with Arterial Pseudoaneurysm. *Pancreatology* 2017, *17*, 658–662. [CrossRef]
30. Sekikawa, Z.; Yamamoto, T.; Aoki, R.; Obara, A.D.; Furugori, S.; Sugimori, K.; Takebayashi, S. Prophylactic Coil Embolization of the Vessels for Endoscopic Necrosectomy in Patients with Necrotizing Pancreatitis. *J. Vasc. Interv. Radiol.* 2019, *30*, 124–126. [CrossRef]

31. Honta, S.; Hayashi, T.; Katanuma, A. Coil Embolization of Artery in Advance Endoscopic Necrosectomy for Walled-off Necrosis Can Prevent Arterial Bleeding. *Dig. Endosc.* **2021**, *33*, e8–e9. [CrossRef] [PubMed]
32. Facciorusso, A.; Amato, A.; Crinò, S.F.; Sinagra, E.; Maida, M.; Fugazza, A.; Binda, C.; Repici, A.; Tarantino, I.; Anderloni, A.; et al. Nomogram for Prediction of Adverse Events after Lumen-Apposing Metal Stent Placement for Drainage of Pancreatic Fluid Collections. *Dig. Endosc.* **2022**, *34*, 1459–1470. [CrossRef] [PubMed]
33. Holmes, I.; Shinn, B.; Mitsuhashi, S.; Boortalary, T.; Bashir, M.; Kowalski, T.; Loren, D.; Kumar, A.; Schlachterman, A.; Chiang, A. Prediction and Management of Bleeding during Endoscopic Necrosectomy for Pancreatic Walled-off Necrosis: Results of a Large Retrospective Cohort at a Tertiary Referral Center. *Gastrointest. Endosc.* **2022**, *95*, 482–488. [CrossRef] [PubMed]
34. Uraoka, T.; Ochiai, Y.; Fujimoto, A.; Goto, O.; Kawahara, Y.; Kobayashi, N.; Kanai, T.; Matsuda, S.; Kitagawa, Y.; Yahagi, N. A Novel Fully Synthetic and Self-Assembled Peptide Solution for Endoscopic Submucosal Dissection-Induced Ulcer in the Stomach. *Gastrointest. Endosc.* **2016**, *83*, 1259–1264. [CrossRef]
35. White, K.; Henson, C.C. Endoscopically Delivered Purastat for the Treatment of Severe Haemorrhagic Radiation Proctopathy: A Service Evaluation of a New Endoscopic Treatment for a Challenging Condition. *Frontline Gastroenterol.* **2021**, *12*, 608–613. [CrossRef]

Disclaimer/Publisher's Note: The statements, opinions and data contained in all publications are solely those of the individual author(s) and contributor(s) and not of MDPI and/or the editor(s). MDPI and/or the editor(s) disclaim responsibility for any injury to people or property resulting from any ideas, methods, instructions or products referred to in the content.

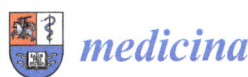

Article

Factors Predicting Malignant Occurrence and Polyp Recurrence after the Endoscopic Resection of Large Colorectal Polyps: A Single Center Experience

Olga Mandic [1], Igor Jovanovic [1], Mirjana Cvetkovic [1], Jasmina Maksimovic [1], Tijana Radonjic [1], Maja Popovic [2], Novica Nikolic [3] and Marija Brankovic [1,4,*]

[1] Department of Gastroenterology and Hepatology, University Hospital Medical Center Bezanijska Kosa, 11000 Belgrade, Serbia
[2] Department of Radiology, University Hospital Medical Center Bezanijska Kosa, 11000 Belgrade, Serbia
[3] Department of Anesthesiology and Reanimation, University Hospital Medical Center Bezanijska Kosa, 11000 Belgrade, Serbia
[4] Faculty of Medicine, University of Belgrade, 11000 Belgrade, Serbia
* Correspondence: marijasbrankovic@gmail.com

Citation: Mandic, O.; Jovanovic, I.; Cvetkovic, M.; Maksimovic, J.; Radonjic, T.; Popovic, M.; Nikolic, N.; Brankovic, M. Factors Predicting Malignant Occurrence and Polyp Recurrence after the Endoscopic Resection of Large Colorectal Polyps: A Single Center Experience. *Medicina* 2022, 58, 1440. https://doi.org/10.3390/medicina58101440

Academic Editors: Andrea Anderloni and Cecilia Binda

Received: 19 August 2022
Accepted: 8 October 2022
Published: 13 October 2022

Publisher's Note: MDPI stays neutral with regard to jurisdictional claims in published maps and institutional affiliations.

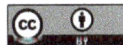

Copyright: © 2022 by the authors. Licensee MDPI, Basel, Switzerland. This article is an open access article distributed under the terms and conditions of the Creative Commons Attribution (CC BY) license (https://creativecommons.org/licenses/by/4.0/).

Abstract: *Background:* The aim of this study was to identify risk factors contributing to the malignancy of colorectal polyps, as well as risk factors for recurrence after the successful endoscopic mucosal resection of large colorectal polyps in a referral center. *Materials and Methods:* This retrospective cohort study was performed in patients diagnosed with large (≥20 mm diameter) colorectal polyps and treated in the period from January 2014 to December 2019 at the University Hospital Medical Center Bezanijska Kosa, Belgrade, Serbia. Based on the endoscopic evaluation and classification of polyps, the following procedures were performed: en bloc resection, piecemeal resection or surgical treatment. *Results:* A total of 472 patients with large colorectal polyps were included in the study. The majority of the study population were male (62.9%), with a mean age of 65.7 ± 10.8 years. The majority of patients had one polyp (73.7%) less than 40 mm in size (74.6%) sessile morphology (46.4%), type IIA polyps (88.2%) or polyps localized in the descending colon (52.5%). The accessibility of the polyp was complicated in 17.4% of patients. En bloc resection was successfully performed in 61.0% of the patients, while the rate of piecemeal resection was 26.1%. Due to incomplete endoscopic resection, surgery was performed in 5.1% of the patients, while 7.8% of the patients were referred to surgery directly. Hematochezia ($p = 0.001$), type IIB polyps ($p < 0.001$) and complicated polyp accessibility ($p = 0.002$) were significant independent predictors of carcinoma presence in a multivariate logistic regression analysis. Out of the 472 patients enrolled in the study, 364 were followed after endoscopic resection for colorectal polyp recurrence, which was observed in 30 patients (8.2%) during follow-up. Piecemeal resection ($p = 0.048$) and incomplete resection success ($p = 0.013$) were significant independent predictors of polyp recurrence in the multivariate logistic regression analysis. *Conclusions:* Whenever an endoscopist encounters a complex colorectal lesion (i.e., a polyp with complicated accessibility), polyp size > 40 mm, the Laterally Spreading Tumor nongranular (LST-NG) morphological type, type IIB polyps or the presence of hematochezia, malignancy risk should be considered before making the decision to either resect, refer to an advanced endoscopist or perform surgery.

Keywords: colorectal polyp; endoscopic mucosal resection; malignancy; recurrence

1. Introduction

Colorectal cancer is the third most common cancer, as well as the second leading cause in terms of cancer-related deaths worldwide [1]. With 5989 new cases and 3356 registered deaths from colorectal cancer in 2020, data from the International Agency for Research on Cancer (IARC) put Serbia in fifth place in the world in terms of the number of deaths caused by colorectal cancer [2]. Although every colorectal neoplasia has malignant potential, polyps classified as large colon polyps (≥ 2 cm) carry an even greater risk for carcinoma development [3–7]. In order to avoid unnecessary surgery, many large colon polyps are removed endoscopically, making endoscopic resection the most effective strategy for the prevention and decline of colorectal cancer mortality, morbidity and cost [8]. Data from the literature show that up to 11% of colorectal polyps that are endoscopically removed are already malignant [9]. In addition, it was shown in one study that 15% of local recurrences of adenoma occurred after an endoscopic resection procedure and about 88% of recurrences were detected after the first follow-up colonoscopy [10]. In most cases, these local recurrences can be managed endoscopically [11]; however, rigorous surveillance is needed in order to detect them early on. Therefore, the recognition of factors contributing to malignancy as well as local recurrence predictive factors may enhance the prevention of this disease, primarily through the stratification of patients according to their individual risk profile and polyp-related characteristics.

The aim of this study was to identify risk factors contributing to the malignancy of colorectal polyps, as well as risk factors for recurrence after the successful endoscopic mucosal resection of large colorectal polyps in a referral center.

2. Materials and Methods

This retrospective cohort study was performed on patients diagnosed with large (≥ 20 mm diameter) colorectal polyps and treated in the period from January 2014 to December 2019 by an expert endoscopist in the referral University Hospital Medical Center Bezanijska Kosa, Belgrade, Serbia. Patients who were positive for fecal occult blood test (FOBT) as a part of a National Screening Program were also assessed in the study. Basic demographic and clinical data were obtained for all patients (age, gender, comorbidities, previous history of carcinoma and indications for colonoscopy). In addition, polyp characteristics, including number, size, morphology, pit pattern classification and location, were documented. The accessibility of polyps was defined as complicated if the polyps were located in difficult sites, such as the appendiceal orifice, ileocecal valve or anorectal junction, or if they were located behind haustral folds. The Paris Classification System for Superficial Neoplastic Lesions in the Digestive Tract and the classification for Laterally Spreading Tumors (LST) were used to define polyp morphology. The Japan NBI Expert Team (JNET) Classification was used to describe the characteristics of the mucosal surface. The inclusion criteria were patients ≥ 18 years and the presence of one or more polyps, over 20 mm in diameter. The absence of a pathological evaluation of the polyp was the exclusion criterion.

A colonoscopy was performed using an Olympus CF-H170L video colonoscope. Based on the endoscopic evaluation and classification of polyps, the following procedures were performed: en bloc resection, piecemeal resection or surgical treatment due to incomplete endoscopic mucosal resection or the presence of a likely malignant alteration. While performing the endoscopic mucosal resection, a saline solution of adrenaline at a concentration of 1:10,000 was injected into the base of the polypoid change until an adequate elevation of the change was achieved. After the elevation, the polypoid change was removed with a hexagonal loop, en bloc or piece by piece, with the help of an electrocoagulation unit. The evaluation of the endoscopic resectability was based on the presence of a "lifting" sign after the submucosal injection.

The study was approved by the Institutional Research Ethic Committee and informed consent was obtained from all patients.

Statistical Analysis

Numerical data were presented as mean values with standard deviation for numerical variables, or as absolute numbers with percentages for categorical variables. Differences according to the presence of carcinoma or polyp recurrence in patients' sociodemographic and polyp characteristics and were analyzed using Student's t and Chi-square tests for the numerical and categorical data, respectively. Univariate and multivariate logistic regression models were used to assess the predictors of carcinoma and polyp recurrence (as dependent variables). In all analyses, the significance level was set at 0.05. Statistical analysis was performed using the IBM SPSS statistical software (SPSS for Windows, release 25.0, SPSS, Chicago, IL, USA).

3. Results

A total of 472 patients with endoscopically resected colorectal polyps were included in the study. The majority of the study population were male (62.9%) with a mean age of 65.7 ± 10.8 years. The patient characteristics are summarized in Table 1.

Table 1. Characteristics of the study population.

Variable	n (%)
Gender	
Male	297 (62.9)
Female	175 (37.1)
Age, mean ± sd	65.7 ± 10.8
Comorbidities, yes	325 (68.9)
Previous history of carcinoma, yes	28 (5.9)
Indication for colonoscopy	
Symptoms	131 (27.9)
Fecal occult blood test positive	113 (24.0)
Hematochezia	98 (20.9)
Family history	45 (9.6)
Polyp surveillance	33 (7.0)
Anemia	28 (6.0)
Combination of two or more indications	22 (4.7)

The majority of patients had one polyp (73.7%) less than 40 mm in size (74.6%), sessile morphology (46.4%), IIA type (88.2%) and localized in the descending colon (52.5%). The accessibility of the polyp was complicated in 17.4% of patients (Table 2).

Table 2. Polyp characteristics of the study population. Abbreviations: LST-NG, Laterally Spreading Tumor nongranular; LST-G, Laterally Spreading Tumor granular).

Polyps	n (%)
Number	
One	240 (50.8)
More than one	232 (49.2)
Size	
<40 mm	352 (74.6)
≥40 mm	120 (25.4)
Morphology	
Sessile	219 (46.4)
LST-NG	100 (21.2)
LST-G	69 (14.6)
Pedunculated	44 (9.3)
Flat	39 (8.3)
Hyperplastic	1 (0.2)
Pit pattern classification according to JNET *	
IIA	411 (88.2)
IIB	55 (11.8)

Table 2. Cont.

Polyps	n (%)
Location	
Cecum	40 (8.5)
Ascending colon	57 (12.1)
Transverse colon	37 (7.8)
Descending colon	248 (52.5)
Rectum	90 (19.1)
Accessibility	
Non-complicated	366 (82.6)
Complicated	77 (17.4)

* JNET—Japan NBI Expert Team Classification.

En bloc resection was successfully performed in 61.0% of the patients, while the rate of piecemeal resections performed was 26.1%. Due to incomplete endoscopic resection, surgery was performed in 5.1% of the patients, while 7.8% of the patients were referred to surgery directly.

The characteristics of the study population and polyps according to carcinoma presence are presented in Table 3. Patients with hematochezia, polyps ≥ 40 mm in size, LST-NG morphology, type IIB, localized in the cecum and polyps with complicated accessibility were more frequently diagnosed with carcinoma, while patients with an FOBT-positive indication, pedunculated polyps and polyps localized in the transverse colon were diagnosed with carcinoma less frequently (Table 3).

Table 3. Characteristics of the study population and polyps according to carcinoma presence.

Variable	Carcinoma		p
	No (n = 404)	Yes (n = 68)	
Characteristics of the study population, n%			
Gender			
Male	258 (63.9)	39 (57.4)	0.304
Female	146 (36.1)	29 (42.6)	
Age, mean ± sd	65.5 ± 10.8	66.8 ± 10.6	0.357
Comorbidities, yes	273 (67.6)	52 (76.5)	0.143
Indication for colonoscopy			
Symptoms	114 (28.2)	17 (25.0)	0.584
Fecal occult blood test positive	104 (25.7)	9 (13.2)	**0.025**
Hematochezia	73 (18.1)	25 (36.8)	**<0.001**
Family history	42 (10.4)	3 (4.4)	0.120
Polyp surveillance	29 (7.2)	4 (5.9)	0.698
Anemia	24 (5.9)	4 (5.9)	0.985
Combination of two or more indications	16 (4.0)	6 (8.8)	0.078
Polyp characteristics, n%			
Number			
One	206 (51.0)	34 (50.0)	0.880
More than one	198 (49.0)	34 (50.0)	
Size			
<40 mm	321 (79.5)	31 (45.6)	**<0.001**
≥40 mm	83 (20.5)	37 (54.4)	

Table 3. Cont.

Variable	Carcinoma		p
	No (n = 404)	Yes (n = 68)	
Morphology			
Sessile	190 (47.0)	29 (42.6)	0.503
LST-NG	79 (19.6)	21 (30.9)	0.034
LST-G	57 (14.1)	12 (17.6)	0.445
Pedunculated	44 (10.9)	0 (0.0)	0.004
Flat	33 (8.2)	6 (8.8)	0.856
Hyperplastic	1 (0.2)	0 (0.0)	0.681
Pit pattern classification according to JNET *			
IIA	379 (95.2)	32 (47.1)	<0.001
IIB	19 (4.8)	36 (52.9)	
Location			
Cecum	30 (7.4)	10 (14.7)	0.046
Ascending colon	53 (13.1)	4 (5.9)	0.090
Transverse colon	36 (8.9)	1 (1.5)	0.035
Descending colon	211 (52.2)	37 (54.4)	0.739
Rectum	74 (18.3)	16 (23.5)	0.311
Accessibility			0.311
Non-complicated	334 (85.9)	32 (59.3)	<0.001
Complicated	55 (14.1)	22 (40.7)	

* JNET—Japan NBI Expert Team Classification. Abbreviations: LST-NG, Laterally Spreading Tumor nongranular; LST-G, Laterally Spreading Tumor granular).

The results from univariate and multivariate logistic regression analyses with carcinoma as the dependent variable are presented in Table 4. Hematochezia ($p = 0.001$), polyp size over 40 mm ($p < 0.001$), morphological type LST-NG ($p = 0.036$), type IIB polyps ($p < 0.001$) and complicated accessibility ($p < 0.001$) were significant predictors of carcinoma presence in the univariate logistic regression analysis. Hematochezia ($p = 0.001$), type IIB polyps ($p < 0.001$) and complicated accessibility ($p = 0.002$) were significant independent predictors of carcinoma presence in the multivariate logistic regression analysis (Table 4).

Table 4. Univariate and multivariate logistic regression analyses with carcinoma presence as the dependent variable.

Variable	Univariate			Multivariate		
	p	OR	95%CI for OR	p	OR	95%CI for OR
Hematochezia	0.001	2.636	1.514–4.589	0.001	3.173	1.578–6.377
Size of polyps	<0.001	4.616	2.704–7.880			
LST-NG	0.036	1.838	1.039–3.251			
Pit pattern classification according to JNET *	<0.001	22.441	11.568–43.532	<0.001	12.505	5.710–27.386
Accessibility of polyp	<0.001	4.175	2.261–7.708	0.002	3.020	1.478–6.169

* JNET—Japan NBI Expert Team Classification. Abbreviations: LST-NG, Laterally Spreading Tumor nongranular).

Out of the 472 patients enrolled in the study, 364 were followed after endoscopic resection for colorectal polyp recurrence, which was observed in 30 patients (8.2%) during follow-up. Patients who had polyp recurrence more often had previous surgery for colorectal carcinoma, had a single polyp over 40 mm in size, morphologically sessile polyps, LST-NG and LST-G, type IIB, or had polyps localized in the rectum, descending colon or ascending colon. In addition, patients who had polyp recurrence were more often treated via piecemeal resection with incomplete resection success, had complicated accessibility, had a tubulovillous adenoma according to the pathological diagnosis, or were less likely to have a clip placed than patients who did not have polyp recurrence (Table 5).

Table 5. Characteristics of the study population and polyps according to polyp recurrence.

Variable	Polyp Recurrence		p
	No (n = 334)	Yes (n = 30)	
Characteristics of the study population, n%			
Gender			
Male	219 (65.6)	20 (66.7)	0.903
Female	115 (34.4)	10 (33.3)	
Age, mean ± sd	65.40 ± 10.33	68.60 ± 9.82	0.104
Indication for colonoscopy			
Symptoms	88 (26.3)	9 (30.0)	0.655
Fecal occult blood test positive	87 (26.0)	5 (16.7)	0.257
Hematochezia	60 (18.0)	5 (16.7)	0.859
Family history	33 (9.9)	3 (10.0)	0.983
Polyp surveillance	24 (7.2)	6 (20.0)	**0.014**
Anemia	23 (6.9)	1 (3.3)	0.453
Combination of two or more indications	18 (5.4)	1 (3.3)	0.628
Polyp characteristics, n%			
Number			
One	162 (48.5)	21 (70.0)	**0.024**
More than one	172 (51.5)	9 (30.0)	
Size			
<40 mm	246 (73.7)	12 (40.0)	**<0.001**
≥40 mm	88 (26.3)	18 (60.0)	
Morphology			
Sessile	215 (49.2)	4 (11.4)	**<0.001**
LST-NG	83 (19.0)	17 (48.6)	**<0.001**
LST-G	58 (13.3)	11 (31.4)	**0.003**
Pedunculated	43 (9.8)	1 (2.9)	0.172
Flat	37 (8.5)	2 (5.7)	0.569
Hyperplastic	1 (0.2)	0 (0.0)	0.777
Pit pattern classification according to JNET *			
IIA	384 (89.1)	27 (77.1)	**0.035**
IIB	47 (10.9)	8 (22.9)	
Location			
Cecum	77 (17.6)	13 (37.1)	**0.005**
Ascending colon	239 (54.7)	9 (25.7)	**0.001**
Transverse colon	36 (8.2)	1 (2.9)	0.254
Descending colon	49 (11.2)	8 (22.9)	**0.042**
Rectum	36 (8.2)	4 (11.4)	0.514
Accessibility			
Non-complicated	346 (84.4)	20 (60.6)	**0.001**
Complicated	64 (15.6)	13 (39.4)	
Type of treatment			
En bloc resection	205 (61.4)	2 (6.7)	**<0.001**
Piecemeal resection	79 (23.7)	25 (83.3)	
Surgery due to incomplete endoscopic resection	19 (5.7)	2 (6.7)	
Patients referred directly to surgery	31 (9.3)	1 (3.3)	

Table 5. Cont.

Variable	Polyp Recurrence		p
	No (n = 334)	Yes (n = 30)	
Resection success			
Complete	346 (84.4)	20 (60.6)	0.001
Incomplete	64 (15.6)	13 (39.4)	
Pathological diagnosis			
Tubular adenoma	105 (31.4)	7 (23.3)	0.357
Tubulovillous adenoma	166 (49.7)	21 (70.0)	0.033
Hyperplastic	6 (1.8)	0 (0.0)	0.459
Villous adenoma	2 (0.6)	0 (0.0)	0.671
Peutz–Jeghers	1 (0.3)	0 (0.0)	0.764
Intramucosal carcinoma (Tis)	15 (4.5)	1 (3.3)	0.767
Submucosal carcinoma (T1)	34 (10.2)	0 (0.0)	0.066
Carcinoma T2 or more	7 (2.1)	1 (3.3)	0.658
Clip placement, yes	208 (62.3)	10 (33.3)	0.002

* JNET—Japan NBI Expert Team Classification. Abbreviations: LST-NG, Laterally Spreading Tumor nongranular; LST-G, Laterally Spreading Tumor granular).

The results from univariate and multivariate logistic regression analyses with polyp recurrence as the dependent variable are presented in Table 6. Single polyp ($p = 0.028$), size over 40 mm ($p < 0.001$), morphological types LST-G ($p = 0.003$), LST-NG ($p < 0.001$), complicated accessibility ($p = 0.001$), piecemeal resection ($p < 0.001$), incomplete resection success ($p < 0.001$) and polyps localized in rectum ($p = 0.003$) and ascending colon ($p = 0.014$) were significant predictors of polyp recurrence, while sessile polyp morphology ($p = 0.001$) and polyps localized in the descending colon ($p < 0.001$) represented protective factors for polyp recurrence in the univariate logistic regression analysis. Piecemeal resection ($p = 0.048$) and incomplete resection success ($p = 0.013$) were significant independent predictors of polyp recurrence in the multivariate logistic regression analysis (Table 6).

Table 6. Univariate and multivariate logistic regression analyses with polyp recurrence as the dependent variable. Abbreviations: LST-NG, Laterally Spreading Tumor nongranular; LST-G, Laterally Spreading Tumor granular).

Variable	Univariate			Multivariate		
	p	OR	95%CI for OR	p	OR	95%CI for OR
Number of polyps	0.028	0.404	0.180–0.907			
Size of polyps	<0.001	4.193	1.942–9.056			
LST-G	0.003	3.367	1.510–7.510			
LST-NG	<0.001	4.302	1.999–9.257			
Sessile	<0.001	0.076	0.018–0.323			
Accessibility of polyp	0.001	3.925	1.782–8.642			
Piecemeal resection	<0.001	16.139	5.980–43.556	0.048	3.870	1.011–14.819
Resection success	<0.001	17.098	5.808–50.332	0.013	6.363	1.478–27.385
Location (rectum)	0.003	3.240	1.479–7.096			
Location (descending colon)	<0.001	0.159	0.059–0.426			
Location (ascending colon)	0.014	3.010	1.249–7.257			

4. Discussion

The results of our study showed that hematochezia, type IIB polyps, and complicated accessibility were significant independent predictors of carcinoma development, while piecemeal resection and incomplete resection success were significant independent predictors of polyp recurrence in a multivariate logistic regression analysis. Protective factors for polyp recurrence were sessile polyp morphology and polyps localized in the descending colon.

In 2021. Cazacu et al. [12] performed a retrospective study of patients with colonoscopic polypectomy during a 13-year period; out of 905 patients with colonoscopic polyps, pathological examination showed polyps with malignant cells in 109 patients. The results of this study showed that the frequency of male patients with malignant polyps was similar to the group of patients with benign polyps, and that the mean age of the patients was 62.6 years. In addition, the prevalence of the malignant polyps in male patients varies across the literature, with 51 to 88% of male patients having carcinoma and a mean age between 60 and 73 years [13–19]. These results are in agreement with our study results, where 57.4% of male patients with mean age of 66.8 years had malignant polyps upon pathological examination. No statistical significance was found between gender or age and carcinoma diagnosis in our study; however, in the study by Cazacu et al. [12], older patients ($\geq$65 years) had a higher rate of carcinoma in comparison to the younger population.

In the study by Cazacu et al., statistical significance was reported for the mean diameter between benign and malignant polyps [12], which is similar to our study results, where patients with polyps $\geq$ 40 mm in size were more frequently diagnosed with carcinoma. Our study results showed that most of the pathologically examined polyps were sessile, LST-NG and LST-G in the group of patients with carcinoma. The predominance of sessile polyps was found in other studies [12,17], in line with our study results. However, a meta-analysis conducted by Hassan et al. [20] revealed the predominance of pedunculated polyps in patients with colorectal polyps; in our study, only 9.3% of patients had pedunculated polyps. Statistical significance was found for the frequency of pedunculated polyps between the groups of patients with and without carcinoma, where patients with pedunculated polyps were less frequently diagnosed with carcinoma. Traditionally, pedunculated malignant polyps are considered to prevent recurrent disease and have a better prognosis in comparison to sessile lesions [21,22].

The results reported by Cazacu et al. [12] showed that the rate of malignancy in colorectal polyps was higher in patients with two or more polyps, patients with polyps larger than 10 mm in size, in polyp types 0-Ip and 0-Isp (according to JNET classification), in lateral spreading lesions (as compared with flat and sessile lesions) and polyps localized on the left-side, as well as in the rectum. Our study results were similar, where hematochezia, polyp size over 40 mm, morphological type LST-NG, type IIB polyps (according to JNET classification) and complicated accessibility were significant predictors of carcinoma development in the univariate logistic regression analysis. In addition, in the multivariate logistic regression analysis, hematochezia, polyp type IIB (according to JNET classification) and complicated accessibility were significant independent predictors of carcinoma development.

In a study conducted by Nanda et al. [23], lesions considered to be challenging for the technical success of EMR procedure were discussed. The results of their study showed that polyps localized at the ileocecal valve were more challenging to position and access for resection, making resection more complicated as well as the duration of the procedure longer. Moss et al. [24] showed that 7.9% of their study cohort had polyps that were difficult to reach and were located in a difficult position for resection. In addition, Moss et al. [24] assessed risk factors for EMR failure, where the independent predictors in a multivariate regression analysis were polyps located in the ileocecal valve and a difficult position of the polyp. According to Sidhu et al. [25], polyp access may be considered difficult depending on the location of the lesion or whether a stable position is unable to be maintained by the endoscopist when performing EMR. In addition, the assessment of polyp access may not be mentioned specifically by the referring endoscopist. However, Sidhu et al. [25] found that short-term and procedural outcomes were significantly correlated with the size, morphology, site and access (SMSA) score level, even with lesions marked as "easy access". The results of our study showed that complicated accessibility represented a significant predictor of carcinoma development in both univariate and multivariate regression analyses. The complicated accessibility of polyps could affect their early and accurate morphological evaluation, thus prolonging timely endoscopic mucosal resection and increasing the chance of carcinoma development. Future studies concerning the relationship between polyp accessibility and its malignant potential are needed in order to facilitate early identification, better management and the provision of future directions for how to achieve the best optimal outcome for patients with large polyps.

In the case of malignant colorectal polyps, a consensus was reached concerning several carcinogenic factors contributing to colorectal polyps; however, it remains unclear which factors contribute to the recurrence of colorectal polyps and whether these factors are similar to the factors that contribute to carcinogenesis [9,26–28]. In 2017, the European Society of Gastrointestinal Endoscopy (ESGE) Clinical Guideline by Ferlitsch et al. [29] recommended that features related to the recurrence of polyps should include polyps over 40 mm in size, polyps localized on the ileocecal valve, prior failed attempts at resection as well as size, morphology, site and access (SMSA) level 4. Apart from the ESGE guidelines, SMSA score was shown to predict the outcomes of endoscopic mucosal resection in the colon [25]. In a study by Chlebowski et al., the rate of polyp recurrence was shown to be higher in male patients than in female patients [30]. In another study conducted by Saiken A et al. [31], patients over 60 years old had higher rates of colorectal recurrence in comparison to younger patients. Gender and age were not found to be predictive risk factors of colorectal polyp recurrence in the study by Chaoui et al. [32], which is in agreement with our study results. In terms of polyp characteristics, several factors can contribute to local recurrence risk. A greater tendency of recurrence was shown for colorectal polyps located in the proximal and ascending colon in a study by Atkin et al. [33]. The results of our study showed that polyps localized in the rectum and ascending colon were significant predictors of polyp recurrence, while polyps localized in the descending colon represented protective factors for polyp recurrence in the univariate logistic regression analysis. In addition, a potential risk factor for the recurrence of adenoma is the size of colorectal polyp; the results of a meta-analysis conducted in 2016 showed that endoscopic recurrence occurred in 13.8% of patients with large colorectal polyps ($\geq$20 mm in size) [34]. In the study conducted by Zhan et al., polyp size was significantly associated with the risk for polyp recurrence in a multivariable regression analysis [35]. Other studies have also demonstrated that a predictor of polyp recurrence is large polyp size [24,36,37]; this is in agreement with our study results, where polyp size over 40 mm was a significant predictor of polyp recurrence.

A growing number of studies have shown that although it is considered to be a safe and effective endoscopic treatment for large colorectal polyps, recurrence after EMR has been a point of contention since this technique emerged [11,34,38]. A meta-analysis conducted by Belderbos et al. showed that after a piecemeal resection, the recurrence rate of colorectal polyps was higher than after en bloc resection [10]. Additionally, the results of a study conducted by Moss et al. [11] showed that en bloc resection was associated with lower rates of recurrence than piecemeal resection. Our study results are in agreement with the abovementioned findings, where piecemeal resection was shown to be a significant predictor of polyp recurrence in both univariate and multivariate logistic regression analyses. In the last two decades, management strategies for colonic neoplasia have evolved considerably, leading to a paradigm shift from surgery to endoscopic resection. Due to an improved understanding of the pathophysiology of polyps, as well as ongoing advancements in technology, such as the development of novel endoscopic techniques and tools, clinical predictors of malignant colonic neoplasia have been well studied, yet factors that contribute to improved clinical decision making are still lacking. Most large ($\geq$20 mm diameter) colorectal polyps can be removed with advanced endoscopist techniques; however, these procedures require a center with the proper equipment and trained staff, specifically an endoscopic expert in the field. Whenever an endoscopist encounters a complex colorectal lesion (with complicated accessibility), a polyp size > 40 mm, the morphological type LST-NG, a type IIB polyp or the presence of hematochezia, malignancy risk should be considered before making the decision to either resect, refer the patient to an advanced endoscopist or perform surgery.

Our study has several limitations. Despite the prospective enrollment of the patients, the data were collected and analyzed retrospectively. Second, the performed procedures were supervised by experienced endoscopists, thus making the results non-generalizable to centers where these procedures are performed by less advanced endoscopists. Furthermore, considering the small number of patients with malignancy and the recurrence of disease, as well as incomplete patient medical histories, any additional risk factors might not have been detected. Therefore, future prospective studies with larger patient cohorts using a longer surveillance period are needed in order to validate our findings.

5. Conclusions

In lesions without overt evidence of colorectal carcinoma, an evidence-based risk estimation approach may be used to choose the correct resection modality for large colorectal polyps. In order to optimize clinical outcomes and minimize the rate of adverse events, endoscopic resection should be performed based on patient-specific characteristics, local availability and expertise.

Author Contributions: Conceptualization, O.M. and M.B.; methodology O.M. and M.B.; software, O.M.; validation, O.M., I.J., M.C., J.M., T.R., M.P., N.N. and M.B.; formal analysis, O.M. and M.B.; investigation, O.M., I.J., M.C., J.M., T.R., M.P., N.N. and M.B.; resources, O.M., I.J., M.C., J.M., T.R., M.P., N.N. and M.B.; data curation, O.M., I.J., M.C., J.M., T.R., M.P., N.N. and M.B.; writing—original draft preparation, O.M., I.J., M.C., J.M., T.R., M.P., N.N. and M.B.; writing—review and editing, O.M., I.J., M.C., J.M., T.R., M.P., N.N. and M.B.; visualization, O.M. and M.B.; supervision, O.M. and M.B.; project administration, O.M. and M.B.; funding acquisition, O.M., I.J., M.C., J.M., T.R., M.P., N.N. and M.B. All authors have read and agreed to the published version of the manuscript.

Funding: This research received no external funding.

Institutional Review Board Statement: This study was conducted in accordance with the Declaration of Helsinki and approved by the Ethics Committee of University Hospital Medical Center Bezanijska Kosa, Belgrade, Serbia (no. 5451/1) for studies involving humans.

Informed Consent Statement: Informed consent was obtained from all subjects involved in the study.

Data Availability Statement: The data that support the findings of this study are available on request from the corresponding author.

Conflicts of Interest: The authors declare no conflict of interest.

References

1. Bray, F.; Ferlay, J.; Soerjomataram, I.; Siegel, R.L.; Torre, L.A.; Jemal, A. Global cancer statistics 2018: GLOBOCAN estimates of incidence and mortality worldwide for 36 cancers in 185 countries. *CA Cancer J. Clin.* **2018**, *68*, 394–424. [CrossRef] [PubMed]
2. IARC. Global Cancer Observatory. 2020. Available online: https://www.iarc.who.int/faq/latest-global-cancer-data-2020-qa/ (accessed on 10 July 2022).
3. Siegel, R.L.; Miller, K.D.; Jemal, A. Cancer statistics, 2019. *CA Cancer J. Clin.* **2019**, *69*, 7–34. [CrossRef] [PubMed]
4. Heitman, S.J.; Ronksley, P.E.; Hilsden, R.J.; Manns, B.J.; Rostom, A.; Hemmelgarn, B.R. Prevalence of Adenomas and Colorectal Cancer in Average Risk Individuals: A Systematic Review and Meta-analysis. *Clin. Gastroenterol. Hepatol.* **2009**, *7*, 1272–1278. [CrossRef] [PubMed]
5. Ahlawat, S.K.; Gupta, N.; Benjamin, S.B.; Al-Kawas, F.H. Large colorectal polyps: Endoscopic management and rate of malignancy: Does size matter? *J. Clin. Gastroenterol.* **2011**, *45*, 347–354. [CrossRef]
6. Church, J.M. Experience in the endoscopic management of large colonic polyps. *ANZ J. Surg.* **2003**, *73*, 988–995. [CrossRef]
7. Binmoeller, K.F.; Bohnacker, S.; Seifert, H.; Thonke, F.; Valdeyar, H.; Soehendra, N. Endoscopic snare excision of "giant" colorectal polyps. *Gastrointest. Endosc.* **1996**, *43*, 183–188. [CrossRef]
8. Worland, T.; Cronin, O.; Harrison, B.; Alexander, L.; Ding, N.; Ting, A.; Dimopoulos, S.; Sykes, R.; Alexander, S. Clinical and financial impacts of introducing an endoscopic mucosal resection service for treatment of patients with large colonic polyps into a regional tertiary hospital. *Endosc. Int. Open* **2019**, *7*, E1386–E1392. [CrossRef]
9. Bujanda, L.; Cosme, A.; Gil, I.; Arenas-Mirave, J.I. Malignant colorectal polyps. *World J. Gastroenterol.* **2010**, *16*, 3103–3111. [CrossRef]

10. Belderbos, T.D.; Leenders, M.; Moons, L.M.G.; Siersema, P.D. Local recurrence after endoscopic mucosal resection of nonpedunculated colorectal lesions: Systematic review and meta-analysis. *Endoscopy* **2014**, *46*, 388–402. [CrossRef]
11. Moss, A.; Williams, S.J.; Hourigan, L.F.; Brown, G.; Tam, W.; Singh, R.; Zanati, S.; Burgess, N.; Sonson, R.; Byth, K.; et al. Long-term adenoma recurrence following wide-field endoscopic mucosal resection (WF-EMR) for advanced colonic mucosal neoplasia is infrequent: Results and risk factors in 1000 cases from the Australian Colonic EMR (ACE) study. *Gut* **2014**, *64*, 57–65. [CrossRef]
12. Cazacu, S.M.; Săftoiu, A.; Iordache, S.; Ghiluși, M.-C.; Georgescu, C.V.; Iovănescu, V.F.; Neagoe, C.D.; Streba, L.; Calița, M.; Burtea, E.D.; et al. Factors predicting occurrence and therapeutic choice in malignant colorectal polyps: A study of 13 years of colonoscopic polypectomy. *Rom. J. Morphol. Embryol.* **2022**, *62*, 917–928. [CrossRef] [PubMed]
13. Naqvi, S.; Burroughs, S.; Chave, H.S.; Branagan, G. Management of colorectal polyp cancers. *Ann. R. Coll. Surg. Engl.* **2012**, *94*, 574–578. [CrossRef]
14. Backes, Y.; Moons, L.M.; Novelli, M.R.; van Bergeijk, J.D.; Groen, J.N.; Seerden, T.C.; Schwartz, M.P.; de Vos Tot Nederveen Cappel, W.H.; Spanier, B.W.; Geesing, J.M.; et al. Diagnosis of T1 colorectal cancer in pedunculated polyps in daily clinical practice: A multicenter study. *Mod. Pathol.* **2016**, *30*, 104–112. [CrossRef] [PubMed]
15. Brown, I.S.; Bettington, M.L.; Bettington, A.; Miller, G.; Rosty, C. Adverse histological features in malignant colorectal polyps: A contemporary series of 239 cases. *J. Clin. Pathol.* **2016**, *69*, 292–299. [CrossRef] [PubMed]
16. Cooper, G.S.; Xu, F.; Barnholtz-Sloan, J.; Koroukian, S.; Schluchter, M.D. Management of malignant colonic polyps: A population-based analysis of colonoscopic polypectomy versus surgery. *Cancer* **2011**, *118*, 651–659. [CrossRef] [PubMed]
17. Jang, E.J.; Kim, D.D.; Cho, C.H. Value and Interpretation of Resection Margin after a Colonoscopic Polypectomy for Malignant Polyps. *J. Korean Soc. Coloproctology* **2011**, *27*, 194–201. [CrossRef]
18. Butte, J.M.; Tang, P.; Gonen, M.; Shia, J.; Schattner, M.; Nash, G.M.; Temple, L.K.F.; Weiser, M.R. Rate of Residual Disease After Complete Endoscopic Resection of Malignant Colonic Polyp. *Dis. Colon Rectum* **2012**, *55*, 122–127. [CrossRef]
19. Kawachi, H.; Eishi, Y.; Ueno, H.; Nemoto, T.; Fujimori, T.; Iwashita, A.; Ajioka, Y.; Ochiai, A.; Ishiguro, S.; Shimoda, T.; et al. A three-tier classification system based on the depth of submucosal invasion and budding/sprouting can improve the treatment strategy for T1 colorectal cancer: A retrospective multicenter study. *Mod. Pathol.* **2015**, *28*, 872–879. [CrossRef]
20. Hassan, C.; Zullo, A.; Risio, M.; Rossini, F.P.; Morini, H. Histologic Risk Factors and Clinical Outcome in Colorectal Malignant Polyp: A Pooled-Data Analysis. *Dis. Colon Rectum* **2005**, *48*, 1588–1596. [CrossRef]
21. Freeman, H.J. Long-term follow-up of patients with malignant pedunculated colon polyps after colonoscopic polypectomy. *Can. J. Gastroenterol.* **2013**, *27*, 20–24. [CrossRef]
22. Lopez, A.; Bouvier, A.-M.; Jooste, V.; Cottet, V.; Romain, G.; Faivre, J.; Manfredi, S.; Lepage, C. Outcomes following polypectomy for malignant colorectal polyps are similar to those following surgery in the general population. *Gut* **2017**, *68*, 111–117. [CrossRef] [PubMed]
23. Nanda, K.S.; Tutticci, N.; Burgess, N.G.; Sonson, R.; Williams, S.J.; Bourke, M.J. Endoscopic mucosal resection of laterally spreading lesions involving the ileocecal valve: Technique, risk factors for failure, and outcomes. *Endoscopy* **2015**, *47*, 710–718. [CrossRef] [PubMed]
24. Moss, A.; Bourke, M.J.; Williams, S.J.; Hourigan, L.F.; Brown, G.; Tam, W.; Singh, R.; Zanati, S.; Chen, R.Y.; Byth, K. Endoscopic Mucosal Resection Outcomes and Prediction of Submucosal Cancer from Advanced Colonic Mucosal Neoplasia. *Gastroenterology* **2011**, *140*, 1909–1918. [CrossRef] [PubMed]
25. Sidhu, M.; Tate, D.J.; Desomer, L.; Brown, G.; Hourigan, L.F.; Lee, E.Y.T.; Moss, A.; Raftopoulos, S.; Singh, R.; Williams, S.J.; et al. The size, morphology, site, and access score predicts critical outcomes of endoscopic mucosal resection in the colon. *Endoscopy* **2018**, *50*, 684–692.
26. Fragaki, M.; Voudoukis, E.; Chliara, E.; Dimas, I.; Mpitouli, A.; Velegraki, M.; Vardas, E.; Theodoropoulou, A.; Karmiris, K.; Giannikaki, L.; et al. Complete endoscopic mucosal resection of malignant colonic sessile polyps and clinical outcome of 51 cases. *Ann. Gastroenterol.* **2019**, *32*, 174–177. [CrossRef]
27. Geramizadeh, B.; Marzban, M.; Owen, D.A. Malignant Colorectal Polyps; Pathological Consideration (A review). *Iran. J. Pathol.* **2017**, *12*, 1–8. [CrossRef]
28. Hao, Y.; Wang, Y.; Qi, M.; He, X.; Zhu, Y.; Hong, J. Risk Factors for Recurrent Colorectal Polyps. *Gut Liver* **2020**, *14*, 399–411. [CrossRef]
29. Ferlitsch, M.; Moss, A.; Hassan, C.; Bhandari, P.; Dumonceau, J.-M.; Paspatis, G.; Jover, R.; Langner, C.; Bronzwaer, M.; Nalankilli, K.; et al. Colorectal polypectomy and endoscopic mucosal resection (EMR): European Society of Gastrointestinal Endoscopy (ESGE) Clinical Guideline. *Endoscopy* **2017**, *49*, 270–297. [CrossRef]
30. Chlebowski, R.T.; Wactawski-Wende, J.; Ritenbaugh, C.; Hubbell, F.A.; Ascensao, J.; Rodabough, R.J.; Rosenberg, C.A.; Taylor, V.M.; Harris, R.; Chen, C.; et al. Estrogen plus Progestin and Colorectal Cancer in Postmenopausal Women. *N. Engl. J. Med.* **2004**, *350*, 991–1004. [CrossRef]
31. Saiken, A.; Gu, F. Lifestyle and lifestyle-related comorbidities in dependently associated with colorectal adenoma recurre elderly Chinese people. *Clin. Interv. Aging* **2016**, *11*, 801–805. [CrossRef]
32. Chaoui, I.; Demedts, I.; Roelandt, P.; Willekens, H.; Bisschops, R. Endoscopic mucosal resection of colorectal polyps: Results, adverse events and two-year outcome. *Acta Gastroenterol. Belg.* **2022**, *85*, 47–55. [CrossRef] [PubMed]

33. Atkin, W.S.; Valori, R.; Kuipers, E.J.; Hoff, G.; Senore, C.; Segnan, N.; Jover, R.; Schmiegel, W.; Lambert, R.; Pox, C.; et al. European guidelines for quality assurance in colorectal cancer screening and diagnosis. First edition: Colonoscopic surveillance following adenoma removal. *Endoscopy* **2012**, *44* (Suppl. 3), SE151–SE163. [CrossRef] [PubMed]
34. Hassan, C.; Repici, A.; Sharma, P.; Correale, L.; Zullo, A.; Bretthauer, M.; Senore, C.; Spada, C.; Bellisario, C.; Bhandari, P.; et al. Efficacy and safety of endoscopic resection of large colorectal polyps: A systematic review and meta-analysis. *Gut* **2016**, *65*, 806–820. [CrossRef]
35. Zhan, T.; Hielscher, T.; Hahn, F.; Hauf, C.; Betge, J.; Ebert, M.P.; Belle, S. Risk Factors for Local Recurrence of Large, Flat Colorectal Polyps after Endoscopic Mucosal Resection. *Digestion* **2016**, *93*, 311–317. [CrossRef] [PubMed]
36. Longcroft-Wheaton, G.; Duku, M.; Mead, R.; Basford, P.; Bhandari, P. Risk Stratification System for Evaluation of Complex Polyps Can Predict Outcomes of Endoscopic Mucosal Resection. *Dis. Colon Rectum* **2013**, *56*, 960–966. [CrossRef] [PubMed]
37. Lee, T.J.W.; Rees, C.J.; Nickerson, C.; Stebbing, J.; Abercrombie, J.F.; McNally, R.; Rutter, M.D. Management of complex colonic polyps in the English Bowel Cancer Screening Programme. *Br. J. Surg.* **2013**, *100*, 1633–1639. [CrossRef]
38. Khashab, M.; Eid, E.; Rusche, M.; Rex, D.K. Incidence and predictors of "late" recurrences after endoscopic piecemeal resection of large sessile adenomas. *Gastrointest. Endosc.* **2009**, *70*, 344–349. [CrossRef]

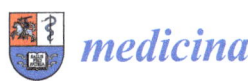

Case Report

Solitary Rectal Ulcer Syndrome Is Not Always Ulcerated: A Case Report

Yi Liu [1,†], Zhihao Chen [1,†], Lizhou Dou [1,†], Zhaoyang Yang [2] and Guiqi Wang [1,*]

1. Department of Endoscopy, National Cancer Center/National Clinical Research Center for Cancer/Cancer Hospital, Chinese Academy of Medical Sciences and Peking Union Medical College, Beijing 100021, China
2. Department of Pathology, National Cancer Center/National Clinical Research Center for Cancer/Cancer Hospital, Chinese Academy of Medical Sciences and Peking Union Medical College, Beijing 100021, China
* Correspondence: wangguiq@126.com
† These authors contributed equally to this work.

Abstract: Solitary rectal ulcer syndrome (SRUS) is a benign and chronic disorder well known in young adults that is characterized by a series of symptoms such as rectal bleeding, copious mucus discharge, prolonged excessive straining, perineal and abdominal pain, a feeling of incomplete defecation, constipation and, rarely, rectal prolapse. The etiology of this syndrome remains obscure, and the diagnosis is easily confused with that of other diseases, contributing to difficulties in treatment. We present a case of a 37-year-old male with a nonulcerated rectal lesion grossly resembling a superficial depressed rectal cancer misdiagnosed in another hospital and describe its appearance on endoscopy and in the analysis of its pathological manifestations. The aim of this case report is to report an easily misdiagnosed case of SRUS, which needs to be distinguished from superficial rectal cancer, which should be educational for endoscopists.

Keywords: solitary rectal ulcer syndrome; endoscopy; magnifying narrow-band imaging (magnifying NBI)

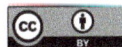

1. Introduction

Solitary rectal ulcer syndrome (SRUS) is a rare benign rectal disease that is characterized by a combination of symptoms, clinical findings and histological abnormalities [1]. However, SRUS is an infrequent disease that is easily underdiagnosed, with an estimated annual prevalence of one in 100,000 persons. It occurs most commonly in the third decade in men and in the fourth decade in women [2]. Patients mainly exhibit intestinal symptoms, such as constipation, feelings of incomplete defecation, bloody or purulent stools, discomfort with a falling anus and rectal ulcers. Physical examination usually reveals some thickening or a mass typically on the anterior rectal wall. Endoscopy often reveals a discrete, punched-out ulcer. Analysis of the tissue biopsy can confirm the diagnosis. Meanwhile, some medical treatments, including sucralfate, salicylate, corticosteroids, sulfasalazine, mesalazine and topical fibrin sealant, have been reported to be effective [3]. Apart from local medication, the treatment of SRUS also includes the improvement of bowel defecation habits, biofeedback and surgical operation [4]. We report, herein, the case of a 37-year-old male with a nonulcerated rectal lesion grossly resembling a superficial depressed rectal cancer but microscopically proving to be an SRUS. The purpose of publishing this case is to report and discuss the diagnosis of SRUS by magnifying narrow-band imaging endoscopy.

2. Case Report

A 37-year-old male had recurrent abdominal pain, diarrhea and hematochezia for 1 year. The patient had several bad habits such as tobacco use, alcohol consumption and betel quid chewing, and had no previous family history of cancer or special sexual behavior. This patient was recommended to receive endoscopy. Regrettably, he was diagnosed with superficial depressed rectal cancer in other two hospitals. He was then transferred to our hospital in preparation for surgery. The preoperative endoscopy discovered a reddish and irregular but well-defined 0-IIc lesion in the anterior wall of the rectum 4–6 cm from the anal margin (Figure 1a). Magnifying narrow-band imaging revealed fine reticulated vessels with a uniform thickness and distribution (Figure 1b,c). Some irregular pit patterns were observed after crystal violet staining (Figure 1d). Endoscopic ultrasonography (EUS) showed thickening of the mucosal layer at the lesion, and the submucosa was still intact (Figure 1e). Although the morphology of the pit patterns was disordered (Figure 1d), we suspected it not to be an infiltrative tumor, taking the magnifying endoscopic characteristics into account. Thus, we suggested this patient undergo a re-biopsy. Interestingly, histopathological examination at our hospital revealed that the lamina propria was filled with muscle fibers (Figure 2d). However, when pathologists consulted the biopsy results of the external hospital, they found that the glands were highly distorted and enlarged, accompanied by atypical changes in glandular epithelial cells (Figure 2a–c). Therefore, the diagnosis of the patient remained controversial after discussions among experts, with some experts suggesting only inflammatory changes and others suggesting the possibility of high-grade intraepithelial neoplasia. In light of the above situation, we advised the patient to first receive conservative treatment such as a high-fiber diet, reducing irregular stool habits and biofeedback training. The patient still strongly demanded endoscopic submucosal dissection (ESD) for a definitive diagnosis. Finally, the postoperative pathological results supported the diagnosis of SRUS (Figure 3). The wounds recovered well without recurrence, and the symptoms of hematochezia disappeared (Figure 1f).

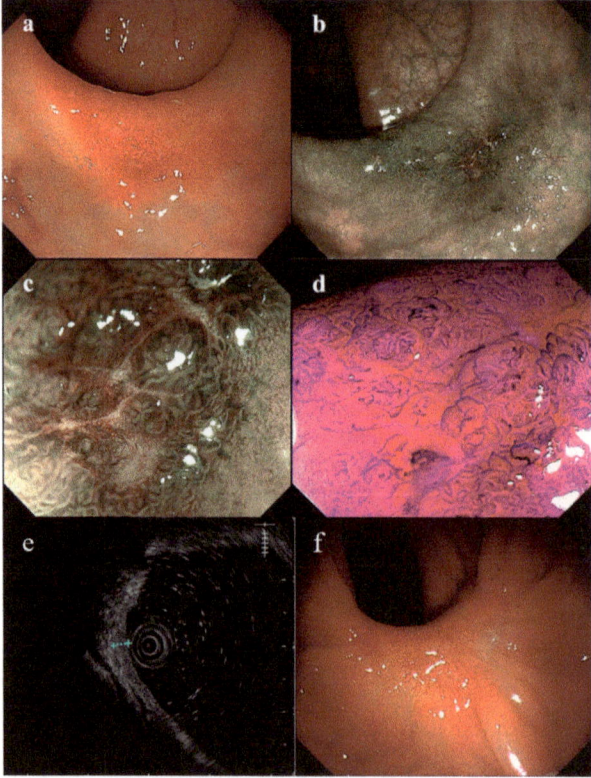

Figure 1. Endoscopic view of rectal lesion: (**a**) white-light endoscopy; (**b**) narrow-band imaging; (**c**) magnified version of the image in (**b**); (**d**) magnified endoscopic view after crystal violet staining; (**e**) the ultrasound image; (**f**) the white-light image of the scar.

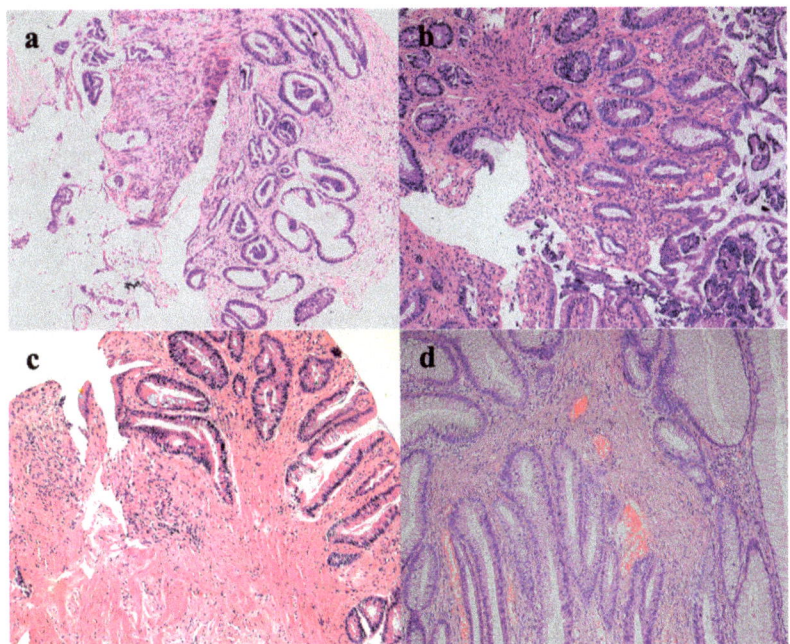

Figure 2. Histologic examination: (**a**–**c**) histologic biopsy in other hospitals: highly distorted and expanded glandular bodies with atypical changes in glandular epithelial cells (magnification: ×100); (**d**) histologic biopsy in our hospital: microvascular hyperplasia and musculomucosal hyperplasia.

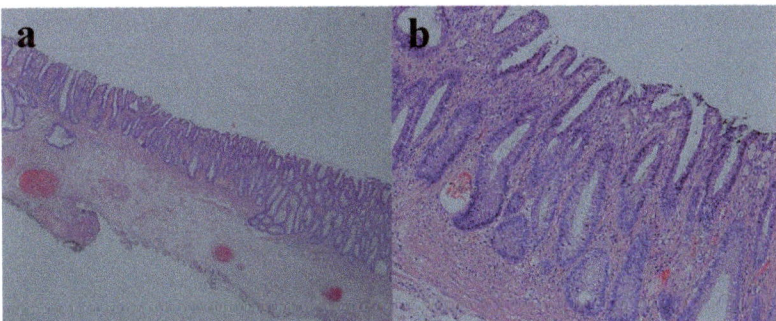

Figure 3. Resection histology: microvascular hyperplasia and musculomucosal hyperplasia. (**a**) Magnification: ×10; (**b**) magnification: ×200.

3. Discussion

SRUS is an unusual benign rectal disorder [4,5]. Several etiologies of SRUS have been proposed. This syndrome may have various factors that simultaneously cause the lesions, including rectal prolapse and chronic and severe constipation. Rectal ulcers are frequently described as always being found as single or multiple ulcers located on the anterior wall of the rectum within 10 cm of the anal margin [4]. A relevant study considered that rectal intussusception could lead to localized vascular trauma and, consequently, the onset of solitary local ulceration [6], while other studies showed that uncoordinated muscle contraction in the puborectalis muscle may be associated with increased intra-rectum pressure and pressure in the anal canal, which resulted in ulceration [7,8]. The clinical symptoms include abdominal pain, bleeding, mucus discharge, and chronic and severe constipation, among others. The histological features of SRUS are characterized by a thickening mucosal layer, fibromuscular obliteration, mucous cell proliferation, mucosal gland distortion, etc. [5]. SRUS is easily misdiagnosed as rectal cancer, based on the similarity in the symptomatic profiles and endoscopic features, which include bleeding, mucus discharge, and chronic and severe constipation. To date, these histological features have been helpful in distinguishing SRUS from malignancies. There are few reports about the diagnosis of SRUS by magnifying narrow-band imaging endoscopy.

In this case, the lesion appeared as a nonulcerated rectal lesion, with a superficial depressed area. The patient was misdiagnosed with superficial depressed rectal cancer in other two hospitals. Related studies reported that superficial depressed cancers arose through the de novo pathogenic sequence and had a higher tendency for early invasions [9,10]. As a result of the misdiagnosis, the patient came to our hospital seeking surgery. However, we found that magnifying narrow-band imaging revealed fine reticulated vessels with a uniform thickness and distribution, although some irregular and disordered pit patterns were observed after crystal violet staining. We highly suspected it to be SRUS according to the histopathological examination. We advised the patient to receive conservative treatment, but the patient still strongly demanded endoscopic submucosal dissection (ESD) for a definitive diagnosis. Finally, the postoperative pathological results supported the diagnosis of SRUS.

SRUS is an already well-known but easily misdiagnosed condition; the proper diagnosis and treatment of SRUS remain important challenges. It is worth noting that its rare occurrence usually leads to the fact that it is not properly diagnosed due to the lack of knowledge or lack of experience of doctors. The diagnosis of SRUS can usually be performed by a combination of symptomatology, endoscopy and histology. However, patients sometimes have typical symptoms without typical endoscopic findings. As mentioned above, this lesion did not present with typical ulcerative changes, but presented with superficial depressed changes. We used magnifying NBI and chromoendoscopy to observe this lesion and biopsied again, thus ruling out the possibility of rectal cancer, and finally reached the correct diagnosis. Although there is a little regret due to the fact that the patient strongly demanded ESD for a definitive diagnosis, we believe this is the most fortunate outcome for the patient, as he avoided surgery or even the risk of a permanent fistula.

We consider this case to be a good learning opportunity for gastroenterologists, as when they encounter similar cases, SRUS should be one of the options in the differential diagnosis list.

4. Conclusions

Not all SRUS cases present ulcers. Patients with typical symptoms and nonulcerated rectal lesions should be differentiated from those with superficial rectal cancer. Magnifying NBI and chromoendoscopy are useful, and histopathological examination should be performed to confirm the diagnosis.

Author Contributions: Conceptualization, G.W.; methodology, Y.L. and Z.C.; software, Y.L. and L.D.; validation, Y.L., Z.C. and L.D.; formal analysis, Y.L. and Z.Y.; investigation, Y.L. and Z.C.; resources, G.W.; data curation, Y.L. and G.W.; writing—original draft preparation, Y.L.; writing—review and editing, Z.C., L.D. and Z.Y.; visualization, Y.L. and Z.C.; supervision, G.W.; project administration, G.W.; funding acquisition, G.W. All authors have read and agreed to the published version of the manuscript.

Funding: This work was supported by grants from the Beijing Science and Technology Planning Project (CN) (D17110002617002), National Key Research and Development Program of China (2016YFC1302800), CAMS Innovation Fund for Medical Sciences (CIFMS) (2016-I2M-1-001), CAMS Innovation Fund for Medical Sciences (CIFMS) (2017-I2M-1-006), and Sanming Project of Medicine in Shenzhen (No. SZSM201911008).

Institutional Review Board Statement: The surgical procedure was approved by the Department of Endoscopy at the National Cancer Center/Cancer Hospital, Chinese Academy of Medical Sciences

(CICAMS), and the Ethics Committee of the National Cancer Center/Cancer Hospital, Chinese Academy of Medical Science and Peking Union Medical College (Approval Number: 18-002/1466). Written informed consent was obtained from the patient for the surgery and for the publication of this cohort study and any accompanying images.

Informed Consent Statement: Informed consent was obtained from all subjects involved in the study.

Acknowledgments: We gratefully acknowledge the work of past and present members of the Department of Endoscopy/Pathology, National Cancer Center/National Clinical Research Center for Cancer/Cancer Hospital, Chinese Academy of Medical Science and Peking Union Medical College, Beijing, China.

Conflicts of Interest: There are no potential conflict of interest (financial, professional or personal) relevant to the manuscript. All the authors confirm no conflict of interest for this work.

References

1. Felt-Bersma, R.J.F.; Tiersma, E.S.M.; Cuesta, M.A. Rectal Prolapse, Rectal Intussusception, Rectocele, Solitary Rectal Ulcer Syndrome, and Enterocele. *Gastroenterol. Clin. N. Am.* **2008**, *37*, 645–668. [CrossRef] [PubMed]
2. Martin, C.; Parks, T.; Biggart, J. Solitary rectal ulcer syndrome in Northern Ireland. 1971–1980. *Br. J. Surg.* **1981**, *68*, 744–747. [CrossRef] [PubMed]
3. Edden, Y.; Shih, S.; Wexner, S. Solitary rectal ulcer syndrome and stercoral ulcers. *Gastroenterol. Clin. N. Am.* **2009**, *38*, 541–545. [CrossRef] [PubMed]
4. Zhu, Q.C.; Shen, R.R.; Qin, H.L.; Wang, Y. Solitary rectal ulcer syndrome: Clinical features, pathophysiology, diagnosis and treatment strategies. *World J. Gastroenterol.* **2014**, *20*, 738–744. [CrossRef] [PubMed]
5. Forootan, M.; Darvishi, M. Solitary rectal ulcer syndrome: A systematic review. *Medicine* **2018**, *97*, e0565. [CrossRef] [PubMed]
6. Nagar, A. Isolated colonic ulcers: Diagnosis and management. *Curr. Gastroenterol. Rep.* **2007**, *9*, 422–428. [CrossRef] [PubMed]
7. Latos, W.; Kawczyk-Krupka, A.; Ledwoń, A.; Sieroń-Stołtny, K.; Sieroń, A. Solitary rectal ulcer syndrome-The role of autofluorescence colonoscopy. *Photodiagn. Photodyn. Ther.* **2007**, *4*, 179–183. [CrossRef] [PubMed]
8. Morio, O.; Meurette, G.; Desfourneaux, V.; D'Halluin, P.N.; Bretagne, J.F.; Siproudhis, L. Anorectal physiology in solitary ulcer syndrome: A case-matched series. *Dis. Colon Rectum* **2005**, *48*, 1917–1922. [CrossRef] [PubMed]
9. Mueller, J.D.; Bethke, B.; Stolte, M. Colorectal de novo carcinoma: A review of its diagnosis, histopathology, molecular biology, and clinical relevance. *Virchows Arch. Int. J. Pathol.* **2002**, *440*, 453–460. [CrossRef] [PubMed]
10. Hurlstone, D.P.; Sanders, D.S.; Thomson, M. Detection and treatment of early flat and depressed colorectal cancer using high-magnification chromoscopic colonoscopy: A change in paradigm for Western endoscopists? *Dig. Dis. Sci.* **2007**, *52*, 1387–1393. [CrossRef] [PubMed]

MDPI
St. Alban-Anlage 66
4052 Basel
Switzerland
www.mdpi.com

Medicina Editorial Office
E-mail: medicina@mdpi.com
www.mdpi.com/journal/medicina

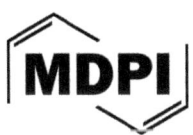

Disclaimer/Publisher's Note: The statements, opinions and data contained in all publications are solely those of the individual author(s) and contributor(s) and not of MDPI and/or the editor(s). MDPI and/or the editor(s) disclaim responsibility for any injury to people or property resulting from any ideas, methods, instructions or products referred to in the content.

www.ingramcontent.com/pod-product-compliance
Lightning Source LLC
LaVergne TN
LVHW070619100526
838202LV00012B/683